Diabetic Athlete's
H A N D B O O K

Sheri R. Colberg, PhD

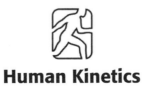

Human Kinetics

Library of Congress Cataloging-in-Publication Data

Colberg, Sheri, 1963-
Diabetic athlete's handbook / Sheri R. Colberg.
p. cm.
Includes bibliographical references and index.
ISBN-13: 978-0-7360-7493-3 (soft cover)
ISBN-10: 0-7360-7493-7 (soft cover)
1. Diabetic athletes--Handbooks, manuals, etc. 2. Diabetes--Exercise therapy--Handbooks, manuals, etc. I. Title.
RC660.C4747 2009
616.4'62--dc22

2008028738

ISBN-10: 0-7360-7493-7 (print)   ISBN-10: 0-7360-8300-6 (Adobe PDF)
ISBN-13: 978-0-7360-7493-3 (print)   ISBN-13: 978-0-7360-8300-3 (Adobe PDF)

This book is a revised edition of *The Diabetic Athlete*, published in 2001 by Human Kinetics.

The Web addresses cited in this text were current as of September 2008, unless otherwise noted.

Acquisitions Editor: Tom Heine; **Developmental Editor:** Kevin Matz; **Assistant Editors:** Laura Koritz, Elizabeth Watson; **Copyeditor:** Bob Replinger; **Proofreader:** Sarah Wiseman; **Indexer:** Craig Brown; **Permission Manager:** Martha Gullo; **Graphic Designer:** Fred Starbird; **Graphic Artist:** Tara Welsch; **Cover Designer:** Keith Blomberg; **Cover Photos (clockwise from left):** © Tom Roberts, courtesy of Missy Foy, © Mark Harmel, courtesy of Kevin Light; **Photos (interior):** © Human Kinetics, unless otherwise noted; **Photo Asset Manager:** Laura Fitch; **Visual Production Assistant:** Joyce Brumfield; **Photo Office Assistant:** Jason Allen; **Art Manager:** Kelly Hendren; **Associate Art Manager:** Alan L. Wilborn; **Illustrator:** Accurate Art; **Printer:** McNaughton & Gunn

Human Kinetics books are available at special discounts for bulk purchase. Special editions or book excerpts can also be created to specification. For details, contact the Special Sales Manager at Human Kinetics.

Printed in the United States of America   10 9 8 7 6 5 4 3 2 1

Human Kinetics
Web site: www.HumanKinetics.com

United States: Human Kinetics
P.O. Box 5076
Champaign, IL 61825-5076
800-747-4457
e-mail: humank@hkusa.com

Canada: Human Kinetics
475 Devonshire Road Unit 100
Windsor, ON N8Y 2L5
800-465-7301 (in Canada only)
e-mail: info@hkcanada.com

Europe: Human Kinetics
107 Bradford Road
Stanningley
Leeds LS28 6AT, United Kingdom
+44 (0) 113 255 5665
e-mail: hk@hkeurope.com

Australia: Human Kinetics
57A Price Avenue
Lower Mitcham, South Australia 5062
08 8372 0999
e-mail: info@hkaustralia.com

New Zealand: Human Kinetics
Division of Sports Distributors NZ Ltd.
P.O. Box 300 226 Albany
North Shore City
Auckland
0064 9 448 1207
e-mail: info@humankinetics.co.nz

This book is dedicated to my wonderful husband, Ray Ochs, who continues to be a ray of sunshine and a blessing in my life, and to my three delightful (and growing) sons—Alex, Anton, and RayJ—who keep me focused on what is really important in life.

Contents

Foreword   vii   Preface   ix   Acknowledgments   xi

Part I   Diabetic Athlete's Toolbox. 1

Basics of exercise, fitness, energy, insulin action, hypoglycemia, blood sugar balance with exercise, insulin and other diabetic medications, dietary practices and supplements, exercise guidelines, glucose monitoring, sport psychology, and athletic injuries

CHAPTER 1   **Training for Fitness and Sports** 3
Exercise training, fitness, and effective workouts (aerobic and resistance)

CHAPTER 2   **Balancing Exercise Blood Sugars** 21
Energy systems, body fuels, hypoglycemia prevention and treatment, insulin action and training effects, female athletes, and pregnancy

CHAPTER 3   **Ups and Downs of Insulin and Other Medications** 45
Circulating insulin and exercise, insulin regimens and pumps, the latest medications, and balancing exercise blood sugars

CHAPTER 4   **Diet and Supplements for Active People** . . 57
Dietary practices for diabetic athletes, carbohydrate loading, sports gels and supplements, and nutritional aids

CHAPTER 5   **Exercise and Blood Glucose Monitoring Guidelines** 81
Current guidelines for type 1 and type 2 diabetic exercisers and concerns about and precautions for exercising with diabetes-related health complications

CHAPTER 6   **Thinking and Acting Like an Athlete** 95
Psychology of being an athlete with diabetes and motivation for exercise and fitness

CHAPTER 7   **Preventing and Treating Athletic Injuries** . . 107
Prevention and treatment of athletic and sports-related injuries and dealing with diabetes-related joint problems

Part II   Guidelines for Specific Activities . .   127

General and specific recommendations for diet and medication changes (for both insulin and oral medication users) for almost 100 sports and activities, along with real-life examples from diabetic athletes and athlete profiles

CHAPTER **8**   **Fitness Activities** **129**

Walking, conditioning machines, resistance training, aerobics and other fitness classes, martial arts, P.E. classes, water aerobics, dance (various types), in-line skating, yard work and gardening, and housework

CHAPTER **9**   **Endurance Sports** **157**

Running, cycling, swimming, marathons, triathlons, cross-country skiing, and other endurance activities

CHAPTER **10**   **Endurance–Power Sports** **187**

Basketball, field hockey, golf, tennis, soccer, ice hockey, gymnastics, competitive cheerleading, indoor racquet sports, rowing, roller derby, water polo, wrestling, and longer track events

CHAPTER **11**   **Power Sports** **215**

Bodybuilding, baseball, softball, volleyball, fencing, sprinting, field events, Olympic weightlifting, and other power sports

CHAPTER **12**   **Outdoor Recreational Activities and Sports** **229**

Kayaking, snorkeling and scuba diving, rock and ice climbing, snowboarding, dog mushing, hiking, mountaineering, mountain biking, skateboarding, skydiving, horseback riding, windsurfing, whitewater sports, motorcycle racing, gaming, adventure racing, yard work and gardening, and many more

Appendix A   Diabetes and Athletic Organizations   261

Appendix B   Diabetes, Sport, and Nutrition Web Sites   263

Suggested Reading   265   Selected Bibliography   266

Index   275   About the Author   284

Foreword

By Matthew Corcoran, MD, CDE

A person does not have to work long in the field of diabetes to recognize the huge void out there in the arena of diabetes and exercise. Most busy physicians do not have the time, energy, or understanding of exercise to provide effective counsel on exercise in the brief time that they have to meet with patients. Insurance does not reimburse for exercise and sports counseling. Fitness and exercise specialists, coaches, and trainers do not have training in the complexities of diabetes, its management, or its management during exercise training. As a result, in the past, when people with diabetes sought out a resource devoted to diabetes and exercise, they often came up empty handed. They, too, had stumbled across the gap that exists between the worlds of fitness, exercise, and sport and the physicians' offices and diabetes centers that have historically been the center of diabetes care in the United States. Thankfully, the times are changing and the void is narrowing a bit each day. Now multiple credible and available resources are available to people with diabetes who are interested in expanding their understanding and knowledge when it comes to managing diabetes, exercise, and sport.

Dr. Sheri Colberg's book *The Diabetic Athlete* (2001) was one of the earlier resources that people could consult to learn more about the management of their diabetes during exercise and sports. *Diabetic Athlete's Handbook*, which you hold in your hands, expands on her earlier book in many wonderful ways. It includes updated sections on the latest and greatest therapeutic tools available, as well as important new chapters on the prevention and treatment of common injuries (especially as they pertain to diabetes) and the psychology of exercise and sport. Again, Colberg successfully taps into one of the greatest resources out there: the wisdom and experience of athletes and exercisers with diabetes from around the world. The sheer number of you who are out their giving it your all every day is one of the most astounding and inspiring aspects of this book. You all are embracing your diabetes and challenging it head on!

But you should not have to go it alone. You deserve to have a team of people surrounding you every step of the way. *Diabetic Athlete's Handbook* starts by building your knowledge base and begins to surround you with a support team of like-minded people from all walks of life. This book provides the basics of the physiology of diabetes and exercise, along with novel diabetes therapies and management tools for both type 1 and type 2 diabetes. A greater understanding of their interplay is necessary for successful management of your diabetes during exercise and sport. You also learn from the experience of people who have done this before you or are out there with you during your times of trial and error. Finally, in each chapter, Colberg introduces you to a variety of useful resources that are available to help you reach your goals and pursue your dreams.

Make no mistake about it: Diabetes is a complex chronic disease, more complicated than most. Exercise and sport involve complicated physiological processes, and doing them with a disease like diabetes makes them that much more challenging. This reality should not stop you from exercising, getting fit, or competing at whatever level you choose. In fact, as Colberg writes, diabetes should be your reason to exercise. The tremendous array of health and mental benefits that exercise and fitness bestow on you usually outweighs the risks, but you need to tackle the challenges with an understanding of what is going on in your body. Your physician and health care team should be part of your support team. You also want to surround yourself with educators, dietitians and nutritionists, sport psychologists, and behavior change specialists, as well as your friends with diabetes who are taking on the challenges with you. With a firm foundation and a solid support team, you will be well on your way to successful completion of your goals.

Ultimately, integrating diabetes and exercise is all about self-management. It is not about relying on a medical system to hold your hand; rather, it mandates continual learning and empowerment to free you from a need to rely on an already overtaxed system of health care delivery. Enjoy reading and rereading this fine book, enjoy learning from one another and the resources that are out there for you, and continue to surround yourself with a health care team that strives to be a valuable resource for you. I believe that you can do whatever you want to do in the face of diabetes, provided that your efforts do not put your health at risk. You can achieve whatever it is that you set your sights on: greater long-term health through increasing fitness, competing in the Olympics, or anything in between. Be smart, understand your disease, and look to your support team and resources for help along the way. Most of all have fun. Best of health and success!

Preface

Diabetes treatment has gone through dramatic changes in the past few decades. I am happy to report for this second edition that although exercise was often overlooked as a cornerstone in diabetes treatment when my first book, *The Diabetic Athlete*, came out, regular physical activity has finally become a tool that many people with diabetes embrace. There is still room for improvement, however, and I hope that this updated book can help many others learn how to exercise safely and without fear of severely upsetting a delicate glucose balance.

Diagnosed with diabetes myself at the age of four in what I call the dark ages of diabetes (1968), I went through childhood, adolescence, and early adulthood without benefit of a blood glucose meter. I still participated in a variety of sports and physical activities over the years: swimming, running, racquetball, soccer, tennis, weight training, gymnastics, volleyball, cycling, aerobics, dancing, stair climbing, hiking and backpacking, canoeing, football equipment managing, snow-shoeing, cross-country and downhill skiing, horseback riding, sailing, snorkeling, skydiving, and child rearing! I did many of these things while feeling less than my physical best because without a meter and the ability to adjust my insulin doses to compensate, my blood sugars were often too high or low.

While I was growing up, exercise of any kind made me feel better overall, although at the time I did not understand the physiology behind it enough to know why. I believed that exercising gave me more control over my diabetes as well. So I began exercising regularly on my own and through team sports as a preteen, and I have continued exercising throughout my adulthood. Not until I had a blood glucose meter did I realize, however, how much better I felt during exercise when my blood sugars were in a more normal range. Keeping them normal with the help of a blood glucose meter has totally been a trial-and-error learning process!

When I got my first meter, few guidelines or books were available to offer me any guidance. I eventually learned to control my blood sugars for various activities, but every time I tried a new or unusual one, it was like starting over again. When I attended my first IDAA (then the International Diabetic Athletes Association but now the Diabetes Exercise & Sports Association, or DESA) meeting in 1990, I met many other active people. It struck me then that I could learn much from others' experiences to ease and shorten my trial-and-error process. From this experience I eventually got the idea and motivation for the book *The Diabetic Athlete*, which included many real-life examples from IDAA members. For this book, I posted my diabetic athlete questionnaire on my Web site—forget snail mail in the new millennium!—and received replies from active people with type 1 and type 2 diabetes of all ages from around the world, more than 360 of them. My question-naire asked them to describe their usual diets, medications, and exercise routines, along with specific alterations that they make for any of a variety of sports and recreational physical activities, as well as their greatest athletic achievements. In addition, for this book I added all new athlete profiles, one per chapter, which highlight the training regimens of athletes of various types and ages. Also new are boxes about diabetic athlete–related organizations, one in each of the first seven chapters. This book is a compilation of those updated experiences, and I hope that you can use this information to attain better blood sugar control while exercising or just being more active in general.

Part I of this book covers the basics about exercise. I have always found that knowledge is power when it comes to managing diabetes. I have researched this topic for years—all through my childhood, while earning a doctoral degree in exercise physiology from the University of California at Berkeley, and ever since. Although you do not need a PhD to understand how your body adapts to exercise, you do need to understand the basics to make safe changes in your diet and medication.

Part II of this book is more experiential in nature and can really help you reduce your trial-and-error time for almost any conceivable sport or physical activity. This second part of the book is arranged into five chapters by type of activity. Each chapter gives general recommendations for diet and medication changes (for both insulin and oral medication users) for each sport or activity, along with real-life examples from diabetic athletes who participate in those sports. No one-size-fits-all solution applies to blood sugar control because everyone's physiology is unique. Although these chapters provide many examples, in the end you'll have to figure out what works best for you using the examples as guidelines or as a starting place.

I believe that combining this basic information (the why of exercise) and experiential information (the how of exercise) can help everyone know how to maintain blood sugars during any physical endeavor. Whether you are interested in just recreating or want to be a serious competitive athlete, it is time to get out there and go for it!

Acknowledgments

I would like to thank all the people who helped me update this book so that I can continue to make a difference in the lives of active people with diabetes. This list includes the wonderful members of my extended, professional diabetes family (you know who you are) who informed active people with diabetes from the United States and abroad about where to go to fill out my online diabetic athlete questionnaire. I also appreciate the input of my friends and colleagues, particularly Missy Foy, Gary Scheiner, Jeff Hitchcock, Rick Philbin, Bill King, Rich Weil, Steve Edelman, and Joe Largay, all of whom took the time to give me their comments about what I could do to make this new edition far better than the first one. I am especially grateful to the diabetic athletes themselves who replied because without their input I would have had a limited number of real-life, sport-specific examples to share. For any of you whose examples I could not fit into the book, I apologize and again thank you for taking the time to tell me about all that you do. My thanks also go to Michael Tamburello, PhD, PT, ATC, who willingly shared his knowledge on the topic of clinical joint disorders in diabetic people that often require physical therapy interventions. Finally, I would like to acknowledge all the hard-working people at Human Kinetics, including Tom Heine, Kevin Matz, Rebecca Lynch, Sue Outlaw, and countless others who work behind the scenes.

PART

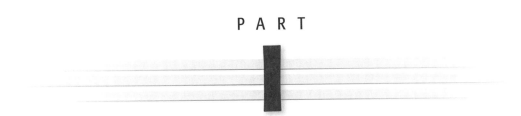

Diabetic Athlete's Toolbox

Training for Fitness and Sports

If you are already an avid exerciser, then you are aware of most of the benefits of exercise for your physical health and your diabetes control. If you are thinking about getting serious about sports or fitness activities, then you have a lot of positive changes to look forward to. Besides perhaps allowing you to have treats afterward, exercise can help you build muscle and lose body fat, suppress your appetite, eat more without gaining fat weight, enhance your mood, reduce stress and anxiety levels, increase your energy level, improve your immune system, keep your joints and muscles more flexible, and improve the quality of your life. For many with diabetes, being physically active has made all the difference between controlling diabetes or letting it control them.

DIABETES: THE BASICS

If you have diabetes, your body lacks the capacity to control your blood glucose, the primary sugar circulating in your blood. Normally, after you eat a meal, it gets digested and broken down into easily absorbed molecules, glucose being one of them. A simple sugar that comes mostly from the carbohydrate that you eat, glucose must be present in your blood in sufficient quantity that your brain and nervous system can take it up and use it as their primary fuel. If you've ever experienced a low blood sugar reaction, otherwise known as hypoglycemia or a low, which can happen when your blood sugars drop below 65 milligrams per deciliter (mg/dl), or 3.6 millimolar (mmol/L) if you live outside the United States, you're familiar with the effect that it has on your ability to think straight and react normally! For instance, if you ever find yourself thinking, "Gee, I know what 2 + 2 equals, but I just can't figure it out right now," you're probably low.

In a nondiabetic person, when blood glucose levels start to rise above normal (70 to 99 mg/dl fasting, or 3.9 to 5.5 mmol/L), the pancreas senses the increase and releases a hormone called insulin to help lower them. Insulin works by binding to receptors on cells in muscle and fat tissues, the primary places where glucose can be stored. In the case of diabetes, either your pancreas has a greatly reduced capacity to release insulin (resulting in insulin deficiency) or the insulin that you release doesn't work effectively enough in removing excess glucose from your

3

blood (meaning that you're insulin resistant). In either case, or often when both scenarios are in effect, your blood sugars rise too high after you eat, when you're stressed out, or when you're ill. Your liver is the organ responsible for making sure that you have enough glucose in your blood. In some people with diabetes, it becomes insulin resistant and releases too much glucose, especially overnight when they go for long periods without eating.

Although functioning is usually easier with your blood glucose a little too high (compared with too low), the long-term health problems that may be caused by elevated blood sugars related to poorly controlled diabetes are best avoided. Among the list of nasty possibilities are heart disease, premature death, nerve damage (both central and peripheral), amputations, joint problems, vision loss, kidney failure, birth defects in your offspring (if you're female), and more. We know by now that keeping blood sugars as close to normal as possible is the best way to prevent many, if not all, of these potential health problems. That's where regular exercise, a good diet, effective use of medications, and a blood glucose meter come in handy.

DOES THE TYPE OF DIABETES YOU HAVE MATTER?

Regardless of what type of diabetes you have been diagnosed with, exercise can throw you a curveball when it comes to blood glucose management. The risks and precautions vary somewhat with the type, so understanding the differences among them is important before we get into the nitty-gritty of exercise and specific recommendations for regimen changes.

Type 1: Always Insulin Requiring

Type 1 diabetes is less common than type 2; the former comprises only about 5 to 10 percent of all cases. Type 1 has an autoimmune basis—meaning that an immune system gone awry is responsible for destroying most or all of the insulin-making capacity of the pancreatic beta cells. Having this type means that you have to take insulin to survive. If you developed type 1 rapidly during your childhood or adolescence, you are not alone; the teen years are when type 1 diabetes is most commonly diagnosed. Its usual symptoms include the "polys" (polyuria, polydipsia, and polyphagia, otherwise known as excessive urination, thirst, and hunger), unexplained weight loss, and unusual fatigue, all of which are related to having an elevated blood glucose level caused by lack of insulin in the body.

Requiring daily insulin also means that balancing your blood sugar levels when you exercise is going to be tricky because both insulin and physical activity can independently (but additively) lower your blood glucose. You may need to alter your insulin and your carbohydrate intake before, during, and after exercise to stay in balance because hypoglycemia commonly results from being physically active.

Type 1.5, or LADA: Adult-Onset Type 1

If you have LADA (latent autoimmune diabetes of the adult), sometimes called type 1.5 or slow-onset type 1, you still have a form of type 1 diabetes and will be insulin requiring at some point. More than half of all cases of type 1 diabetes are now being diagnosed in adults of all ages, so it's not surprising that the American Diabetes Association stopped calling it juvenile-onset diabetes more than a decade ago. The onset of LADA is generally much slower in adults than it is in youngsters, and the symptoms may be controllable much longer without going on insulin. If you have LADA, you may still be making some of your own insulin for a while, which makes controlling your blood sugars much easier. After you eventually lose your glucose control even when you're still exercising like a fiend, it's time to consider insulin injections (or an insulin pump) your friend and not your foe.

If you're an extremely athletic adult (age 25 or older) and you were diagnosed with type 2 while regularly active and at normal or near-normal body weight, you likely have LADA instead. Up to 20 percent of people with type 2 diabetes actually have LADA. Being misdiagnosed with type 2 because of your age is common, and you may initially respond well to oral diabetes medications (which further confuses the diagnosis). But you're not likely to be insulin resistant as a true type 2 person is. If desired, you can get antibody tests done to help make the diagnosis of LADA, mainly because you need to start your insulin therapy (rather than diabetes pills); early treatment with insulin injections may actually help preserve your remaining pancreatic beta cells for a little longer.

Type 2: Insulin Resistant With an Overworked Pancreas

Although many consider it a more easily managed condition, type 2 diabetes should not be taken lightly. It often goes undiagnosed for five or more years, so when you are diagnosed with it, you may already be experiencing some diabetes-related health problems. Generally, its onset is caused by insulin resistance (meaning that your insulin doesn't work effectively) and loss of insulin production over time, the combination of which leaves your beta cells unable to keep up with insulin demands. The good news is that becoming more physically active makes your insulin work better, which explains why exercise and dietary changes early on are often effective in controlling it. Unfortunately, about 40 percent of people with type 2 diabetes end up eventually needing some supplemental insulin to control their blood sugars. A related type, gestational diabetes, which is commonly diagnosed during the last trimester of a woman's pregnancy, usually goes away after she gives birth, but having it greatly increases her risk for later developing type 2 diabetes.

GETTING PHYSICALLY FIT IS THE BEST THING YOU CAN DO

Physical fitness has undeniable health benefits for everyone. If you exercise regularly, you will have lower risk for many health problems including heart disease, obesity, hypertension, type 2 diabetes, certain cancers, and other metabolic disorders. The usual health benefits of exercise apply to people with diabetes, probably even more than they do to those without diabetes. Enhanced insulin action is a key benefit, because this effect will make all types of diabetes easier to manage. The improvements that you'll experience in your cholesterol levels (e.g., higher HDL cholesterol, the good type; lower bad, LDL, cholesterol; and lower blood fats called triglycerides) will greatly lower your heart disease risk, which is elevated by diabetes. Regular exercise can lower your level of systemic inflammation, which in turn reduces your blood platelet stickiness and lessens the chances that blood clots will form, thereby lowering your risk for heart attack or stroke. If nothing else, being active will help improve your ability to cope with stress and enhance your outlook on life and diabetes management.

Much of what we attribute to getting older—such as muscle atrophy or loss of flexibility in joints—really results from disuse over time. Diabetes, especially when your blood sugars are poorly controlled, can cause premature aging, accelerated heart disease, and other illnesses. Thus, regular exercise can keep you looking and feeling younger for longer and even greatly lower your risk of getting any diabetes-related complications. By continuing to enjoy your favorite physical activities, you can help maintain your long-term health—now there's a win–win situation!

> *Regular exercise is the most important activity that you can do to slow the aging process, manage your blood sugars, and reduce your risk of diabetic complications.*

WHAT DOES IT MINIMALLY TAKE TO GET FIT?

How much and what types of exercises do you need to do to reach an acceptable minimal level of fitness? According to updated physical activity guidelines released jointly by the American College of Sports Medicine (ACSM) and the American Heart Association (AHA) in August 2007 (shown in table 1.1), all healthy adults ages 18 to 65 years need to engage in moderate-intensity aerobic physical activity (e.g., brisk walking or bicycling on level terrain) for at least 30 minutes on 5 days each week or vigorous-intensity aerobic activity like running or uphill bicycling for at least 20 minutes on 3 days. In addition, the ACSM and AHA state that adults will benefit from performing activities that maintain or increase muscular strength and endurance for at least two days each week. You should do these planned activities in addition to performing routine, light-intensity activities of daily living, such as self-care, casual walking, grocery shopping, or any physical activities that last less than 10 minutes like walking to the parking lot or taking out the trash.

The ACSM and AHA also released separate, updated recommendations for adults over 65 or anyone between 50 and 64 years old with chronic conditions or physical functional limitations (e.g., arthritis) that affect their ability to move or their physical fitness. Older adults should meet or exceed 30 minutes of moderate physical activity on most days of the week, but more humble goals may be necessary for anyone with a physical impairment like arthritic joints. They also recognize that just maintaining functionality is an important benefit for older people and that maintaining some level of fitness makes it easier to do everyday activities, such as gardening, walking, or cleaning the house. For older people or those with limitations, strength training is especially important to prevent loss of muscle mass and bone strength, and working on flexibility will additionally help prevent limitations in such activities. Finally, as people age they must work on maintaining balance and staying on their feet.

Table 1.1   ACSM and AHA 2007 Recommendations for Physical Activity

Guidelines for healthy adults under age 65

- Do moderately intense cardio 30 minutes a day, five days a week.
    - or
- Do vigorously intense cardio 20 minutes a day, three days a week.
    - and
- Do 8 to 10 strength-training exercises, 8 to 12 repetitions of each exercise, twice a week.

Guidelines for adults over age 65 (or age 50 to 64 with chronic health conditions)

- Do moderately intense aerobic exercise 30 minutes a day, five days a week.
    - or
- Do vigorously intense aerobic exercise 20 minutes a day, three days a week.
    - and
- Do 8 to 10 strength-training exercises, 10 to 15 repetitions of each exercise, twice to three times per week.
    - and
- If you are at risk of falling, perform balance exercises.
    - and
- Have a physical activity plan.

COMPONENTS OF AN EXERCISE TRAINING PROGRAM

Whether you are already a regular exerciser or just a beginner, several basic guidelines apply to improving your fitness level and controlling your blood sugar levels. Keep in mind that fitness can be defined many different ways. Your overall health benefits from aerobic or cardiovascular fitness, or what we think of as physical conditioning resulting from prolonged aerobic activities such as brisk walking, jogging, cycling, swimming, rowing, and aerobic dance. Another form of fitness is muscular, related to both muscular strength and muscular endurance, which you would do well not to neglect. Particularly if you're just getting started, your physician or exercise professional should help you develop an exercise prescription with careful consideration of your diabetes control, complications, and other health problems; risk factors for cardiovascular disease; personal goals; and exercise preferences.

An exercise program incorporates the type of exercise that you choose to do (mode), how hard you perform it (intensity), how long you engage in it (duration), how often you exercise (frequency), and how quickly you advance with your training (progression).

Mode: Picking Aerobic and Anaerobic Activities

If your main goal is to increase your maximal oxygen consumption ($\dot{V}O_2$max) and your endurance capacity, your training should be aerobic in nature, involving the large-muscle groups performing rhythmic, prolonged activities like walking,

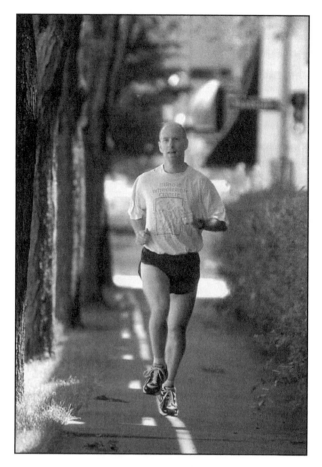

Aerobic activities like running increase your endurance capacity.

running, swimming, cycling, rowing, in-line skating, and cross-country skiing. Anaerobic resistance training is not a usual means to increase $\dot{V}O_2max$, but it is effective in increasing muscular strength and muscular endurance and preventing the loss of lean muscle mass that normally occurs with aging and disuse. Any gains in your muscle mass from either type of training can increase your daily caloric needs and improve your insulin sensitivity and blood glucose control. Thus, to achieve optimal cardiovascular fitness, your exercise program must include an aerobic component, and to preserve your muscle mass and strength, you should incorporate regular resistance training into your exercise routine as recommended.

Another simple way to become more fit is simply to do a variety of activities, an approach known as cross-training. For example, you could run for 30 minutes and do some resistance training on Monday, Wednesday, and Friday; swim for 45 minutes on Tuesday; and take dance classes on Saturday. Cross-training is really the key to avoiding overuse injuries, keeping your exercise fresh and fun, and achieving maximal fitness. When it comes to managing your blood sugars, this approach is also effective. Each activity uses muscles differently, recruiting either different muscles altogether or the same ones in different patterns, which results in wider use and enhanced fitness of your whole body. The only downside is that because you do each activity less frequently when you vary them, you will likely not experience a training effect as pronounced as it otherwise would be.

Intensity: How Hard Are You Working Out?

How hard you work out should reflect your training goals, such as whether you want to maximize your endurance performance or just expend some calories, but for improvements in cardiovascular fitness, you'll need to do exercise of either moderate or vigorous intensity. Vigorous activities should challenge you, resulting in rapid breathing and a greatly elevated heart rate. Some examples are race walking, jogging or running, water jogging, bicycling uphill, gardening with a shovel, or playing competitive sports like soccer or lacrosse. Moderate-intensity activities still make you feel as if you're exerting yourself, but your breathing will be less labored and your pace slower. Such activities include brisk walking, swimming at a moderate pace, or bicycling on level terrain.

Intensity and Interval Training

Intensity and duration of exercise are interrelated. Usually when you're doing higher-intensity exercise, you can't keep going as long as you can during lower-intensity activities, but the greater overload that the harder exercise provides leads to greater gains in performance. If your goal is weight loss, doing an activity at a lower intensity for a longer duration may work better for you. In either case, you need to consider your initial fitness level, exercise goals, risk for orthopedic or cardiovascular problems, diabetes-related complications, and personal preferences. If your workouts are too hard, you may stop doing them because of injuries (more on potential injuries and prevention in chapter 7) or loss of motivation.

If you can't maintain a higher intensity to start, you can increase your fitness by doing intervals. During any activity, simply increase the intensity of your exercise for short periods (interval training) to gain more from it. For example, if you are out walking, speed up slightly for a short distance (such as between two light poles or mailboxes) before slowing back down to your original pace. During your workouts, continue to include these short, faster intervals occasionally and, as you are able to, lengthen the intervals so that they last two to five minutes at a time. Performing intervals will not only improve your fitness and use up extra calories but also will likely cause you to feel more tired when you finish. Over the course of several weeks, you will be able to move faster and sustain a quicker pace for longer as a result of this extra conditioning from your interspersed bouts of faster activity. In one study, when unfit men and women in their 30s and 40s trained just twice a week doing only three to four minutes of aerobic exercise at high intensity, preceded and followed by three-minute warm-up and cool-down periods, they increased their maximal aerobic capacity by more than 13 percent in 12 weeks even though most people can't increase their maximal capacity by more than 25 percent total, no matter how much or how long they train. These fitness gains came from doing only six to eight minutes of harder exercise a week. The same intensity principle applies to almost every kind of exercise that you do, from walking to cycling to gardening. In fact, even competitive athletes generally reach a plateau at a certain level unless they do some type of more intense interval training from time to time.

Monitoring Exercise Intensity

You can choose to monitor exercise intensity in various ways. You can use your heart rate as a measure of intensity because it is linearly related to oxygen consumption ($\dot{V}O_2max$), although it declines as you age. To be effective, your exercise should maintain your heart rate in a target training range. For maximal fitness gains, you should work at 60 to 90 percent of your maximum heart rate, or 50 to 85 percent of $\dot{V}O_2max$ or heart rate reserve (HRR). Direct measurement of your maximal heart rate is best, but you can also estimate it fairly accurately using either of the following formulas (valid for adults). Generally, the first works well on college-aged people, and the second one is better for master athletes:

$$\text{Max HR} = 220 - \text{age}$$

$$\text{Max HR} = 208 - 70\% \text{ of age}$$

Using this estimating technique, a 45-year-old athlete would have a maximal heart rate of 177 beats per minute (208 minus 31). Target heart rate ranges will generally be more accurate and individualized using the HRR method, estimated as your maximal heart rate minus your resting heart rate. You should measure your resting heart rate upon waking before you get out of bed. Multiply your estimated reserve first by 50 percent and then by 85 percent before adding each back to your resting heart rate to determine your lower and upper limits (a range of 50 to 85 percent of HRR).

$$\text{Lower range of HR } (50\%) = 0.50 \ (\text{max HR} - \text{rest HR}) + \text{rest HR}$$

$$\text{Upper range of HR } (85\%) = 0.85 \ (\text{max HR} - \text{rest HR}) + \text{rest HR}$$

For example, if our 45-year-old athlete has a resting heart rate of 72, her HRR is 105 beats per minute (177 minus 72). Her range is 50 to 85 percent of HRR added to her resting value, or 125 to 161 beats per minute. See table 1.2 to look up these

Table 1.2 Target Heart Rate Training Zones

RHR	Age							
	15-19	**20-24**	**25-29**	**30-34**	**35-39**	**40-44**	**45-49**	**50-54**
45	125-180	123-175	120-171	118-167	115-163	113-158	110-154	108-150
50	127-181	125-176	122-172	120-168	117-164	115-159	112-155	110-151
55	130-181	128-176	125-172	123-168	120-164	118-159	115-155	113-151
60	132-182	130-177	127-173	125-169	122-165	120-160	117-156	115-152
65	135-183	133-178	130-174	128-170	125-166	123-161	120-157	118-153
70	137-184	135-179	132-175	130-171	127-167	125-162	122-158	120-154
75	140-184	138-180	135-176	133-172	130-168	128-163	125-159	123-155
80	142-185	140-181	137-177	135-173	132-169	130-164	127-160	125-156
85	145-186	143-181	140-177	138-173	135-169	133-164	130-160	128-156
90	148-186	145-182	142-178	140-174	138-170	135-165	132-161	130-157

RHR = Resting heart rate (HR), which ideally you should measure first thing in the morning before you eat, drink, or move around. HR values are estimated as a target zone of 50 to 85 percent of your heart rate reserve (HRR). Your HRR is simply the difference between your highest and lowest HRs (i.e., your estimated maximal HR minus your RHR). To find a target range, multiply your HRR by 50 percent for the low end and by 85 percent for the highest value. The table gives you those ranges based on the median age for each range.

values if you prefer not having to calculate them yourself. A person with a very low fitness level should start exercising at a lower range of HRR using 40 percent rather than 50 percent.

Another method to monitor intensity is by using a rating of perceived exertion (RPE) scale. This scale allows you to measure how hard you believe you are working overall. The number you choose should reflect how heavy and strenuous the exercise feels to you, encompassing your overall physical stress, effort, and fatigue rather than a single factor like leg pain or shortness of breath. The recommended range of RPE for optimal fitness gains is 12 to 16 ("somewhat hard" to "hard") on the Borg category (original) scale that ranges from 6 to 20. Working out below the range of 12 to 16 may not overload your cardiovascular system enough, and working above that range may limit how long you can keep going and may make your session more anaerobic than aerobic. A simpler method to ensure that your exercise intensity is in the appropriate range is to use the talk test; if you are breathing too hard to carry on a conversation with an exercise partner, then your intensity is higher than necessary or recommended. And if you can sing a few phrases without breathing hard, you are exercising at too low an intensity.

Hard and Easy Days

You may benefit from purposefully varying your exercise intensity from day to day, such as by doing hard and easy days of training. By alternating workout intensities (mild, moderate, and heavy), your body will gain both the enhanced fitness and

Age							
55-59	**60-64**	**65-69**	**70-74**	**75-79**	**80-84**	**85-89**	**90-94**
105-146	103-141	100-137	98-133	95-128	93-124	90-120	88-116
107-147	105-142	102-138	100-134	97-129	95-125	92-121	90-117
110-147	108-142	105-138	103-134	100-129	98-125	95-121	93-117
112-148	110-143	107-139	105-135	102-130	100-126	97-122	95-118
115-149	113-144	110-140	108-136	105-131	103-127	100-123	98-119
117-150	115-145	112-141	110-137	107-132	105-128	102-124	100-120
120-151	118-146	115-142	113-138	110-133	108-129	105-125	103-121
122-152	120-147	117-143	115-139	112-134	110-130	107-126	105-122
125-152	123-147	120-143	118-139	115-134	113-130	110-126	108-122
128-153	125-148	122-144	120-140	118-135	115-131	112-127	110-123

strength benefits of hard workouts and the healing effects of greater recuperative time between intense workouts. Varying intensity in this manner also helps prevent overuse syndrome, which results from overstressing your body with repeated heavy workouts and manifests itself as frequent colds, chronic tiredness, and joint and muscle injuries. A day of rest at least once a week is vitally important, even if on that day you do a different or low-intensity activity. But don't allow more than two days to elapse between workouts if you want to maintain your heightened insulin action, as discussed further in the next chapter.

Precompetition Tapers

As you near an athletic competition or event (like a road race, even if you're doing it recreationally), you will want to think about how to cut back on your training to optimize how well you do and how good you feel when the big day arrives. How hard you work out is probably the most important factor in improving performance and maintaining your fitness level even when you cut your frequency or duration of exercise. Preevent tapers (i.e., decreased training volume) can last from one day up to a week or more and are most effective if you maintain the intensity of your workouts while cutting their duration. With diabetes, although you may effectively maintain your fitness levels during preevent tapering, be prepared to increase your insulin doses or reduce your food intake during a taper because you'll be expending fewer calories and using less muscle glycogen and blood glucose. If you decrease your exercise intensity as well, you may need even greater regimen changes to keep your blood sugars from rising.

Duration: Length of Your Workouts

The updated guidelines now recommend that the minimal length of your workout be based on its intensity: 30 minutes of moderate-intensity work or 20 minutes of vigorous-intensity work. Although some improvements in endurance have been shown with extremely intense exercise (more than 90 percent of $\dot{V}O_2max$) lasting only 5 to 10 minutes, this type of exercise adds significantly to the risk for injuries and cardiovascular events and therefore is less often recommended for most people.

Also, you will generally expend more calories by exercising over a longer duration at a lower, more sustainable intensity. The new recommendations emphasize that although relatively modest amounts of physical activity will improve health, for weight loss and greater health benefits you may have to do more than the minimum of 30 minutes of moderate activity most days of the week. Your risk of getting an athletic injury increases, however, when your intensity and duration of exercise go up. The risk of injury has been found to be as high as 55 percent among joggers. So keep in mind that although more is often better, too much may result in injury. You should respect your personal limits.

You can also break up your aerobic activity into smaller bouts during the day—as long as you are active at least 10 minutes at a time—and achieve almost the same fitness gains. If you can't currently work out for 20 to 30 minutes at a time without stopping, you can start with shorter bouts and work up to doing longer ones. On the other hand, if you are training for a prolonged event like a marathon, you undoubtedly will need to do some longer workouts, although not necessarily of marathon length. Similarly, an athlete training to participate in a 5K run (3.1 miles) may not benefit from workouts longer than an hour. Usually, increasing your exercise duration beyond 60 minutes doesn't increase your fitness gains enough to offset your greater risk of developing overuse or other orthopedic injuries resulting from longer-distance training.

Frequency: Are You Exercising Often Enough?

Frequency is interrelated with both intensity and duration of exercise. As mentioned earlier, five days per week is now the recommended minimum unless your exercise is considered vigorous, in which case you can get by with three. You can even mix it up; for example, you can meet the recommended guidelines by walking briskly for 30 minutes twice during the week and then jogging for 20 minutes on two other days. Athletes who train for a specific event or sport, however, may work out more often to get ready for an event even if their workouts are high intensity. Moreover, the recommendations emphasize that doing more physical activity than the recommended minimum amount provides even greater health benefits. The point of maximum benefit for most health benefits has not been established, but it likely varies with genetic endowment, age, sex, health status, body composition, and other factors. But without a doubt, doing more than the minimum (in frequency, intensity, and duration) further reduces your risk of developing inactivity-related chronic diseases.

Generally, when you have diabetes your blood sugars will benefit from nearly daily and more consistent exercise. But with blood glucose monitoring and other methods of glycemic control available nowadays, you can still control your blood sugars even if you choose not to exercise every day. Besides, taking at least one day a week to rest (or at least to do easier activities) allows your body time to recuperate and may prevent overuse injuries, such as tendinitis and stress fractures (see chapter 7). In any case, you can maintain your current fitness level with a minimum of two days per week of appropriately intense activity.

The ACSM also recommends engaging in resistance training, along with flexibility training, a minimum of two to three days per week. You can gain or maintain strength by doing anywhere from 3 to 15 repetitions per set on each resistance exercise and one to three sets with at least two minutes of rest between multiple sets. Generally, doing 8 to 12 repetitions and two to three sets is recommended. Resistance training is essential to prevent loss of muscle tissue over time. Having more muscle will increase your metabolism and daily calorie use and can prevent fat weight gain while improving your insulin sensitivity. Proper training techniques for resistance work are discussed later in this chapter. Flexibility training is also essential in maintaining joint mobility and preventing injuries.

Progression: How to Move Forward With Your Training

How fast you progress should be an individual choice. If you are just starting an exercise program, you will benefit from doing an initial conditioning phase lasting four to six weeks before moving on to an improvement phase lasting four to five months and then to a maintenance phase from six months on. If you already have a higher level of fitness, you may shorten or skip the initial stage altogether. Keep in mind that you will make fitness gains more rapidly if you work out at the higher end of your intensity range (closer to 85 percent of heart rate reserve than to 50). After you reach the maintenance stage, your progress will slow unless you continue to overload yourself by increasing your exercise intensity, duration, frequency, or a combination of these. According to the overload principle of training, you must continue to challenge your muscles and cardiovascular system appropriately to have any further fitness improvements.

RESOURCES FOR ACTIVE PEOPLE WITH DIABETES

DESA

The original organization for active people with diabetes, the Diabetes Exercise and Sports Association (DESA, formerly IDAA), has as its stated mission to enhance the quality of life for people with diabetes through exercise and physical fitness. Their goals range from educating people about the benefits of physical activity, to creating opportunities for active people with diabetes to participate in recreational, sport, and athletic activities (through their local chapters), to promoting networking and forums for exchange of information, to acting as experts in diabetes and exercise.

Founded by Paula Harper in 1985, DESA has both local chapters throughout the United States and international affiliates abroad. To promote its goals, this organization holds annual educational conferences open to everyone in both North America and abroad. Their quarterly newsletter profiles diabetic athletes around the world and features stories about a variety of athletic endeavors. For more information, visit DESA's Web site at diabetes-exercise.org or call them at 800-898-4322.

COMPONENTS OF AN AEROBIC WORKOUT

Having reviewed what components you need to consider in your exercise program, you next need to consider what to include in each workout. An exercise session should consist of a warm-up, an aerobic exercise, and a cool-down (see figure 1.1). The warm-up and cool-down periods should consist of an aerobic activity similar to the one that you will perform as the main element of the workout but at a lower intensity, such as a slow jog before and after a faster run. A good warm-up comprises at least five minutes of an activity before the intensity is increased to meet the guidelines to improve aerobic fitness. An appropriate cool-down is five minutes of the same activity after the more intense activity.

Your workout session should also include a period of 5 to 10 minutes of static or dynamic stretching of the major muscle groups, the purpose of which is to facilitate movement throughout the full range of motion of each of your joints (which can be limited by aging-related changes in joint structures but worsened by elevations

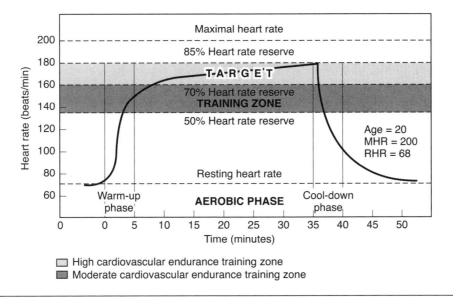

Figure 1.1 Example of an appropriate aerobic workout for a 20-year-old person with a resting heart rate of 68 beats per minute.

in blood sugar levels). You can stretch before and after exercise. The key in static stretching is to stretch to the point of discomfort, back off just a little bit, and then hold the stretch at that point for 10 to 30 seconds without bouncing. Bouncing elicits the muscles' stretch reflexes, and you may end up contracting the muscle or muscles that you are trying to relax. Stretching is usually easier after you have warmed up the muscles and joints and have increased blood flow to those areas, which is more the idea behind dynamic stretching. This type of stretching includes active movements like lunges, knee bends, and arm circles that work the full range of motion around your joints actively. Some studies have shown dynamic stretching to be more effective at preventing injuries than the more traditional static type.

People with diabetes form more glycated end products than people without diabetes do; that is, glucose molecules adhere to various structures in the body including cartilage and collagen, causing them to stiffen and lose their usual range of motion around joints. Although all people lose joint and muscular mobility with age, diabetes accelerates the usual loss of flexibility, especially when blood sugar levels are higher and greater glycation of bodily structures occurs. The result is that people with diabetes are usually more prone to overuse injuries such as tendinitis (inflammation of the tendons connecting muscle to bone) and diabetic frozen shoulder, a condition characterized by limited and painful movement of the shoulder (see chapter 7), and it may also take longer for joint injuries to heal properly if injured.

When you have diabetes, you must take the time to warm up, cool down, and stretch properly.

Thus, when you have diabetes, you really need to take the time to warm up for at least five minutes before your aerobic exercise session, cool down for five minutes, and stretch the major muscle groups involved in your activity either statically or dynamically. Diabetic people are at higher risk for heart disease and silent heart attacks, and proper warm-ups and cool-downs can help prevent cardiac arrhythmias (abnormal heartbeats) or sudden cardiac events during and following exercise. A proper cool-down is important as well to prevent blood from pooling in the extremities. You're more prone to dehydration when your blood sugars run above normal, especially while exercising in the heat. The reduced blood volume resulting from a combination of sweating and preexisting dehydration can cause fainting if you stop exercising abruptly without cooling down and allowing your body to redirect blood flow away from your muscles and back to your central circulation.

GETTING THE MOST OUT OF RESISTANCE TRAINING

Muscle-strengthening activities include a progressive weight-training program, weight-bearing calisthenics, stair climbing, and similar resistance exercises that use the major muscle groups. Ideally, you should do 8 to 10 exercises using your major muscle groups (in the upper body, thighs, and torso) on two or more non-consecutive days a week. Some examples of traditional strength-training exercises are overhead (military) press, bench press, biceps and triceps curls, leg presses, leg extensions and curls, calf raises, and abdominal crunches.

> *You will definitely benefit from working on maintaining or increasing your muscular strength and endurance at least two days each week.*

Your strength gains will be maximized by doing 8 to 12 repetitions of each exercise (usually 8 to 10 of them) until you're fatigued. If you are a novice at resistance work, you can start out with lighter weights or more flexible resistance bands that enable you to complete one or two sets of 12 to 15 repetitions on each exercise, but you should use enough weight or resistance to feel fatigued by the end of the last set. Although focusing on more reps using lower weights increases muscular endurance more effectively, lifting a greater resistance for fewer reps generally produces more of an overload on the muscle fibers and greater gains in muscular strength; consequently, all your muscle fibers will be engaged and increase in size faster, and you'll add more muscle mass. As a result, your muscles will then use more calories even at rest, your resting metabolism will increase, and your insulin sensitivity will improve.

The current recommendations don't state how many sets of repetitions you should do on each exercise. Previous studies showed that you can gain strength by doing only one set but that you'll likely gain more strength by performing two or three sets of each. Alternatively, when doing more than one set per exercise, you can increase the weight or resistance on each successive set, slightly decreasing the number of reps each time the load increases (for example, from 15 reps on the

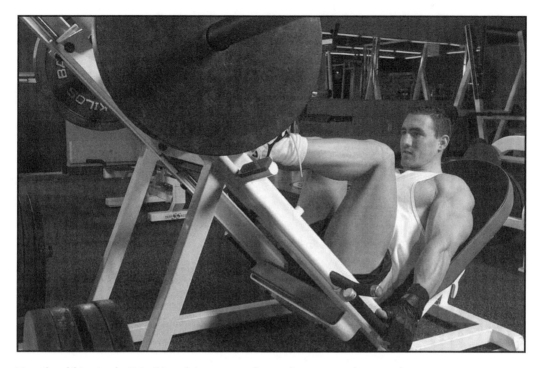

You should try to do 8 to 10 resistance exercises using your major muscle groups on two or more nonconsecutive days a week.

first set to 10 on the second, harder set). If you have time for only one set, make it an intense, nearly maximal set that fully fatigues your muscles by the time you reach the last repetition in your desired range.

You may even decide to vary between easy days, when you do more reps with lighter weights, and hard days, when you lift heavier weights fewer times, depending on how motivated you feel on a given day and how much time you have to train. The only resistance-training principles that you absolutely need to follow are to work a particular area of your body (i.e., upper body) no more frequently than every other day and to train muscles with opposite actions on a joint equally, such as the biceps and triceps muscles of your upper arm or the quadriceps and hamstring muscles of your thigh. The last point to keep in mind is that if you stop overloading your muscles, your strength gains will reach a plateau or start to reverse. After you can do more than the number of reps that you're aiming for (i.e., if you can do 13 or more reps on your hardest set when your goal is 8 to 12), then you can increase the weight or resistance. If you do resistance training correctly your workout will never feel any easier, but you will know that you're getting stronger because you can lift more weight.

As you can see from this first chapter, you can undeniably benefit by getting and staying as fit as you possibly can. The health rewards of your regular workouts will far outweigh any potential problems of having to consider exercise as an added (and often unpredictable) variable in managing your diabetes.

*A*thlete *P*rofile

Name: Chris Jarvis

Hometown: Victoria, British Columbia, Canada

Diabetes history: Type 1 diabetes diagnosed in 1994 (at age 14)

Sport or activity: My primary sport is rowing, but I also do marathons, cycling, triathlons, dance, and yoga (although in high school I played hockey, football, and soccer).

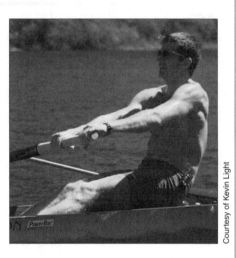

Courtesy of Kevin Light

Greatest athletic achievement: In 2002 I was struggling with my health and diabetes management so much that both my coach and I though I might let my rowing teammates down by being in the varsity boat (at Northeastern University in Boston). At that point, I decided I wanted to be an athlete whom others could count on no matter what. Two years later, I broke into the two-time world champion men's eight and helped my team take their undefeated winning streak from 11 to 17, including the final two World Cups. My most memorable moment was when my coach, Mike Spracklen, remarked that he had altogether forgotten that I had diabetes. I am also proud of competing in the 2004 Olympic Games, rowing for my home country of Canada.

Current insulin and medication regimen: Insulin pump

Training tips: I think that there are two key aspects for success with diabetes in sport. The first is to accept the challenge of diabetes, and the second is to challenge it back! A big factor in my training is to be proactive. Just as good training habits in sports lead to success, diabetes management skills will pay off too. It takes training, though, and a few practices of intensive monitoring and record keeping can teach you where your problem areas are and what to watch for or how to prevent them. I watch my glucose trends and am always aware of active insulin in my body, carbohydrates on board, most certainly what type of exercise I am doing, and the effects of the mental stress that comes along with race days. I use what I observe to make a plan, but I stay flexible. The biggest challenge I have experienced with diabetes and exercise is realizing when I am insulin sensitive. With my continuous glucose monitoring system (CGMS), I can quickly adjust diabetes management to reduce or save me from low blood sugar reactions.

Typical daily and weekly training and diabetes regimen:

▶ **Monday:** Train from 7:30 to 9:30 a.m. (rowing), stretch at 10:00 a.m., row or run from 11:00 a.m. to noon, and do weights and ergometer (erg, or rowing machine) training from 3:00 to 5:00 p.m.

▶ **Tuesday:** Row from 7:30 to 9:30 a.m., from 11:00 a.m. to noon, and again from 3:00 to 5:00 p.m.

▸ *Wednesday:* Row two hours in the morning, stretch, and then do weights and erg training from 11:00 a.m. to 1:30 p.m.

▸ *Thursday:* Repeat of Tuesday's training

▸ *Friday:* Repeat of Monday's training

▸ *Saturday:* Row from 7:30 a.m. to 9:30 a.m., stretch, and then row again from 11:00 a.m. to 1:00 p.m.

▸ *Sunday:* Rest or recreational exercise (hiking, biking, swimming) only

Insulin adjustments for one sample day: When I wake, I take insulin 15 minutes early and reduce the amount I take for the food I eat then to 0.5 unit per 125 grams of carbohydrate and 0.6 unit of basal (baseline coverage) insulin per hour. During warm-up, I either remain at that basal or lower it. From time to time, I'll need a Power Gel to prevent a low. At 9:00 a.m. I bring basal up to 1.25 units per hour and give a bolus (an insulin dose to cover my food intake) after competitive work is finished at 9:30 (usually 1 to 3 units), wait 30 to 45 minutes, and then eat breakfast (bolus typically only 1 to 2 units for 130 grams of carbohydrate).

Before my next workout at 11:00, I reduce my basal to 0.8 unit per hour 20 minutes beforehand. At 11:30, my basal returns to 1.25. Based on my glucose trends, I adjust timing and ratio of insulin, but it's roughly 4 units for a lunch of 90 grams of carbohydrate. For my final workout of the day, my basal shifts 45 minutes before 3:00 to 0.35, and I'll eat a PowerBar if necessary. I then raise my basal rate to 1.3 after practice and bolus with 1 unit per 28 grams. I do a two-step progression for my basal dose at bedtime; at 10:00 p.m. it goes down to 0.8 unit per hour and at midnight lowers to 0.6. My heightened insulin sensitivity can be masked by large, slow-absorbing dinners.

Other hobbies and interests: I am interested in cooking, dancing, running marathons, and social change.

Good diabetes and exercise story: I raced at the Medtronic Twin Cities Marathon on October 7, 2007, as part of a group of people connected through diabetes. We were a collection of people from completely different backgrounds. Some were Boston Marathon qualified, and others were out for their first race. One was a teenager, and a few were near retirement. Some I had known for a long time, and others I met there for the first time. But we had gathered together to collectively declare, "I challenge diabetes." This initiative made the race particularly special for me. It imposed additional challenges when we went to work with my craft kit to make our shirts. With our differences, some of us had plain shirts with just the slogan, others had sparkles and stars, others had fire, and still another had the slogan surrounded by a smile.

One aspect that made this a great opportunity was our discussions of diabetes strategies and tactics. We shared how to secure our pumps and transmitters, what insulin adjustments we make, and even what our favorite flavors of gels and bars are and how we use them to fuel us during our training and races. We learned a lot from one another through the online forum and even more in person. If a similar opportunity for such interaction ever presents itself to you, I suggest that you embrace it.

Even more special during this run was the feeling of representing a challenge to diabetes. It was invigorating to hear the cheers of people reading my shirt, which really helped after I had been running for a couple of hours! I realize that although diabetes can (and does) always challenge me, every challenge comes with possibilities of reward. In this case there were several. The obvious health benefits that our training efforts afforded us were extended even further as we encouraged one another in our diabetes management. The teamwork also turned into some wonderful friendships, which were strengthened all the more by the similar challenges we all faced. The feeling of accomplishment permeated the group so thoroughly that some people have already started planning it again for next year! I think the greatest reward we experienced was the postrace walk. When else can you limp, hobble, stumble, and climb or descend stairs while clutching the banister for dear life with a legitimate reason?

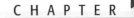
Balancing Exercise Blood Sugars

As all people with diabetes know, a constant balancing act is required to keep blood sugars in a normal range. Exercise presents its own special set of problems for control. The challenge of adding exercise into the mix as one more variable to figure out can feel overwhelming at times. The more you understand about what makes your blood sugars go down (or sometimes up) during exercise, the easier it becomes to control and the more confident you can be about doing activities and staying in control of your diabetes.

EXERCISE AS AN ADDED VARIABLE

Any muscular activity increases your body's use of blood glucose, which can cause you to develop hypoglycemia more readily during or following exercise. Much of your blood sugar response has to do with how much insulin is in your bloodstream, along with how well that insulin is working. If your insulin levels are high during an activity, your muscles will take up more blood glucose and you're more likely to end up with low blood sugars. You can even end up with late-onset hypoglycemia, which can occur for up to 48 hours after you exercise (more on this topic later in this chapter).

On the other hand, doing any exercise when your blood sugars are too high—especially when you have ketones, produced as a by-product whenever your body tries to use stored fat as an alternative fuel, which indicates a lack of insulin in your body—can cause them to go even higher. Exercising under those conditions can put you into diabetic ketoacidosis (DKA), a condition that results from the combination of elevated blood sugars and insulin deficiency. DKA causes your liver to produce ketones that make your blood too acidic, which can be life threatening and land you in the hospital. Certain types of exercise, such as intense resistance workouts, can also raise your blood glucose levels (as explained in the following section), regardless of whether you have diabetes.

Because so many variables can potentially affect your blood sugar responses to exercise, especially if you use insulin or certain other diabetic medications, on some days you may feel like giving up! Don't, though, because regardless of any frustration that you may feel from time to time, the health benefits of being active

The best way to deal with the multitude of variables that can affect you during exercise is to learn your unique responses to all of them by checking your blood glucose levels before, (occasionally) during, and after exercise.

far outweigh the drawbacks. Table 2.1 is a short list of some of the more important of these variables. After you learn to control some of them and anticipate their effects, a somewhat predictable pattern will emerge over time to help you better predict your blood sugar responses to similar exercise.

Table 2.1   Variables Affecting Blood Glucose Responses to Exercise

• Energy system used (exercise intensity and duration)	• Type of exercise that you do
• Blood sugars at start of activity	• Time of day that you exercise
• Training status (i.e., new versus usual activity)	• Previous episode of hypoglycemia
• Prior exercise (same day or day before)	• Timing of last insulin dose (circulating insulin levels)
• Types of insulin you use	• Other glucose-lowering medications that you take
• Time you last ate	• Type of food that you ate
• Temperature and other environmental conditions	• Level of hydration
• Recent or current illness	• Pregnancy (women only)
• Phase of menstrual cycle (women only)	

HORMONAL RESPONSES TO EXERCISE

Studies of people with type 1 and type 2 diabetes have shown that extremely intense exercise like resistance training, weight lifting, or near-maximal anaerobic workouts can actually cause an immediate rise in your blood sugar levels, primarily resulting from your body's hormonal response. Intense exercise causes the release of several hormones that increase the production of glucose by your liver and reduce your muscular uptake of it. These hormones include epinephrine (more commonly known as adrenaline) and norepinephrine, which are released by the sympathetic nervous system (the one that allows your body to respond to physical or mental stressors with an increased heart rate), as well as glucagon, growth hormone, and cortisol (see table 2.2). The effects of these glucose-raising hormones can easily exceed your body's immediate need for glucose, especially because exercise done at high intensity can't be sustained for long. The result is an immediate rise in your blood sugars during and following short bouts of intense exercise.

Intense exercise can cause a large increase in blood sugars because of your body's exaggerated release of glucose-raising hormones, such as adrenaline and glucagon.

Table 2.2   Hormones With Glucose-Raising Effects During Exercise

Hormone	Source	Main actions during exercise
Glucagon	Pancreas	Stimulation of liver glycogen breakdown and new glucose production from precursors to increase glucose output; large effect of changes in the insulin-to-glucagon ratio
Epinephrine (adrenaline)	Adrenal medulla	Stimulation of muscle and, to a lesser extent, liver, glycogen breakdown, and mobilization of free fatty acids from adipose (fat) tissues
Norepinephrine	Adrenal medulla, sympathetic nerve endings	Stimulation of liver to produce new glucose from available precursors; "feed-forward" control of glucose during intense exercise along with epinephrine
Growth hormone	Anterior pituitary	Direct stimulation of fat metabolism (release of free fatty acids from adipose) and indirect suppression of glucose use; stimulation of amino acid storage
Cortisol	Adrenal cortex	Mobilization of amino acids and glycerol as precursors for glucose production by the liver and release of free fatty acids for muscle use in lieu of glucose

You may experience some insulin resistance immediately after intense exercise, which can last for a few hours. For instance, after doing near-maximal cycling to exhaustion, one group of people with type 1 diabetes using insulin pumps experienced elevated blood glucose levels for two hours following the activity. Your body will likely need some supplemental insulin to bring your blood sugar levels back to normal. Similarly, in type 2 diabetic exercisers, blood glucose levels also rose for one hour in response to maximal cycling, as did their levels of circulating insulin because they were still making their own. Even if you don't have diabetes, your body will increase its release of insulin following such workouts. After these hormonal effects wane, your blood sugars can easily drop later on while your body is working hard to restore the muscle glycogen that you used during the activity.

ENERGY SYSTEMS AND ATP USE

The way that your muscles make and use energy during physical activities, including how fast you move, how much force your muscles produce, and how long the activity lasts, can also affect your blood sugar levels. Your body has three distinct energy systems to supply your muscles with ATP (adenosine triphosphate), which is a high-energy compound found in all cells that directly fuels muscular work. The three systems can best be considered a continuum, with one, then the next, and finally the third being recruited to produce ATP as exercise continues. If you exercise long enough (even for just a minute), you will end up using all three to some extent.

All the systems work by causing increased production of ATP, the only direct source of energy that your muscles can use; its breakdown directly fuels all contractions, as shown in figure 2.1. When a nerve impulse initiates a muscle contraction, calcium is released within your recruited muscle cells, ATP "energizes" the muscle fibers, and they go into action. Without ATP, your muscles can't contract and you won't be able to exercise.

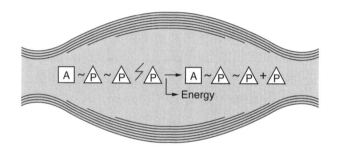

Figure 2.1 ATP directly provides all energy for muscular contractions by removing its last high-energy phosphate group.

Muscle cells contain only small quantities of ATP ready for use when you start, enough to fuel any activity for about a second, at best. If you want to keep going longer, your muscles need to get ATP from another source right away. Although all the systems can supply additional ATP, the rate at which they supply it varies. The fuels used to make the ATP and the amount of time needed to produce it also differ by system. Keep in mind that because of differences in how your energy systems work, the type of exercise that you do can affect your blood sugar responses differently.

ATP–CP System: Short and Intense

For short and powerful activities, one energy system primarily provides all the requisite energy: the ATP–CP system. Also known as the phosphagen system, it consists of ATP that is already stored in muscle and creatine phosphate (CP), which rapidly replenishes ATP. This system requires no oxygen for energy production, making it anaerobic in nature (see figure 2.2). CP can't fuel an activity directly, but the energy released from its rapid breakdown is used to resynthesize ATP for an additional five to nine seconds following depletion of the muscles' initial one-second supply of ATP.

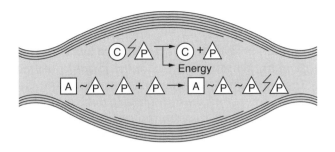

Figure 2.2 Creatine phosphate (CP) provides energy to replenish ATP rapidly during 6 to 10 seconds of all-out effort.

In total, all of your body's phosphagen stores (ATP and CP) can fuel an all-out effort for only about 10 seconds before being depleted. Thus, any activity that you do that lasts less than 10 seconds is fueled mainly by phosphagens, including a power lift, 40-meter sprint, pole vault, long jump, baseball pitch, or basketball dunk. Generally, these types of activities don't lower your blood sugar levels because glucose isn't used to produce the energy. In fact, they can raise your glucose levels because of an exaggerated release of glucose-raising hormones.

Lactic Acid System: Muscle Glycogen and Glucose Use Only

The second energy system, the lactic acid system, supplies the additional energy for activities that last longer than 10 seconds and up to about 2 minutes. The lactic acid system also produces energy anaerobically (without using oxygen) through the breakdown of muscle glycogen (a storage form of glucose in the muscle), a process called glycogenolysis. After it has been released from storage, glycogen produces energy through the metabolic pathway of glycolysis, which forms lactic acid as a by-product (as shown in figure 2.3). When you're resting, your muscle cells do some glycolysis, but because you are not using up much ATP, carbohydrates are processed aerobically (using oxygen) and not much lactic acid builds up.

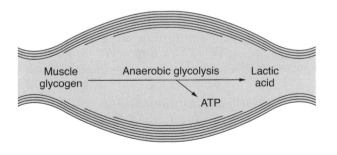

Figure 2.3 The breakdown of muscle glycogen results in ATP and lactic acid production and provides energy for activities lasting 20 seconds to 2 minutes.

Because your muscles' immediate need for additional energy when your exercise continues beyond 10 seconds, glycolysis proceeds rapidly to provide more ATP, and the system soon becomes limited by the accumulation of lactic and other acids. When large quantities are present in muscle, lactic acid drops the pH of muscle and blood, causing the associated "burn" in those muscles and fatigue. This system can make only 3 ATP from each glucose molecule derived from muscle glycogen, which is a relatively small amount compared with the 37 to 39 ATP that may be made through aerobic means. Consequently, this system can't supply enough energy for prolonged periods of exercise. Activities that primarily depend on this energy system include 800-meter runs, 200-meter swimming events, and stop-and-start activities like basketball, lacrosse, field hockey, and ice hockey.

Aerobic System: Using Carbohydrate, Fat, and Protein With Oxygen

The other end of the spectrum is the aerobic energy system used for prolonged endurance or ultraendurance exercise. Because of their duration, these activities mainly depend on aerobic production of energy by the oxygen system (depicted in figure 2.4). Your muscles require a steady supply of ATP during sustained activities like walking, running, swimming, cycling, rowing, and cross-country skiing, which you usually do for longer than two minutes. Running a marathon or ultramarathon, doing an Ironman triathlon, or participating in successive full days of long-distance cycling or backpacking are extreme examples of prolonged aerobic activities.

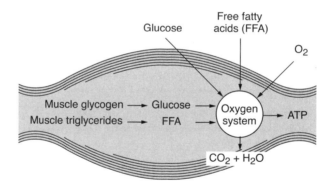

Figure 2.4 The aerobic system supplies ATP for longer-duration activities from carbohydrate and fat sources, plus a little protein.

The fuels for these activities are mainly a mix of carbohydrate and fat, more of the latter than the former during rest and greater carbohydrate use during exercise. Protein can be used to fuel an activity, but it usually contributes less than 5 percent of the total energy. Your body may use slightly more (up to 15 percent) protein during extremely prolonged endurance activities like running a marathon.

At rest, your diet and how recently you last exercised affect the mix of fuels that your body uses, but most people use about 60 percent fat and 40 percent carbohydrate.

Your body will rapidly begin to use more carbohydrate as soon as you start to exercise, and its contribution rises further during harder exercise intensity. High-intensity or near-maximal activities use 100 percent carbohydrate. Muscle glycogen provides more—usually close to 80 percent—than blood glucose, unless you are already glycogen depleted from long-duration exercise or from being on a low-carbohydrate diet. The actual aerobic fuels that your body uses during the activity depend on your training status, your diet before and during the activity, the intensity and duration of the activity, and your circulating levels of insulin.

Circulating hormones like adrenaline mobilize fats from fat cells (adipocytes), and those fats then circulate in your blood as free fatty acids that active muscles can take up and use during less intense activities. Your body will be able to use fats more during mild and moderate activities, along with some carbohydrates. The fats stored in the muscles themselves (intramuscular triglycerides) become more important in fueling your recovery from exercise or during prolonged exercise sessions (greater than two to three hours in length).

Remember that reaching the aerobic system requires that you first use the other two. Both of your anaerobic energy systems (the phosphagens and the lactic acid system) are important at the beginning of any longer-duration exercise before your aerobic metabolism gears up to supply enough ATP (as shown in figure 2.5). These first two systems are also important whenever you have to pick up the pace or work harder, such as when you begin to run uphill or sprint to the finish line of a 10K race.

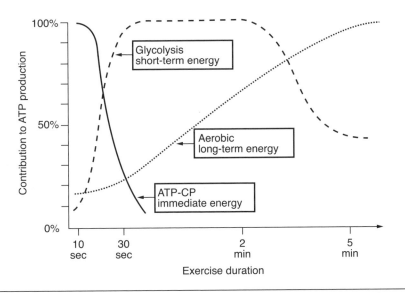

Figure 2.5　Exercise duration largely determines the overall contribution of the three energy systems during an activity.

WHY YOUR BODY ALWAYS USES CARBOHYDRATE DURING EXERCISE

At rest, you're already using about 40 percent carbohydrate to fuel your body's energy needs under normal circumstances, but as soon as you start to do any exercise, your carbohydrate use increases. Usage depends on intensity, so harder workouts will always require greater use of blood glucose and glycogen than easier ones will, but even the easiest workouts will use some. Muscle contractions stimulate the breakdown of glycogen in your muscles, along with glucose uptake from your bloodstream. Carbohydrate is more fuel efficient, meaning that your body gets more ATP out of it for a given amount of oxygen, so for that reason and others it is your body's number one choice of fuels.

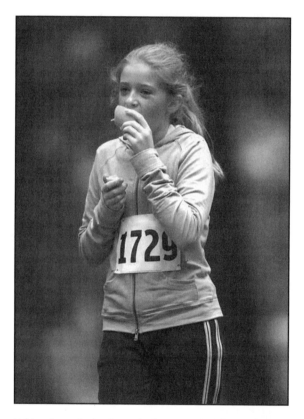

Taking in carbohydrate during exercise, by eating an orange, for example, keeps your blood sugars higher for longer and prevents fatigue.

Fatigue (defined as the inability to continue exercising at the same intensity) is often caused by depletion of glycogen stores in the muscles that you're using, resulting in the phenomenon of "hitting the wall" that is common in longer-distance events. Reaching that point when you're exercising at a moderate pace usually takes longer than 90 minutes, but it can take less time during intense or near-maximal activities. Your muscles use some blood glucose along with the glycogen, sometimes more depending on your insulin levels (more on this topic in the next chapter), but you'll also start using glucose at a faster rate when glycogen stores start to get low—that's when you really have to watch out for low blood sugars! You can deplete muscle and liver glycogen, especially if you haven't eaten much for a while, and then you'll really be in trouble.

If you exercise long enough, your body will use a lot of carbohydrate, so starting with adequate muscle glycogen stores to prevent both early fatigue and hypoglycemia is critical.

By taking in carbohydrate during exercise, you can keep your blood sugars higher for longer and prevent fatigue. They are digested and absorbed more quickly than either protein or fat; carbohydrate usually starts to hit your bloodstream within five minutes. The amount of carbohydrate that you need to take in depends on how long and hard you're exercising, what time of day it is, and how much insulin is in your system. You will need to monitor your blood sugars to figure out the appropriate amount (if any) for each different activity that you do. Refer to table 2.3 for some general guidelines for increasing your carbohydrate intake for aerobic exercise.

Table 2.3 General Carbohydrate Increases for Endurance Sports

Duration	Intensity[1]	Blood sugar before exercise in mg/dl (mmol/L)			
		<100 (5.6)	100–150 (5.6–8.3)	150–200 (8.3–11.1)	>200 (11.1)[2]
15 min	Low	0–5	None	None	None
	Moderate	5–10	0–10	0–5	None
	High[3]	0–15	0–15	0–10	0–5
30 min	Low	5–10	0–10	None	None
	Moderate	10–25	10–20	5–15	0–10
	High	15–35	15–30	10–25	5–20
45 min	Low	5–15	5–10	0–5	None
	Moderate	15–35	10–30	5–20	0–10
	High	20–40	20–35	15–30	10–25
60 min	Low	10–15	10–15	5–10	0–5
	Moderate	20–50	15–40	10–30	5–15
	High	30–45	25–40	20–35	15–30
90 min	Low	15–20	10–20	5–15	0–10
	Moderate	30–60	25–50	20–35	10–20
	High	45–70	40–60	30–50	25–40
120 min	Low	15–30	15–25	10–20	5–15
	Moderate	40–80	35–70	30–50	15–30
	High	60–90	50–80	40–70	30–60
180 min	Low	30–45	25–40	20–30	10–20
	Moderate	60–120	50–100	40–80	25–45
	High	90–135	75–120	60–105	45–90

Note: The recommended quantity is given in grams of rapidly absorbed carbohydrate. One fruit or one bread exchange equals 15 grams of carbohydrate.

[1]Low-intensity activities are done at less than 50%, moderate activities at 50 to 70%, and high-intensity activities at 70 to 85% of heart rate reserve (refer to chapter 1).

[2]For blood sugars above this level, or when ketones are present, an additional dose of rapid-acting insulin may be required to reduce these levels during an activity, and the recommended carbohydrate intake may be higher than actually needed.

[3]Intense (near-maximal), short-duration exercise may actually cause blood sugar levels to increase.

HOW MUCH INSULIN YOU HAVE ON BOARD MATTERS

In people without diabetes and in most people with type 2 diabetes, insulin levels in the blood fall during exercise, and the rise in glucagon release from the pancreas stimulates the liver to produce more glucose. If you have to inject insulin, however, your body can't lower your circulating levels when you start to exercise. Having too much insulin under those circumstances is bad news because it stimulates your muscles to take up glucose from your bloodstream. Muscle contractions do the same thing, and the effect is additive, meaning that higher insulin levels can result in double the glucose-lowering effect and rapid-onset lows. Insulin excesses also keep your fat cells from releasing free fatty acids, lowering the amount of fat available as an alternative fuel for muscles. Note that if you exercise with higher blood sugars, you may use slightly more glucose and less glycogen as fuel.

The amount of insulin that is circulating in your bloodstream during exercise is critical in determining how well you perform and whether you fatigue early from hypoglycemia.

But you need to have some insulin in your body. If you have too little, your body will be missing the normal counterbalance to the rise in your glucose-raising hormones, and you could end up hyperglycemic instead. A fine balance is required because if your insulin levels are too high, they can severely inhibit the release of these hormones and you can end up low. You need some of these hormones because adrenaline mobilizes stored fat and causes muscle glycogen breakdown, and glucagon increases glucose production by your liver. Without these, your muscles can take up more glucose than your liver produces, as shown in figure 2.6. In one study, intense cycling done with extremely low circulating insulin caused hyperglycemia and exaggerated lipolysis (mobilization of fat), whereas the same exercise with too much insulin resulted in hypoglycemia and reduced release of fat. To perform optimally, you need some insulin in your body to counterbalance the release of glucose-raising hormones, but not so much insulin that your blood sugars drop excessively.

Plasma insulin level during exercise	Liver glucose production	Muscle glucose uptake	Blood glucose
Normal exercise level	⇧	⇧	→
Markedly decreased	⇧	↑	↑
Above normal	↑	⇧	↓

Figure 2.6 Your blood glucose response to exercise is greatly affected by circulating plasma insulin levels, which can alter liver production and muscle uptake of blood sugar.

Timing of Exercise and Insulin Levels

The timing of exercise may also play a big role in your body's responses. For instance, you're less likely to experience low blood sugars if you exercise before breakfast, especially before taking any insulin. At that time of day, you have only your basal insulin (the insulin that covers your body's need for insulin at rest separate from food intake) on board, so your circulating levels will generally be low, but you usually have higher levels of cortisol, a hormone that increases your insulin resistance, to compensate.

If you exercise after breakfast and a quick-acting insulin injection, your insulin dose may affect whether you get low because the dose will impact your levels of circulating insulin. In one study, exercisers with type 1 diabetes did 60 minutes of moderate cycling starting 90 minutes after taking their regular dose with an insulin pump and eating breakfast. To prevent lows, they reduced their rapid-acting insulin boluses by 50 percent and took no basal insulin. Their morning insulin reductions, however, turned out to be less than afternoon ones made for a similar workout. Thus, if you often develop hypoglycemia during exercise, you might be better off exercising before taking any insulin to cover breakfast instead of afterward or later in the day.

Anyone with type 2 diabetes who still makes insulin is also more likely to have glucose levels drop if exercising after breakfast or another meal (as opposed to before) because of the insulin that is released in response to eating. Keep in mind, though, that if you exercise long enough without eating, whether you have diabetes or not, you can develop hypoglycemia because of running low on fuels and liver glycogen after not eating overnight, so running a marathon without eating anything beforehand isn't a good idea.

> *You are likely to develop hypoglycemia when you exercise moderately early in the morning before breakfast or whenever your insulin levels are lower.*

Regulating Insulin Levels During Exercise

Physical activity is one of the main causes of hypoglycemia in people with tightly controlled diabetes. Exercising with low levels of insulin is indeed a much more normal physiological response. To lower yours, you may need to lower (if possible) your premeal insulin doses. Table 2.4 gives some general recommendations for insulin changes but refers primarily to rapid- or short-acting insulins, not basal ones. (Basal insulins can also be reduced, but for guidelines on doing so, refer to the recommendations for individual sports in part II.)

How much insulin you have in your system between your exercise sessions can also affect how well you do during the next workout. You may end up restoring less muscle glycogen after exercise (or any time) if you don't have enough insulin or your insulin action is diminished. Although your muscles can take up glucose and restore glycogen mostly without insulin for the first hour following an intense or long bout of exercise, after that time, you need to have enough insulin available to continue stimulating glucose uptake and glycogen storage. If you end up not

Table 2.4 General Insulin Reductions for Endurance Sports

Duration	Low intensity	Moderate intensity	High intensity
	Insulin reductions[1]		
15 min	None	5–10%	0–15%[2]
30 min	None	10–20%	10–30%
45 min	5–15%	15–30%	20–45%
60 min	10–20%	20–40%	30–60%
90 min	15–30%	30–55%	45–75%
120 min	20–40%	40–70%	60–90%
180 min	30–60%	60–90%	75–100%

Note: These insulin recommendations assume that no additional food is eaten before or during the activity to compensate. For insulin pump users, basal rate reductions during an activity may be greater or lesser than these recommendations, and they may be done alone or along with reduced bolus amounts.

[1]These insulin reductions apply to the specific insulin peaking during exercise (usually rapid-acting ones). A lesser insulin reduction may be needed if exercise occurs more than three hours following the last injection of rapid-acting insulin. Postexercise insulin reductions may also be necessary.

[2]For intense, near-maximal exercise, an actual increase in rapid-acting insulin (rather than a decrease) may be necessary to counter the glucose-raising effects of hormones released during exercise.

storing as much glycogen, the next time you exercise your body may depend on greater use of fat, which will lower your ability to exercise and likely cause you to fatigue much more quickly, especially if having low glycogen levels causes you to take up more blood glucose. Keeping your blood sugars closer to normal after exercise also helps you restore glycogen more effectively than if your sugars run high during that time. So, you'll likely need some insulin after exercise for any carbohydrate that you eat, albeit a reduced amount.

HOW TRAINING AFFECTS THE FUELS THAT YOUR BODY USES

Physical training improves the capacity of your body to metabolize fat, which generally results in greater use of it, slower depletion of muscle glycogen, and reduced reliance on blood glucose during an activity after your muscles have adapted. The training effect on fuel utilization is evident when you have diabetes because you'll find that you either need to take in less carbohydrate for the same activity after several weeks or need to lower your insulin less to compensate.

Some of these training adaptations occur because of a lesser release of your glucose-raising hormones when you're exercising at moderate or lower intensity. People without diabetes experience the same training effect, but it may be harder for them to see it because their blood glucose levels hardly fluctuate. Insulin release usually goes down during exercise (if you make some or all of your own), but training actually causes it to go down less. As a result, after training, your body uses less glucose and muscle glycogen and slightly more fat when you do the same intensity of exercise—all of which result in more normal (higher) blood sugar levels and reduced risk of getting low.

This change in fuel use explains why you may need more carbohydrate to maintain your blood sugar levels when you first start doing an activity but less after doing the same activity for several weeks. But if you work out harder to reach the same relative intensity (e.g., if reaching 80 percent of your maximal after training requires you to do a harder workload than at the start), your carbohydrate use during the activity will likely be just as high as before. In addition, the training effect is sport specific, which means that if you've been running and then decide to try a new activity like swimming, your blood sugars will probably drop more during swimming until you're trained in that sport as well.

You may find that after training for several weeks, your blood glucose does not drop as significantly as it did when you first started.

RESOURCES FOR ACTIVE PEOPLE WITH DIABETES

DSWF

The mission of the Diabetes Sports and Wellness Foundation (DSWF) is to inspire and empower people living with type 1 diabetes to embrace health, fitness, and well-being through an active lifestyle. Their stated goal is to give people with diabetes the practical tools, programs and resources, and confidence to start living an active lifestyle. With diabetes as the opponent, the challenges of taking the first step to better health are no different for a beginning walker than they are for an experienced triathlete, according to founder and President Jay Handy, who started the organization in 1999. He and his organization have coached countless diabetic athletes who aspired to complete marathons or 100-mile (160-kilometer) bike rides.

Currently, besides providing an online forum for type 1 diabetic athletes, the DSWF offers annual snowboarding camps for children and adults living with type 1 diabetes (and their friends and families). You can learn more about this organization and its activities at www.dswf.org, or by e-mailing Jay Handy (jay@dswf.org) or Vice-President Bobby Heyer (bob@dswf.org).

HOW EXERCISE AFFECTS INSULIN ACTION

When you're physically trained, you will likely have heightened sensitivity to insulin, which allows your muscles to take up glucose more easily despite having lower levels of insulin. This effect is especially evident in people with type 2 diabetes or anyone else who is more resistant to insulin (such as those with type 1 who have "double diabetes," or symptoms of both types).

Regular physical activity improves blood glucose control by increasing your insulin action, both right afterward, for up to a day or two, and overall.

Right after you work out, your insulin action increases mainly because you're taking up glucose to restore the muscle glycogen that you used. You may need to reduce your basal levels of insulin and doses for meals to compensate for this effect and lower your risk of postexercise lows. By measuring your blood sugars, you're likely to be more aware of changes in your insulin action than anyone without diabetes. You will need less insulin not only during exercise but also afterward, particularly during the window of opportunity for maximal rates of glycogen repletion that occur during the first half hour to two hours after exercise.

Over the long haul, though, training helps with insulin action by increasing your muscle mass, in effect giving you a larger "glucose sink" in which to put excess glucose after meals. Trained athletes generally have low levels of circulating insulin despite being extremely insulin sensitive. Insulin action, though, begins to decline after a period with no exercise, in as little as one to two days, even if you're normally active. Many athletes report that their total insulin requirements increase after two to three days without their regular exercise (such as when they're too busy to exercise, injured, or sick). By way of example, Peter Nerothin of San Diego, California, notices that when he hasn't trained for a few days, he doesn't get nearly the same blood glucose responses to meals. To adjust for periods of less activity, he has to take more insulin up front for his carbohydrate, along with possibly giving himself some extra units in a dual wave using his insulin pump to cover the three to four hours after eating and waiting longer before starting to eat to lower his postmeal spikes.

Although insulin action can stay higher for 24 to 48 hours (or more) after an activity, a study of type 1 diabetic runners found no change in insulin sensitivity following a marathon. In spite of 50 percent glycogen depletion in these athletes, they were no more insulin sensitive on the day after the marathon than they were on a resting day before it, and they had increased utilization of fat. These findings are similar to those in nondiabetic people after a marathon. The cause is likely muscular damage from long-distance events that reduces a person's ability to restore glycogen until the muscles are repaired.

As you can see, many factors affect your blood sugar control during and after a workout. Keep in mind that you will tend to lower your blood sugars more when participating in new or unusual activities, but the intensity and duration of your exercise will also affect glucose use. Intense activities may temporarily raise your blood sugar levels but can cause them to fall later when your muscle glycogen is being restored, so be vigilant then to prevent postexercise lows. The reward of exercise training, though, is that you will lower your overall insulin needs with regular workouts of any type.

EXERCISE AND HYPOGLYCEMIA: THEIR EFFECT ON HORMONAL RESPONSES

Just in the past 5 years or so some new research has finally looked at the physiology behind why low blood sugars can sneak up on you at some times more than at others. Not surprising to most athletes, exercise can have a lot to do with it. Unfortunately, if you've had diabetes for longer than 10 years, you likely have a blunted release of glucose-raising hormones (e.g., glucagon and adrenaline) in response to hypoglycemia, meaning that your body will release less of these hormones than it used to and your blood sugars may stay or go lower than before.

Prior Hypoglycemia Increases Risk of Hypoglycemia During Exercise

Having an episode of hypoglycemia may blunt your body's hormonal response the next time you do any exercise within a day or so. For instance, in one study, volunteers with type 1 diabetes underwent two 2-hour periods of hypoglycemia (experimentally induced) with glucose levels clamped at about 50 milligrams per deciliter (mg/dl), or 2.8 millimolar (mmol/L). The next day, they did 90 minutes of cycling exercise and experienced an extremely blunted release of glucose-raising hormones, which shows that having a bad low the day before may make it harder for your body to keep your glucose levels up when you exercise the next day. However, women's hormonal responses appear to be better preserved during exercise the day after a low compared with men's, making the fairer sex better able to respond to exercise-induced lows. Having a prior bad low blood sugar reaction makes your hormones less able to respond to the next low when it comes along.

Finally, how low you go also appears to make a difference in your ability to respond the next time. In another recent study, different levels of hypoglycemia were induced: 70 (3.9), 60 (3.3), and 50 mg/dl (2.8 mmol/L). After undergoing two 2-hour periods at one of these levels versus a more normal blood glucose level, volunteers did 90 minutes of moderate-intensity cycling exercise the next day. When their glucose levels had remained normal the previous day, they had perfect hormonal responses to exercise, but any hypoglycemia, even just down to 70 mg/dl (3.9 mmol/L), blunted their hormonal responses. In fact, the lower they had been kept the previous day, the worse their responses were during their next-day workouts. These results give you just one more reason to try to prevent lows, especially bad ones, if you want to keep from having low blood sugars during your next exercise session.

Prior Exercise Decreases Hormonal Responses to the Next Low

Along a similar vein, two 90-minute bouts of either low- or moderate-intensity cycling blunt the release of key glucose-raising hormones in response to next-day hypoglycemia, which means that you're more likely to develop bad lows the day after you exercise. This exercise-induced effect appears to occur rapidly—within a couple of hours—and can increase your risk of getting low for the rest of the day after you worked out and the following one.

DEALING WITH EXERCISE-INDUCED HYPOGLYCEMIA

Experiencing bad low blood sugar reactions is one of the main factors that lowers the quality of life of those with diabetes. Even the fear of such lows is enough to increase your anxiety levels. You can do several things, however, to lower your risk, including becoming more aware of the possible symptoms of hypoglycemia.

Recognizing the Symptoms of Hypoglycemia

You really need to know all the possible symptoms of lows, both at rest and during exercise, to detect and treat them early. As you know, normal fasting blood sugars range from 70 to 99 mg/dl (3.9 to 5.5 mmol/L). Although hypoglycemia is technically any blood sugar below 70 (3.9 mmol/L), how low it has to go to cause symptoms of hypoglycemia varies. For instance, if you have been in poorer control, sometimes you will get symptoms while your blood sugars are still normal if they drop rapidly, without ever getting as low as 70 (3.9 mmol/L). If you're in really tight control, your symptoms may not start until you reach 55 mg/dl (3.1 mmol/L) or lower. Some people have hypoglycemic unawareness, which means that they either don't have or fail to recognize the usual symptoms. This condition appears to be more common in people with tight control or frequent lows (more on this later).

The hormones that your body releases during exercise result in some of the same symptoms as hypoglycemia, which can sometimes make it hard to distinguish between the onset of hypoglycemia and the normal physical sensations associated with exercising, such as fatigue, especially during exercise in cold weather. Typical symptoms of hypoglycemia include shakiness, hand trembling, tingling of your hands or tongue, sweating, mental confusion, irritability, poor physical coordination (i.e., clumsiness), and visual changes; see table 2.5 for a more extensive list.

Table 2.5   Hypoglycemic Symptoms

• Buzzing in ears	• Nausea
• Cold or clammy skin	• Nervousness
• Dizziness or lightheadedness	• Nightmares
• Double or blurred vision	• Poor physical coordination
• Elevated pulse rate	• Restlessness
• Fatigue	• Shakiness
• Hand tremors	• Slurred speech
• Headache	• Sweating
• Inability to do basic math	• Tingling of hands or tongue
• Insomnia	• Tiredness
• Irritability	• Visual spots
• Mental confusion	• Weakness

Symptoms may also vary among people and by type of physical activity. By way of example, one athlete with diabetes reportedly sees a spot develop in one eye while running every time he becomes hypoglycemic, and another exerciser begins kicking the back of one heel with the toe of his other foot while running when he starts to get low. Your symptoms can also change over time when your fitness levels improve or worsen, so you should learn to recognize your unique set. Be aware that the symptoms can also differ from workout to workout depending on the type of exercise that you're doing, the rate of decline of your blood sugars, and the environmental conditions.

Make certain that you carry something with you to treat your lows, such as glucose tablets and gels or hard candy. You may possibly step out of your house and forget to bring something with you, only to have a bad low with nothing available to treat it. One hard-training triathlete who always carries something with her during her long, strenuous workouts often goes out to walk the dog without bringing anything along and has her blood sugars drop like a rock. (Perhaps for her, taking the dog out just doesn't seem like enough exercise to cause low blood sugar, but it certainly can.) The maxim for treating exercise-induced lows should be the same as the Boy Scout motto: "Always be prepared."

Testing for Hypoglycemia

In reality, it's not always easy to tell right away if your blood glucose level is too high or low right when you start feeling funny, especially when you're exercising. In fact, when your blood sugars are changing rapidly—either going up or down—you often can't tell which way they're going until your symptoms progress. If you've been running high for a while or you're exercising hard when your blood sugars

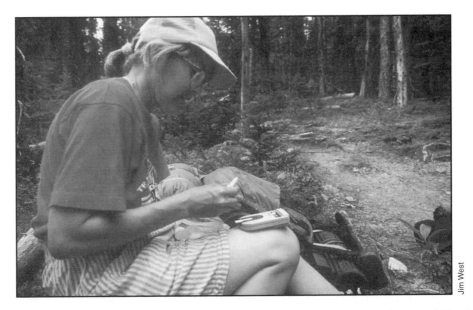

Jim West

Testing your blood sugars frequently, sometimes even during exercise, can help reveal blood sugar trends that might not be apparent with normal testing and can help you anticipate hypoglycemia.

start to decrease rapidly, you may feel hypoglycemic even when your blood sugars are still elevated, or you may not even be able to tell at all.

Regardless of your type of diabetes, testing your blood sugars at different times, more often than just before meals and at bedtime, can help reveal trends that might not be apparent otherwise. Because postmeal glucose excursions may be as important in causing diabetic complications as your overall glucose control, limiting such spikes may be the key to preventing microvascular complications like diabetic retinopathy. Thus, testing not just before meals but also occasionally one hour and two hours afterward can let you know how your various meals are affecting your blood glucose levels and how much variability you are experiencing.

Although the standard recommendation is to check two hours after your first bite of a meal, you may actually peak at 72 minutes after eating and have a variation of 23 minutes either way—based on the results of studies using continuous glucose monitoring. The best idea, then, is to vary your blood glucose testing instead of testing only before meals and at bedtime, especially when you add exercise to the mix. The more you test, the easier it is to figure out what your patterns are, which way your blood glucose levels are going, and when you're likely to drop either during or after exercise. Other keys to preventing lows are given in table 2.6.

Table 2.6 Keys to Preventing Hypoglycemia

- Know yourself—your reaction to specific foods, activities, and stress—by frequently monitoring your blood sugars until you learn your unique patterns and trends.

- Test your blood sugars more frequently whenever you're doing new activities, traveling, or are doing anything outside your usual routine.

- If you dose with rapid-acting insulin for food intake, learn how much insulin you need for a certain intake of carbohydrate so that you don't overdo the insulin.

- Keep the insulin-on-board rules in mind. It takes at least two hours for most rapid-acting insulins to clear your bloodstream; if chasing a high with insulin, wait a while for it to exert its full effects before taking more.

- Never skip meals or food for which you have already taken insulin or medications.

- If you're not sure when you'll eat (like in a restaurant), don't take all your insulin before the food arrives; rather, wait until you have it in front of you.

- Follow your blood sugars for several hours after exercise to catch and prevent postexercise delayed-onset lows.

- Eat a carbohydrate snack (at least 15 grams) within an hour after doing strenuous or prolonged exercise to help restore your muscle glycogen more rapidly. In addition, consume a little protein and fat that will stick around longer.

Preventing Hypoglycemia During and After Exercise

You may be able to prevent, treat, or reverse your impending hypoglycemia during exercise by some novel means. Remember the hormonal effects of intense exercise discussed previously? Some researchers decided to study the effect of doing a short, maximal sprint to counter a fall in blood glucose levels. Some males with type 1 diabetes ate breakfast after injecting their usual insulin dose, waited until their blood glucose levels were no higher than 200 mg/dl (11.1 mmol/L), and then did 20 minutes of easy pedaling on a cycle ergometer. At the end of that, they immediately performed a 10-second cycling sprint. Interestingly, the sprint prevented a further decline in their blood glucose levels for at least 2 hours afterward (compared with when they didn't do it). This technique works anytime during exercise. Although sprinting will have a limited effect if you have extremely high levels of insulin or a blunted hormonal response, it's still beneficial as a short-term means of potentially raising your glucose levels.

> *Whenever you start to feel low, sprint as hard as you can for 10 to 30 seconds to induce a greater release of glucose-raising hormones.*

Along the same lines, another study by the same researchers confirmed that doing the same 10-second sprint, but this time immediately before doing 20 minutes of moderate-intensity cycling, also works to keep blood glucose levels from falling for the 45 minutes after exercise. Levels still fall similarly during 20 minutes of exercise, but the large increase in hormones elicited by the preworkout sprint apparently may keep them from dropping as much afterward.

You can even keep your blood sugars higher during exercise by interspersing 4-second sprints into an easier workout. When diabetic exercisers do a 4-second sprint once every 2 minutes during 30 minutes of otherwise moderate cycling, their glucose-raising hormones again stay higher and their blood sugars decline less. These effects are the result of both greater glucose release (by the liver) during exercise and less glucose uptake during exercise and recovery. Watch out, though, because when the hormonal effects wear off, you may end up more likely to develop hypoglycemia because doing sprints uses up more muscle glycogen.

After exercise, your main concern will be prevention of postexercise, late-onset hypoglycemia, which can occur both because your glycogen levels are low and being replenished (during which time your insulin action is higher) and because hormonal response to low blood sugars diminishes after exercise. Keep in mind two key points to prevent it. First, if you can start to restore your muscle glycogen right after exercise at the fastest rate possible by taking in adequate carbohydrate, you'll be less likely to get as low later on. The first 30 to 60 minutes after exercise is the most critical time when your muscles can take up glucose without much need for insulin. Second, you may have more than one time following a workout when it feels as if your body is rapidly depleting your blood glucose. A recent study showed a biphasic increase in carbohydrate requirements—both right after exercise and again from 7 to 11 hours afterward. Be on the alert for this second wave of potential postexercise hypos and prevent them with adequate food intake and medication changes.

Another study suggested that when it comes to prevention of lows during and after exercise, not all drinks work equally well. Volunteers with type 1 diabetes took in water, whole milk, skim milk, sports drink A (carbohydrate and electrolytes), or sports drink B (carbohydrate, fat, and protein) before, during, and after an hour of moderate cycling in the late afternoon. The number of calories in the drinks averaged around 450, and no insulin adjustments were allowed beforehand. Interestingly, all the drinks except for whole milk and water spiked blood sugars above 200 mg/dl (11.1 mmol/L) during the time between the end of exercise and dinner. Sports drink B (with the extra protein and fat) caused persistently elevated blood glucose levels. Glucose declines after dinner were least in people who drank the whole milk. So, although carbohydrate is most important to replace in the short run, for longer prevention of lows, extra protein and fat intake may also help.

Reversing Hypoglycemic Unawareness

Mild hypoglycemic reactions are not pleasurable, but at least they're easy to treat with carbohydrate intake; however, if your blood sugars drop too low without symptoms or enough time for you to react and treat them, you may become unresponsive or unconscious. If you ever get bad lows without being aware of them, you may have hypoglycemia unawareness, which affects about 20 percent of insulin users. Although it's less common if you have type 2 diabetes, if you do develop it, you're even more likely to experience a higher incidence of severe episodes of hypoglycemia.

If you're hypoglycemic unaware, you may have either milder or missing symptoms due to a blunted hormone release. Because low blood sugars affect the cognitive abilities of your brain, you may test your blood sugars when you're low and not even realize that you need to eat, resist others' help in treating it, or fight off or run from paramedics trying to assist you. Hypoglycemia unawareness can occur at night (because people apparently wake up for less than half of their nighttime lows) as well as during the day. Unless someone is around to recognize that you're very low and help you get treatment, you could even have a grand mal seizure or become unconsciousness.

Fortunately, you may be able to reverse this condition. Although people often experience diminished glucagon release in response to hypoglycemia after 2 to 10 years of diabetes, the most common reason that unawareness develops is frequent low blood sugars. One study found that after people slept through a low during the night (from which they eventually recovered without treatment), they were less likely to recognize another low the next day. You apparently can restore most of your normal hypoglycemic symptoms, however, if you avoid low blood sugars for a 3-week period. If you do have a low, try to avoid having another for at least 2 days to regain better awareness of your next one. You may also be able to do hypoglycemia unawareness training (offered by some diabetes educators), which can teach you to become more cognizant of changes in your blood glucose levels.

BEING FEMALE AND ATHLETIC: SPECIAL CONCERNS FOR WOMEN ONLY

Before the advent of blood glucose meters, discovering how much of an effect female hormones have on insulin action was impossible. If you're female, past puberty, and still young enough to be menstruating, then you'll want to read this section to find out more about factoring your time of the month into your insulin adjustments. Moreover, if you're pregnant, diabetic, and active, you'll also be facing some special circumstances.

How Monthly Cycles Affect Insulin Action

A woman's normal monthly cycle has two phases: (1) follicular, which goes from the start of menses up to ovulation at midcycle, and (2) luteal, spanning the time from ovulation to your next period. We have long known that women are more insulin resistant during the luteal phase because of the greater release of certain female hormones (estrogen and progesterone) during that time. Such changes can also affect female athletes who have this additional factor to work into the equation to achieve balanced blood sugars while having an active lifestyle.

For example, Betty Ferreira, a regular diabetic exerciser from Toronto, Ontario, finds that her blood sugars start to increase gradually 7 to 10 days before her menses and then instantly decrease the day her period starts. To compensate, she has to increase her basal insulin (Levemir) by 1 unit a day starting a minimum of 5 days beforehand, which means that her total basal dose goes from 16 units up to 23 units during that time, including an occasional 1- or 2-unit increase in her night dose. Similarly, Cynthia Fritschi from Chicago, Illinois, finds that she must increase her total insulin by 150 percent 3 days before her menses begin (and she still struggles to maintain control during that time), and the changes she makes for each workout vary. Not all women are affected equally, though, and the differences appear to be tied in with actual increases in estrogen levels; the higher they go, the more effect they have on blood sugars.

Use of oral contraceptives can alter the normal hormonal changes in women as well. Most of these pills or treatments are now made up of low-dose estrogen and progestin. Because they prevent ovulation, insulin action may be somewhat reduced, but at least it remains more balanced over the monthly cycle, leading to greater predictability and easier glucose control for most women who use them.

Being Pregnant, Diabetic, and Active: The Ultimate Challenge for Women

Even if you're athletic and regularly active, the release of the same hormones during pregnancy as you have during the luteal phase of your menstrual cycle ensures that your insulin needs will go up while you're expecting. Raging hormones during the third trimester in particular work to make the mother-to-be insulin resistant and spare glucose for the fetus. Being active, though, will keep you from having to raise your insulin doses as much, even during the last few months of your pregnancy. Being active will also prevent excessive weight gain and keep you from getting out of shape. If you have to stop exercising during your pregnancy for any reason, expect your insulin needs to go up dramatically, both from the hormones released and from the decrease in your insulin action that you will experience from being inactive.

Pregnancy increases the energy costs of doing any activity, so you will be using more calories during all your activities, particularly the weight-bearing ones. Your exercise intensity will likely go down, particularly in the later stages of your pregnancy as Mother Nature takes care of your baby's health by not making it possible for you to work out as hard as normal (even if you try to). You should avoid certain activities when pregnant—contact sports, sports with lots of directional changes (like racquetball), water skiing, and cycling outdoors (when balance becomes an issue)—but you can continue doing most other ones. During the third trimester, consider substituting non-weight-bearing activities like aquatics and stationary cycling for running or doing excessive amounts of walking. Also, don't do any exercises lying flat on your back past the second trimester because doing so can reduce blood flow to your developing baby. Despite all these changes, you will likely find that diabetes control is the least of your problems when you're pregnant, especially if you are able to stay active.

*A*thlete *P*rofile

Name: Scott Dunton

Hometown: Honokaa, Hawaii, USA

Diabetes history: Type 1 diabetes diagnosed in 2002 (at age 16)

Sport or activity: Surfing

Greatest athletic achievement: First diabetic surfer to make the world tour for professional surfing

Current insulin and medication regimen: Medtronic insulin pump

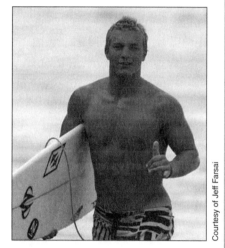

Courtesy of Jeff Farsai

Training tips: I don't really see doing something I love as training. I surf mostly every day when there are waves. I live at one of the prettiest places I have ever been, and it just happens to have my favorite waves on Earth in the same place. I drive my truck down on the sand with my girlfriend and our two dogs, set up the chairs and the BBQ grill, and just surf. I come in when my arms feel like they are going to fall off or I get hungry. I know it's definitely training because if I didn't surf all the time, I wouldn't be at the level I am. Surfing is the best thing for me; it's a time to get away and forget any of life's troubles. That was always what surfing has been for me, although it changed for a while after I was diagnosed.

Diabetes followed me everywhere. I couldn't get any time when I didn't have to worry about what my blood sugar was or if I needed to eat something. So, at first it was really frustrating. Now, with the technology that has come out (like continuous glucose monitors), I have gotten such good control of my blood sugars that I can feel the slightest low or even the smallest high. I can surf and not stress about my diabetes because I know I will feel the changes in my blood sugars. Now when I'm surfing, I am not always so stressed about being diabetic, and when I am doing stuff on dry land like hiking, fishing, or hunting, I wear my continuous glucose monitoring system. That has made everyday life a lot better (knowing my blood sugar every five minutes without having to check all the time), and my day-to-day life and out-of-water activities go a lot smoother.

Typical daily and weekly training and diabetes regimen: Normally, I don't take any different amount of insulin on the days I surf compared with the days I don't. I do, however, like to keep my blood sugar in the range of 120 to 150 before I go surfing just to be safe. I would say that 99 percent of the time it's in that same range when I come in. Even on the days when I surf for three or four hours, it doesn't seem to give me problems when I am in the water. After not being able to surf for a couple of months because of knee surgery, here's an example of one of my first weeks back in the water this winter (2007).

▸ ***Monday:*** I woke up and drove down to surf for about three hours. With a good-sized swell in the water, the waves were pumping across a little sandbar I call Ghost Face. I surfed until about 11:00 and then headed home for lunch. After eating and working in the garden some, I rested. Later, I went back to surf for another couple of hours, but the waves weren't as good, so I got out and just played with the dogs on the beach.

▸ ***Tuesday:*** The wind was up early and ruined the swell. I instantly became lazy because the second that I know the waves are no good, I lose motivation. Finally, around 4:30, the wind died and I went out for a little evening session. The waves were surprisingly good, and I ended up surfing until it was too dark to see the beach.

▸ ***Wednesday:*** The waves weren't cooperating, so I decided to go fishing. I always have fun fishing near home because there are so many fish that I don't have to wait long to catch one.

▸ ***Thursday:*** My neighbor woke me up at 2:30 a.m. to go hunting, so it was an early start for the day. I love walking through the hills getting to see the sun come up over the ocean and everything come to life. After we got back midmorning, I wanted to get in the water even though the waves were small. I had fun trying some new tricks that I have been trying to learn–the days with little waves are perfect for that because it's like skateboarding on a parking curb. I surfed for a little over an hour and then went home to rest from a full day of activities (even though it was only early afternoon).

▸ ***Friday:*** I drove into Hilo to shoot photos with a photographer from town. I don't normally like surfing in town because I'm from the country and I don't really like dealing with the crowds. I surfed with a couple of guys I haven't seen in a while.

▸ ***Saturday:*** Today I decided to go surf one of my favorite waves on the West Side, a bay that has a wave in it that's 200 yards (183 meters) long with a perfect right that has a really fun takeoff section and the best face to just practice about any turn you can think of. I surfed for about three hours, which is a long time because the paddle is so long. I came in and then my good friend Steve showed up and talked me into surfing with him for another half hour, at which point I could hardly stand because my leg muscles were so tired. I went hunting until dark and then made my way back to the house to get dinner.

▸ ***Sunday:*** Today I just stayed home and did stuff around the house.

Other hobbies and interests: I also like doing some dry-land activities, such as hiking, fishing, and hunting. The waves aren't good enough to surf every day!

Good diabetes and exercise story: My doctor, Kevin Kaiserman, MD, has had by far the biggest impact on my diabetes. Without him, I would have never gotten to where I am in surfing or with my diabetes. He persuaded me to reach for my goals and take great care of my diabetes without letting it rule my life. When I was first diagnosed, I was told that being a professional surfer was an unrealistic goal for someone with diabetes and that it was unsafe to be out in the ocean for hours alone. After hearing that, my diagnosis day went from being the worst day of my life to my not caring about life anymore. A surfer was all I had ever wanted to be since the age of five when my uncle taught me to surf. Being told that I couldn't surf anymore because of diabetes really set me back. Dr. Kaiserman inspired me not to let what people say stop me from reaching my goals. A few years later, I was the first diabetic surfer to ever make it onto the world tour. It was the happiest day of my life because I knew that I accomplished it against all odds and set an example for a lot of kids who may have someone tell them that diabetes will keep them from reaching their dreams and goals. I'm glad I didn't listen.

CHAPTER **3**

Ups and Downs of Insulin and Other Medications

At the start of any activity, your body increases the release of glucose-raising hormones to prevent falls in your blood glucose levels. At the same time, your pancreas releases less insulin (if you still make any) during exercise. But if you have to depend on insulin by injections or pump or if you use certain other medications, your body may not be able to respond normally. You can't turn off insulin from an injection site, and exercise can sometimes speed up its absorption somewhat by increasing blood flow to your muscles and skin. As a result, instead of having less insulin circulating around your bloodstream during exercise, you may end up with more than normal, which can easily lower your blood sugars too much. Similarly, certain oral diabetic medicines can also augment the effects of insulin during exercise or cause greater release, potentially resulting in hypoglycemia. The rest of this chapter will let you know what steps you can take to prevent lows, no matter what type of diabetes medications you use.

INSULIN USE: EFFECT ON SPONTANEITY AND MORE

Have you ever felt like jumping on your bike and going for a ride without giving any thought to where you're going or how long you'll be gone? When you have diabetes and you use insulin, the problem with such spontaneity is that your insulin levels during an activity can greatly affect your blood sugar response to exercise (refer to figure 2.6 in chapter 2). To predict your response to a workout, you must take into account what types of insulin you use, when you last took any, and how much is in your bloodstream before, during, and afterward.

Different insulins have varying times to peak action and unique durations, both of which can make activities (especially spontaneous ones) harder to handle. Several types of insulins are now on the market, further complicating matters. In general, insulins are considered rapid or short acting, intermediate acting, or long acting depending on their onset, peak, and duration. Each type of insulin potentially has a different effect on your blood sugar responses to exercise. A fact of life for insulin users is that spontaneity must usually be moderated with extra carbohydrate or immediate insulin changes to prevent hypoglycemia.

> *Knowing when your insulins peaks is crucial to determining your blood sugar responses to exercise and your need for extra carbohydrate or lower insulin doses.*

Short- and Rapid-Acting Insulins: Good for Covering Carbohydrate Intake

As for the shorter-acting insulins, human-synthetic regular insulin (most common trade names: Humulin R, Novolin R, and Actrapid) is still available, but few manufacturers make beef and pork combinations anymore. Insulins of synthetic origin that have the same structure as human ones generally have faster onset, quicker peak time, and shorter duration than their previous animal counterparts and are less likely to cause allergic reactions.

In just the past decade, several rapid-acting insulins have hit and taken over the market from regular insulin, including Humalog (generic name: lispro), NovoLog or NovoRapid (aspart), Apidra (glulisine), and VIAject, an extremely rapid-acting formulation that is absorbed in about half the time as Humalog. These products are actually insulin analogs; they have a structure similar to that of insulin, but the order of the amino acids (i.e., protein building blocks) is slightly modified, which results in faster absorption and shorter duration. The benefit of these analogs for regular exercisers is that they're mostly gone from your circulation within two hours after you take them, lowering your risk of getting low when active later. Most insulin pump users are now using one of these rapid-acting analogs in their pumps for both basal and bolus insulin coverage. For a comparison of the onset, peak, and duration of these and other currently available insulins, refer to table 3.1.

Early in the new millennium, an inhaled insulin called Exubera also received approval for use in the United States. Just recently, though, the manufacturer decided to stop making it because of lackluster sales. Its onset was similar to the rapid-acting insulin analogs, but its duration was more like regular insulin. Although other companies are working on perfecting the delivery of insulin through inhalation or by mouth (orally), the only insulins currently on the market are still the ones that you have to inject with a syringe or infuse with a pump.

Table 3.1   Human Insulin Action Times

Insulin	Onset	Peak	Duration
Humalog, NovoLog, and Apidra	10–30 minutes	0.5–1.5 hours	3–5 hours
Regular (R)	30–60 minutes	2–5 hours	5–8 hours
NPH (N), Protophane	1–2 hours	2–12 hours	14–24 hours
Lantus	1.5 hours	None	20–24 hours
Levemir	1–3 hours	8–10 hours	Up to 24 hours

Note: Individual action times may vary depending on environmental conditions, activity level, injection site, and dosage taken.

Intermediate-Acting Insulins: Not as Widely Used Anymore

Some intermediate-acting insulins are available as well. NPH (trade names: Humulin or Novolin N in the United States and Protophane elsewhere; generic name: isophane) is the most common insulin of this type. Although others are available, they all generally have the same or similar actions as NPH in terms of their onset, peak action, and duration. A usual regimen is NPH at breakfast along with regular or Humalog to cover breakfast, an optional rapid-acting injection at lunch, a mandatory one at dinner, and another dose of NPH at bedtime. An alternative regimen is to take rapid-acting insulin doses during the day with a single bedtime dose of NPH. If you have type 2 diabetes, you may be using NPH alone (usually at bedtime) or a mixture of NPH and with a shorter-acting one (e.g., a 70–30 mix or another mix, a discussion of which is beyond the scope of this book).

Basal Insulins and Basal-Bolus Regimens

Two relatively new basal insulins, Lantus (generic name: glargine) and Levemir (detemir), are now available and have replaced the use of other long-lasting insulins like Ultralente. The main difference between these two newer insulins is that Lantus lasts up to 24 hours and is usually taken once daily, and Levemir requires twice-daily dosing. Both are supposed to be peakless and provide coverage for your basal insulin needs, but you'll likely have to use rapid-acting insulin to cover your meals and snacks effectively if you don't make enough of your own.

The benefit of either of these basal choices is that you can effectively replace just your basal insulin needs and cover meals and snacks solely with rapid- or short-acting insulins. The downside is that basal insulins last 12 to 24 hours, making it harder to implement short-term corrections in basal insulin coverage for unusual or prolonged activities unless you purposefully lower your doses in advance. Also, as mentioned, absorption can be inconsistent because of your choice of injection site, activity level, massaging the area, hot tubbing, or other factors that may speed up how quickly it shows up in your circulation, resulting in basal insulin levels that are first too high and later too low.

Many diabetic athletes have very low basal insulin needs, a scenario that presents a problem when it comes to using Lantus once a day. If you take less than 20 units a day, your basal coverage is unlikely to last a full 24 hours as promised. (Actually, if you read the package insert, you'll see that the duration is quite variable and as short as 12 hours for some people.) In general, with all insulin, even basal ones, the smaller the dose you take, the more rapidly it is absorbed because of the surface area of the insulin depot (the spot where the insulin is injected) under your skin.

For many Lantus users who only need small doses of insulin, coverage lasts significantly less than 24 hours, which may make twice-a-day dosing more effective for basal coverage.

The athletes who have mentioned this problem have found its maximal duration to be about 16 to 22 hours. One way to get around this problem is to give Lantus like Levemir—split into doses that you give twice a day instead of only once—which is what a lot of small-dose Lantus users actually do. Dr. Karen Stark of Saint Louis Park, Minnesota, compared these two basal insulins on herself and found that she has to be more cognizant of taking Levemir at the same time every day because its duration is definitely shorter. On the flip side, she noticed that Lantus has more of a peak than Levemir and that she's likely to experience Lantus-induced lows in the first 6 to 12 hours after taking it, whereas Levemir is absorbed more evenly with less chance of peaking and causing low blood sugars.

A recent study also demonstrated that blood glucose levels in anyone using Lantus usually rise around the time that you're supposed to give your next dose (whether you give it at bedtime, dinner, or lunch). Bedtime injections in particular lead to hyperglycemia in the early part of the night, which is improved if you give your single dose at lunch or dinner instead. Regardless of when you give it, you may need to take extra rapid-acting insulin to cover the rise in your blood sugars when your Lantus dose wears off.

Insulin Pumps: Acting More Like a Pancreas

Whether you have type 1 or type 2 diabetes, if you use insulin, you may choose to give it to yourself using a specialized insulin pump, which nowadays is about the size of a pager or cell phone. Pumps use a subcutaneous (placed under the skin) plastic catheter through which small, basal doses of quick-acting insulin (usually one of the rapid-acting analogs like Humalog) are continually delivered to mimic normal insulin release by the pancreas. You must program the pump to give bolus doses to cover your food (mainly carbohydrate) intake at meals and snacks. Every three days or so, you also have to change the infusion site by putting in a new catheter to avoid excessive buildup of scar tissue that can compromise your insulin delivery.

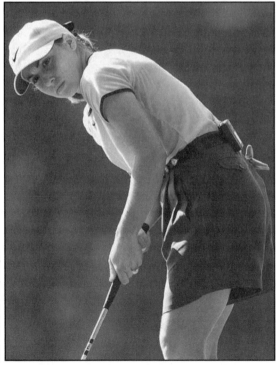

Luke Frazza/AFP/Getty Images

Insulin pumps nowadays are about the size of a cell phone and continually deliver small, basal doses of quick-acting insulin to mimic normal insulin release by the pancreas.

The idea behind insulin pump therapy is to provide insulin just like your body would, that is, in small doses all day long, with bigger doses following food ingestion. Although this physiological pattern can be closely mimicked using any of the newer basal or bolus regimens (e.g., Lantus insulin for basal, Humalog or NovoLog for boluses), insulin pumps make the delivery of that insulin easier and they offer more flexibility by allowing the user to change basal rates of insulin delivery at any time during the day (or set up different preprogrammed profiles of delivery). The exercise responses of people who use either basal insulin or pumps are often similar because both regimens attempt to provide basal insulin levels. Pump users, however, can suspend the pump and immediately reduce basal rates of insulin, which is something that injectable insulin users can't do as easily without planning ahead.

Many insulin pumps are now available, and the features vary by manufacturer and model. For a comparison, see table 3.2. Most of the manufacturers' respective pumps have features like small basal increments (0.05 unit per hour or less), temporary basal rates, menu-driven programming, and various bolus patterns (e.g., normal, extended, and combination). Normal boluses, for instance, give the insulin dose all at once, but extended ones allow a programmed dose to be given over a longer period to avoid peaks and valleys in insulin coverage for foods that are more slowly absorbed; combination boluses simply combine these two strategies for optimal coverage of foods like pizza. At least two even have self-contained food databases or blood glucose meters, and most are now waterproof at shallow depths.

Table 3.2 Features of Some Insulin Pumps

Manufacturer	Latest models	Noteworthy features	More information
Medtronic MiniMed, Inc.	Paradigm 522 and 722	Pumps and real-time continuous glucose monitor can be used together (one screen for both)	www.minimed.com, 800-933-3322
Animas Corporation	IR 1250 and 2020	Smallest basal increments of 0.025 units; automatic bolus calculator; ezCarb 500-item carbohydrate content list, and high-contrast color screen (2020 only)	www.animascorp.com, 877-937-7867
Smiths Medical MD, Inc.	CozMore Insulin Technology System	All-in-one pump (Deltec Cozmo) and glucose monitor (FreeStyle); CoZmanager software; AAA batteries	www.cozmore.com, 800-826-9703
Insulet Corporation	OmniPod	Disposable (three days); no tubing; wireless Personal Diabetes Manager; integrated Freestyle meter; easy cannula insertion	www.myomnipod.com, 800-591-3455
Roche (formerly Disetronic Medical Systems Inc)	AccuChek Spirit	Comes with glucose meter and palm PDA for bolus calculations and easy carbohydrate counting	www.disetronic-usa.com, 800-280-7801
Sooil USA	Dana Diabecare II, S, and SG	Extremely small and lightweight; 20% lower retail price; preset meal boluses; built-in glucose meter (SG model)	www.danapumps.com, 858-404-0659
Nipro Diabetes Systems	Amigo	Built-in bolus estimator (no manual calculations)	www.niprodiabetes.com, 888-651-7867

With all these options, deciding which pump to get can be difficult, so you may want to talk to your health care provider after going to each manufacturer's Web site or calling them for more information. Insulin pumps are not for everyone, though, and the choice to use one (or not) should be an individual one. Their use is not optimal for every sport and activity, but they can help by allowing more rapid alterations in insulin levels during most of them.

WHY INSULIN ABSORPTION MAY BE INCREASED BY EXERCISE

Exercise, as well as other activities like hot tubbing or vigorous massage, can increase the absorption rate of insulin regardless of where you inject it. As a result, your circulating insulin levels may increase during exercise, but then be too low later on, especially with more rapid absorption of rapid-acting insulin analogs. Although exercise can also increase the absorption of Lantus or Levemir, this effect appears to be less significant.

With the rapid-acting insulins, some people use this faster absorption to lower their blood sugar levels rapidly with exercise. For instance, if they start out with elevated blood glucose levels (above about 300 mg/dl, or 16.7 mmol/L), they may take 0.5 to 2.5 units of a rapid-acting insulin like Humalog before exercise to cause a rapid drop into a more normal range. You need to be cautious if you try this, though, because underestimating the amount of insulin that you need is far better than taking too much and having a crashing low blood sugar during your workout. Remember, too, that exercise itself increases your glucose uptake, which can lower your sugars even faster than the insulin alone does, even when it is being absorbed more quickly than usual.

Along those lines, however, some athletes like to correct with intramuscular (IM) injections of rapid-acting insulin to bring their blood sugars back into a desired range more quickly whenever they have hyperglycemia. For example, Garrick Neal of Vancouver, British Columbia (Canada), uses IM injections of Humalog into his calf muscle (where there is not much fat below the skin and the muscle is easier to inject into) to bring his elevated blood sugars down quickly. He finds that an IM injection is usually completely absorbed in about two hours without exercise, but if he gives it and then works out, it's all absorbed within about 40 minutes. Similarly, James Murphy of Valparaiso, Indiana, gives himself 1 unit of Humalog into his arm muscle when his blood sugars are 110 mg/dl (6.1 mmol/L) higher than normal. He then goes for a 30-minute walk with 3-pound (1.4-kilogram) weights in his hands (which increase his overall glucose use by raising his exercise intensity) to bring his sugars back down to normal. Alternatively, he'll give the shot into his leg muscle and bike for a half hour, but he has to be on the lookout for blood glucose drops later on.

ORAL DIABETIC MEDICATIONS: USED BY TYPE 2s (AND SOME TYPE 1.5s)

If you use any of the oral diabetes medications, knowing their potential glucose-lowering effects is important. In general, oral medications for diabetes target one or more of three metabolic disorders found in diabetes: decreased insulin production by the beta cells of the pancreas, elevations in the production of glucose by the liver, or increased insulin resistance in muscle and fat tissues. Their many classes, differing actions, and names are listed in table 3.3. If you ever experience a change in your exercise routine, you may need to consult with your doctor about adjusting the doses of oral medications that you take, particularly if you begin to engage regularly in more physical activity than you did before.

An increase in your activity level may require you to lower your doses, even of oral diabetes medications that do not usually cause exercise-related low blood sugars.

Table 3.3   Oral and Other Diabetic Medications and How They Work

Class of drug	Brand name examples (generic names)	Mechanism of action
Sulfonylureas	Diabinese; Amaryl (glimepiride); Glucotrol and Glucotrol XL (glipizide); DiaBeta, Micronase and Glynase (glyburide)	Promote insulin secretion from the beta cells of the pancreas; some may increase insulin sensitivity
Biguanides	Generic metformin, Glucophage, Glucophage XR	Decrease liver glucose output; increase liver and muscle insulin sensitivity; no direct effect on beta cells
Thiazolidenediones (glitazones or TZDs)	Avandia, Actos	Increase insulin sensitivity of peripheral tissues, such as muscle
Meglitinides	Prandin (repaglinide), Starlix (nateglinide), Glufast (mitiglinide)	Stimulate beta cells to increase insulin secretion but only for a very short duration (unlike sulfonylureas, which have a longer action)
Alpha-glucosidase inhibitors	Precose (acarbose), Glyset (miglitol)	Work in intestines to slow digestion of some carbohydrates to control postmeal blood glucose peaks
DPP-4 inhibitors (gliptins)	Januvia (sitagliptin), Galvus (vildagliptin), and soon others (denagliptin, saxagliptin)	Work by inhibiting DPP-4, an enzyme that breaks down glucagon-like peptide-1 (GLP-1) in the gut; delayed GLP-1 degradation extends the action of insulin while suppressing glucagon release
Amylin (injected)	Symlin (pramlintide)	Works in combination with insulin to control glycemic spikes for three hours after meals
Incretins (injected)	Byetta (exenatide), Byetta LAR (once weekly formula)	Stimulate insulin release; inhibit the liver's release of glucose by glucagon; delay the emptying of food from the stomach

A class of drugs called sulfonylureas was the only one available to treat type 2 diabetes for many years. They work by stimulating insulin release from the pancreas and decreasing insulin resistance. The only first-generation one still on the market is Diabinese (generic name: chloropropamide), which can last for up to 72 hours. Its long duration gives it a greater chance of causing hypoglycemia during or after exercise, especially if you have kidney problems. The more commonly used, second-generation sulfonylureas are more effective at smaller doses and include Amaryl, Glucotrol, DiaBeta, Micronase, and Glynase. Of these, only the latter three (all brand names for generic glyburide) carry a greater risk of causing exercise lows because of their action (24 hours versus only 12 to 16 for Amaryl and Glucotrol), although all of them often contribute to weight gain.

> *In general, oral agents with the longest duration, such as Diabinese, DiaBeta, Micronase, and Glynase have the greatest potential to cause hypoglycemia during and following exercise, especially when you do any unusual or prolonged activity.*

Metformin (marketed both in its generic form and as brands like Glucophage) is in a separate class of drugs called biguanides. Its most important action is to reduce the liver's output of glucose (often elevated in the early morning in people with diabetes), but it has other actions including lowering glucose absorption from the gut and enhancing insulin action. Metformin is, by far, the most prescribed of all oral diabetes drugs. One of its main advantages is that, unlike sulfonylureas, it doesn't contribute to weight gain; it's also unlikely to cause hypoglycemia and can be used in combination with other medications. A recent study investigated using metformin in overweight adults with type 1 diabetes, even though this drug is normally prescribed only to treat type 2. Although not given to normal-weight type 1s, it may prove to be a useful therapy for overweight people with type 1 diabetes who have impaired insulin action that is common to type 2 diabetes (but, of course, regular exercise would also help their insulin action).

Another class of drugs called thiazolidinediones, or TZDs or glitazones for short (including Avandia and Actos), directly enhance peripheral insulin sensitivity without affecting insulin secretion from the pancreas. Although these drugs don't usually cause low blood sugars, Avandia recently received a lot of bad publicity because of its potential to worsen a weakened heart (heart failure); as a result, both medications in this class now have to carry a "black box" warning on them, and many people have chosen to stop taking Avandia or combination drugs containing it like Avandamet and Avandaryl. But their ability to increase insulin action much like exercise does makes them an attractive treatment for those with type 2 diabetes.

Alpha-glucosidase inhibitors, marketed as Precose and Glyset, can prevent increases in blood sugar following meals by delaying carbohydrate digestion in the small intestine. Taking these medications directly before exercise if you eat extra carbohydrate during the activity would slow your absorption of them as well, and they can cause undesirable side effects like flatulence and diarrhea. Exercise itself usually slows the digestion of foods, so if you are exercising after eating you may need lower or no doses of these medications.

Some new classes of meds for people with type 2 diabetes are also being created that target insulin release and insulin action, including Januvia (now approved by the FDA) and Galvus, both of which work with gut hormones, natural enzymes, and the body's own insulin to control blood glucose levels. This class of oral meds works by inhibiting DPP-4, an enzyme that breaks down glucagon-like peptide-1 (GLP-1); delayed GLP-1 degradation extends the action of insulin while suppressing glucagon release. Several other potential classes are also under investigation by pharmaceutical companies.

If a single medication does not adequately control your blood sugars, your doctor may put you on a combination therapy that requires you to take two or more different drugs. Often, you can now get combination drugs that have two of these classes of drugs together, such as Avandia and Amaryl to form Avandaryl, or glyburide and metformin as Glucovance. These combination drugs make taking multiple drugs easier. Such combinations, however, can make the prediction of an exercise response more difficult if you don't know which classes of drugs are in them.

If oral medications, alone or in combination, stop effectively controlling your blood sugars, you may have to change to insulin therapy for better control, often starting with just basal insulin at bedtime. Some studies have shown that starting people on insulin sooner may actually better preserve the remaining beta cell function, so this approach is worth considering. Similarly, if you have LADA (type 1.5 diabetes), its full onset may be delayed enough that taking oral medications may effectively control your blood sugars for a while, but usually you will have to start taking insulin at some point for adequate control.

NEW MEDICATION CHOICES: SYMLIN AND BYETTA

The turn of the millennium brought the first new drug to treat type 1 diabetes in more than 80 years since the discovery of insulin in 1921. The medication is called Symlin (generic name: pramlintide). It is a synthetic form of the body's natural hormone, amylin, normally released along with insulin from pancreatic beta cells. Its main action is to improve the action of insulin after meals by slowing down how quickly the glucose coming from the food that you ate shows up in your circulation. If you normally take or pump insulin to control your postmeal highs, then your body likely is not releasing enough of this hormone naturally. Replacing it will likely even out your blood sugars after eating, make you feel full sooner while eating, and potentially cause weight loss. As an added benefit, Symlin may also reduce oxidative stress and prevent you from developing diabetic complications, although this potential effect needs further study. Its potential side effects are severe hypoglycemia (blood glucose levels below 55 mg/dl, or 3.1 mmol/L, more common in insulin users), nausea, vomiting, abdominal pain, headache, fatigue, and dizziness. Another drawback is that it must be injected.

Many type 1 diabetic exercisers have tried Symlin. Bill King, a marathon runner from Aston, Pennsylvania, has found that using Symlin, taken at the same time as his insulin boluses, helps him correct his blood sugars more rapidly when he becomes hyperglycemic following a big meal. To deal with the nausea that it often causes, some people have tried pumping basal doses of Symlin (using an insulin pump filled with Symlin) instead of giving premeal injections with higher doses and found that this off-label delivery method works better for them. You may need to be careful about taking Symlin before exercising, however, because it can make hypoglycemia harder to treat by slowing the absorption of anything that you eat to raise low blood sugars. Some athletes have complained about getting Symlin-induced lows that they can't easily treat during and following exercise. In addition, if you have gastroparesis (delayed emptying of the contents of your stomach because of damage to the central nerves by diabetes), you may not want to use Symlin at all because it can cause more frequent, severe hypoglycemia by further slowing your already delayed absorption of food.

Another new medication made by the Symlin manufacturers is called Byetta (exenatide), which is an injectable medication mainly intended for the treatment of type 2 diabetes, although some people with slow-onset type 1 in adulthood have used it to try to regenerate their beta cells. Like Symlin, Byetta causes food to empty from the stomach more slowly and blood glucose levels to stay more stable after meals. Byetta also stimulates the pancreas to make more insulin (which will obviously not work in most type 1s), keeps the liver from overproducing glucose, and in most users results in weight loss. This new class of medications effectively replaces natural hormones released by the digestive tract (gut hormones) after meals to spur insulin release and provides another choice for diabetes treatment, particularly if your treatment with oral medications is no longer working effectively. Byetta does have to be injected (rather than ingested) twice a day, which may not appeal to you if you've shied away from insulin therapy to avoid taking shots. Recent studies, however, have suggested that Byetta therapy may be as effective as insulin.

Another potential drawback of Byetta is that it may negatively affect your ability to exercise. Janis Eggleston, a type 2 diabetic athlete from Berkeley, California, reported

---

RESOURCES FOR ACTIVE PEOPLE WITH DIABETES
Diabetes Training Camp

Diabetes Training Camp is a unique clinical resource devoted entirely to diabetes, fitness, and sport. One of its offerings is a fitness and multisport training camp for people with diabetes at all levels of athletic ability. What makes it unique, particularly for adults who don't usually have the opportunity to go to camp, is that it focuses on the athletic part of having diabetes, whether you simply want to become fitter or want to take your triathlon and marathon training to a new level. Diabetes Training Camp's comprehensive, onsite staff consists of an experienced and talented crew of medical and diabetes specialists, exercise scientists, athletic trainers, dietitians, elite coaches, fitness specialists, and sport psychologists. The integrated approach of all these specialists creates a supportive and educational experience.

Founded in 2006 by Dr. Matthew Corcoran, its medical director, this camp is expanding each year to offer more weeklong camps and programs at various locations around the United States. For more information, visit the camp's Web site at www.diabetestrainingcamp.com.

the following: "I have never been able to cycle with Byetta on board without throwing up, feeling weak, losing steam, and having 'no legs' to pedal with. I learned to drop that med early in my training season." In fact, she never takes Byetta when cycling over 65 miles (105 kilometers) in one day because she gets major low blood sugars if she does. Also, she can't take her usual dose of metformin either because it impedes her liver from producing enough glucose to keep her blood sugars stable. When riding long distances, she only takes her evening dose of metformin. Similarly, Tom Seabourne, a type 1.5 diabetic cyclist from Mt. Pleasant, Texas, says, "I have had extreme lows with Byetta, so I dropped to a single dose of 10 units before dinner. I tried Byetta before breakfast for a while, but it turned me into a vegetable until lunchtime. I would never consider taking Byetta before a workout!"

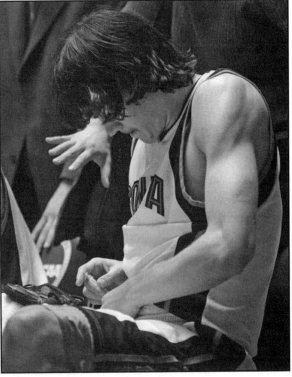

Since everyone's physiology is different, there will be some trial and error to figure out how best to manage all the variables of your medications, their actions, and how they are affected by exercise, but many diabetic athletes do it successfully, and so can you.

KEYS TO MANAGING MEDICATIONS AND PHYSICAL ACTIVITY

As you can see, the more you know about your diabetes medications, their actions, and how they may be affected by exercise, the easier it will be for you to make adjustments to have as normal a physiological response to your physical activities as possible. You will undoubtedly have to suffer through some trial and error to figure out how best to manage all these variables, but many diabetic athletes do it successfully, and so can you. The key things to remember are the following: (1) if you don't have diabetes, your insulin levels go down while the levels of other glucose-raising hormones rise during exercise, more so when you're working out hard; (2) how much insulin you have in your bloodstream during exercise affects whether your blood sugars stay normal, go down too much, or even rise; and (3) certain other diabetic medications like certain sulfonylureas, Symlin, and Byetta also increase your risk for hypoglycemia during exercise and may need to be adjusted for your physical activity.

*A*thlete *P*rofile

Name: Chris Dudley

Hometown: Lake Oswego, Oregon, USA

Diabetes history: Type 1 diabetes diagnosed in 1981 (at age 16)

Sport or activity: Basketball (retired NBA player)

Greatest athletic achievement: My greatest athletic achievement is playing in the NBA for 16 years with type 1 diabetes (in 886 games); apparently, I was the only diabetic basketball player in the entire league during my career. My greatest memory is going to the NBA finals with the New York Knicks.

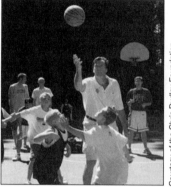

Courtesy of the Chris Dudley Foundation

Training tips: I advise having a good schedule that works for you and then sticking with it.

Typical daily and weekly training and diabetes regimen: On a game day, my typical regimen while playing in the NBA was to test my blood sugars 12 to 14 times. During training days, I would test 8 to 10 times, but only 6 to 8 times on nongame days.

▸ *Typical game day schedule:*

9:30 a.m.	Go to the arena, test
10:00–11:00 a.m.	Shoot around, light practice, test
11:00 a.m.–12:00 p.m.	Lift weights
12:30–2:00 p.m.	Small snack (something with protein), nap, test
2:30 p.m.	Lunch, test
4:30 p.m.	Go to the arena, do warm-ups, shoot around, get taped and stretch, do warm-ups on the court, test three times throughout
7:00 p.m.	Game time: test during the game, at halftime, and afterward (before a late dinner)

▸ *Typical practice day schedule:*

9:30 a.m–1:30 p.m.   Go to the arena, test; practice two hours, do conditioning and weightlifting, test; rest of day could be a travel day depending on the schedule.

▸ *Typical nongame, nonpractice day schedule:*

Test before each meal and supplement two to four times.

Other hobbies and interests: Since retiring from the NBA, I enjoy spending time doing outdoor activities such as wake boarding and snow skiing.

Good diabetes and exercise story: In 1995 my wife and I started the Chris Dudley Foundation Basketball Camp for kids with type 1 diabetes. Kids come from all over the country and Canada to join us for a one-week, once-in-a-lifetime experience. The mission for camp is to walk away with a sense of how to play a vigorous sport while controlling your diabetes. As I always tell the campers, "You've got to embrace your diabetes. You can't hide from it; it's not going to go away. You have to deal with it—and if you do deal with it, you can do whatever you want to do."

CHAPTER 4

Diet and Supplements
for Active People

As a physically active person, you are likely to be bombarded with claims about the superiority of particular diets and guarantees that specific nutritional supplements will enhance your athletic performance. With the fierce competition that exists in sports nowadays, athletes look for any edge to improve their athletic ability. They will try almost any supplement or technique to get it—amino acid supplements, glycerol, sports drinks, creatine, carbohydrate loading, and ginseng, to name just a few. In reality, few of these advertised ergogenic aids (i.e., anything that enhances performance) for athletes are scientifically proved to enhance your physical prowess. Moreover, as an athlete with diabetes, you may have special concerns about the effects of various diets and supplements on your diabetes control, as well as how and what to consume to maintain your blood sugars during exercise.

EFFECTIVE DIETARY PRACTICES OF ACTIVE PEOPLE

The first thing you should know is that active people can eat more than one way and perform effectively in sport and that the best way may be slightly different for everyone. The diets of diabetic athletes are as varied as the sports and activities that they do. No one likes to have to stop exercising because of low blood sugars, though, so preventing hypoglycemia during and after any activity is a high priority for everyone. Becoming low unexpectedly can be especially inconvenient if you're out for a run or a long bike ride and are still a good distance from your destination. Prevention has a lot to do with your food intake both before and during the activity. In general, rapidly absorbed carbohydrate is most effective to take during exercise, but protein and fat can be helpful in preventing lows as well. The following sections include some basic points to remember about the different classes of foods, along with a discussion of nutritional supplements.

Carbohydrate: Critical to Making It to the Finish Line

Carbohydrate is the most important energy source for all types of exercise. Muscle glycogen (the main storage form of carbohydrate) is the primary source of energy for the lactic acid system, along with being the main fuel for moderate and intense aerobic exercise. Whenever you eat carbohydrate, it is broken down by enzymes in your digestive tract, absorbed through the wall of your small intestine, and released as glucose into your blood, making it the main simple sugar found there. Your muscles can take up and use carbohydrate, but they generally use more of the glycogen already stored in them, as long as it's available.

The more intensely you exercise, the greater the rate of muscle glycogen depletion in the muscle fibers that you're using. Your liver also releases its more limited glycogen stores as glucose into the bloodstream to try to maintain your levels during exercise. Glycogen is critical to most activities, so if you deplete your muscle and liver stores during exercise, you will become fatigued and either have to stop exercising or slow down considerably. You've heard of athletes "hitting the wall," often around the 20-mile (32-kilometer) mark of a marathon; they've usually just run out of glycogen at that point.

> *Fat "burns" in a carbohydrate flame, so you can't even use fat effectively as an alternative fuel after you've depleted your carbohydrate (glycogen and glucose) stores.*

In general, most exercisers (even those without diabetes) need to take in some carbohydrate before and during prolonged exercise to help maintain their blood glucose levels, although consuming it usually doesn't slow down the body's use of glycogen, which is primarily driven by the intensity of the workout. Any carbohydrate that you take in during exercise is rapidly metabolized and begins to be available for your body to use within about five minutes. The type of carbohydrate that you need to consume depends on factors such as how long you'll be exercising, the intensity of your workout, and what your blood sugar and insulin levels are before and during the activity, as you will see in the sport-specific examples offered in part II.

Glycemic Effect of Various Carbohydrates

The current dietary recommendations are that 45 to 65 percent of daily calories should be from carbohydrate intake. Whether you eat that amount, more, or less, it is helpful to pay attention to the types of carbohydrate that you're eating when it comes to treating or preventing hypoglycemia, restoring muscle glycogen, keeping your insulin action high, and optimizing your sport performance.

Carbohydrate with a higher glycemic index (GI), by definition, is absorbed more rapidly and has a more immediate effect on your blood sugars. If you're treating hypoglycemia, you need to take in a higher-GI carbohydrate source, such as glucose tablets or gels, regular soda, sports drinks, skim milk, hard candies, and even bagels, bread, crackers, cornflakes, and white potatoes. If you develop low blood sugars during exercise, one of these sources will treat it most rapidly, and you can use them to raise your blood sugars at the start of your exercise. Traditionally, people have used orange and other juices to treat lows, but they really aren't the fastest thing to use because most juices have only a low or moderate glycemic effect.

Glucose tablets, gels, and liquids have some benefits for treating lows that other substances don't have. For starters, glucose is the sugar that ends up in your bloodstream most rapidly and abundantly, and it is the primary fuel for your brain and nerves. By way of comparison, other simple sugars, such as fructose found in fruit, have to be converted into glucose and, therefore, have a lower GI value and a slower effect. Another benefit is that glucose comes in precisely measured amounts—usually 4 grams of glucose per tablet or 15 grams per gel—so you can consume a specific number of grams of rapid-acting carbohydrate without overdoing it. With a little practice, you can easily determine how much each 4-gram glucose tablet or 15-gram gel or liquid is likely to raise your blood glucose level under different circumstances.

What you treat yourself with may need to vary by situation. If you're only slightly low, you may just need a glucose tablet or two. If you're low and likely to keep dropping from whatever insulin you have on board, then you may need to take in some food or a drink with greater staying power, something with some fat or protein to go with the carbohydrate, like peanut butter crackers or Balance Bars. Milk is a good treatment option for that reason, because it contains seven to eight grams of protein, along with some fat depending on what type (e.g., whole, 2 percent, skim, or others) you are drinking. Skim milk works well, but at least one study showed that for prevention of later-onset hypoglycemia following exercise, whole milk is much more effective than skim or even sports drinks, likely because of the extra fat in the whole variety that takes longer to metabolize.

Almost all recommended carbohydrate intake during exercise throughout this book refers to the high-GI carbohydrate for optimal treatment and prevention of hypoglycemia. Although people differ in their glycemic responses, certain foods generally elicit lesser peaks in everyone. For instance, foods with a low GI include high-fiber carbohydrate sources such as apples, cherries, dried beans and legumes (e.g., navy, kidney, chickpeas, and lentils), dates, figs, peaches, plums, whole milk, and yogurt. Medium GI foods include bananas, grapes, oatmeal, orange juice, pasta, rice, yams, corn, and baked beans. Carbohydrate foods with high fat content have slower absorption rates than those with less fat. Regular potato chips and doughnuts are examples of high-carbohydrate, high-fat foods; taken for the treatment of lows, they would definitely not be as rapid or effective. When optimizing your blood sugar control after workouts and restoring glycogen, you can use carbohydrate-rich foods with varying GI values.

Supplementing With Carbohydrate Before, During, and After Exercise

Carbohydrate supplementation is an effective performance enhancer whether or not you have diabetes. In general, taking in extra carbohydrate is not usually necessary for events lasting an hour or less, if you start with normal muscle and liver glycogen stores and moderately low levels of insulin. But you may need to take in carbohydrate for exercise lasting less than an hour, depending on how much insulin is in your system and whether your blood glucose is likely to drop during the event. If you're running low on glycogen for any reason or your insulin levels are too high, your muscles will use more of your blood glucose than normal, and you'll likely have to supplement.

If you train on a regular basis, you will need to take in enough carbohydrate every day to restore your muscle and liver glycogen levels between workouts. When you have diabetes, you have to be especially careful to keep your blood sugars in control before and after exercise so that your glycogen repletion takes place normally. Your body needs adequate insulin levels, especially more than an hour after exercise when glucose uptake into your cells becomes more dependent on insulin. Taking in some carbohydrate immediately after you finish a workout or race will speed up your initial glycogen replacement and help lower your risk of developing low blood sugars later, all with minimal need for insulin during that period. Carbohydrate intake also helps ensure that your glycogen stores are maximally loaded by the time your next workout rolls around. Keep in mind, though, that glycogen repletion can take 24 to 48 hours, and you need to control your blood sugars well during that time for maximal carbohydrate replacement. If you eat a low-carbohydrate diet, full restoration of glycogen will take longer; you may want to consider taking in more carbohydrate of any GI than your normal during that time (at least 100 grams per day) and taking enough insulin (if you use it) to facilitate the storage of carbohydrate as glycogen in your muscles and liver.

The time when your body restores glycogen most rapidly is during the first 30 to 120 minutes after exercise. If you want to minimize your risk of later-onset lows, take in some carbohydrate and keep your blood sugars under control during this time to optimize its repletion.

Particularly during longer workouts or a long sports event, carbohydrate supplementation benefits all athletes. During marathons or triathlons, extra carbohydrate helps maintain your blood sugar levels, enabling you to keep going at a faster pace for longer without fatiguing. Supplementing even works for intermittent, prolonged, high-intensity sports like soccer, field hockey, and tennis. Always take in adequate carbohydrate, along with sufficient (albeit likely reduced) insulin before, during, and after prolonged moderate- or high-intensity workouts to maintain and restore your muscle and liver glycogen and blood glucose, especially during that window of opportunity for glycogen repletion right after you finish exercising. If your blood sugars are normal or slightly low before exercise, you may also want to take in 10 to 15 grams of moderate- or high-GI carbohydrate without any insulin coverage right when you start, especially if your blood glucose levels typically start to drop during the first 30 minutes of an activity.

Fluids, Sport Drinks, Gels, and More

Gatorade, PowerAde, All-Sport, Cytomax, GatorLode, Ultra Fuel, GlucoBurst gels, Power Bars, Clif Bars—with so many sport drinks, gels, and other sport-related supplements to choose from, how can you choose which one to use, if any? Let's start by taking a closer look at sports drinks and other fluids. During exercise, a fluid that is a 5- to 10-percent carbohydrate solution (meaning that it contains 5 to 10 grams of carbohydrate per 100 milliliters of fluid) will empty from your stomach as rapidly as plain water does, can hydrate you effectively, and will provide you with carbohydrate. If you're worrying about maintaining your blood sugars more than your hydration, choose one with a slightly higher carbohydrate content; not surprisingly, taking in a 10-percent carbohydrate sports drink has been shown to keep blood sugars higher than consuming a similar quantity of an 8-percent one.

You should use more concentrated solutions (above 10 percent) only before or after exercise because their emptying from your stomach is somewhat delayed. Fruit juices are usually more concentrated than 10 percent and should be diluted for faster absorption during exercise, but remember that their GI is usually lower than many other choices. You may also want to avoid juice for another reason: Drinks with high amounts of fructose (fruit sugar) may cause abdominal cramps or diarrhea, likely because fructose is absorbed more slowly than glucose is and it pulls water into your stomach and small intestines when consumed in high concentrations.

As far as your hydration status is concerned, whether you can rely on a sports drinks or just plain water depends on how long your activity is going to last. During an exercise session of an hour or less, you can effectively maintain hydration with water alone,

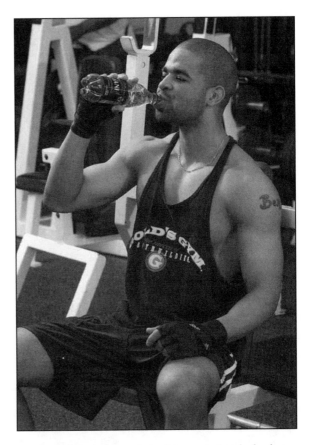

A sport drink that is a 5- to 10-percent carbohydrate solution can hydrate you effectively and will provide you with carbohydrate.

although athletes with diabetes may need the extra carbohydrate in sport drinks for blood sugar maintenance. You don't need to worry about replacing electrolytes (like sodium, potassium, chloride, and magnesium) during shorter events because sweating doesn't immediately unbalance them; sweat is more dilute than blood and contains less sodium and other electrolytes. For longer events, water alone will keep you hydrated, but taking in sports drinks or other substances with carbohydrate will prolong your endurance by preventing drops in blood sugars and providing your muscles with an alternative source of carbohydrate (besides muscle glycogen).

During extremely prolonged activities such as a full Ironman triathlon, you'll need to replace electrolytes lost during the event, especially when you're consuming lots of fluids. Otherwise, you may end up with a dilution of sodium in your blood that causes hyponatremia (low sodium levels), otherwise known as water intoxication. Symptoms include light-headedness, headaches, nausea, repeated vomiting, and malaise. For the most effective hydration, take in fluids before you start, during the activity, and afterward, but don't go overboard on the amount, even if it contains some electrolytes. Too many sports drinks can cause water intoxication despite containing sodium and other electrolytes.

In general, fluids are best drunk cold and with less than 10 percent carbohydrate in them to promote faster emptying from your stomach. Ice-cold water will get into your body more rapidly than a lukewarm drink will, but taking in more than 500 milliliters at a time will slow the rate of emptying and increase your risk for hyponatremia. While exercising you must start drinking before you feel thirsty because thirst is not triggered until you have already lost 1 to 2 percent of your body weight in the form of water. Taking in a large mouthful (1 to 2 ounces, or 20 to 60 milliliters) at a time is usually sufficient.

> *Any drinks that you take in during exercise should ideally contain less than 10 percent carbohydrate, be cold, have a volume of less than 500 milliliters, and contain some replacement electrolytes (during exercise lasting longer than an hour).*

The main benefit of taking in carbohydrate-based gels is that the quantity is measured (e.g., 15 grams) and they don't require you to take in extra fluids if you already are sufficiently hydrated or at risk for hyponatremia. If they're glucose gels or liquids like Dex4 Liquid Blast, one packet equals almost four glucose tablets, and a gel or liquid may be easier to eat while exercising.

For PowerBars, Clif Bars, and other sports bars, you take in some longer-lasting protein and fat along with the carbohydrate, which can help prevent your blood sugars from dropping as much later on during longer workouts or events. A comparison of some of the sports drinks, gels, and other nutritional products for diabetic athletes can be found in table 4.1.

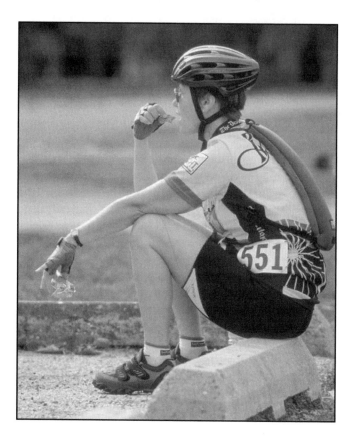

For PowerBars and other sports bars, you take in some longer-lasting protein and fat along with the carbohydrate, which can help prevent your blood sugars from dropping as much later on during longer workouts or events.

Table 4.1 Recommended Sports Drinks, Gels, and Other Carbohydrate Sources

Product	Carbohydrate content	Other ingredients
Gatorade	14 g per 8 oz (240 ml) (6% carbohydrate solution)	Sodium, 110 mg; potassium, 25 mg
PowerAde	21 g per 8 oz (240 ml) (8% carbohydrate solution)	Sodium, 55 mg; potassium, 30 mg
All-Sport	21 g per 8 oz (240 ml) (9% carbohydrate solution)	Sodium, 55 mg; potassium, 55 mg
Cytomax	19 g per 8 oz (240 ml) (8% carbohydrate solution)	Sodium, 10 mg; potassium, 150 mg
Ultra Fuel	50 g per 8 oz (240 ml) (21% carbohydrate solution)	None
Accel Gel	20 g carbohydrate per 41 g pouch	Protein, 5 g (whey protein from milk); fat, 0 g; sodium, 100 mg; potassium, 50 mg; vitamins E and C (100%); various flavors
Gu Energy Gel	25 g carb (85% maltodextrin, 15% fructose) in 1.1 oz (31 g) pouch	Sodium, 50 mg; potassium, 35 mg; vitamins C and E, 100% of daily value
Hammer Gel	23 g carbohydrate per 36 g serving (about 2 tablespoons, or 30 ml)	Amino acids (L-leucine, L-alanine, L-valine, L-isoleucine); sodium chloride; potassium
PowerBar	43 g carbohydrate in one 65 g bar	Protein, 9 g; fat, 2.5 g; fiber, 2 g; sodium, 200 mg; potassium, 115 mg; vitamins; minerals; essential amino acids; various flavors
PowerBar Gel	27 g carbohydrate per 41 g packet	Sodium, 200 mg; potassium, 20 mg; chloride, 90 mg; many flavors with 25 or 50 mg of caffeine added
Clif Bar	45 g carbohydrate per 68 g bar	Protein, 10–11 g; fat, 3–6 g; fiber, 5 g; sodium, 125 mg; potassium, 310 mg; vitamins; minerals; various flavors
Clif Shot Bloks Chews	24 g carbohydrate per three pieces (30 g)	Sodium, 70 mg; potassium, 20 mg; various flavors, some with more sodium or caffeine
GlucoBurst	15 g glucose in 1.3 oz (37 g) pouch	Sodium, 30 mg; potassium, 10 mg
Dex4 Glucose Gel or liquid	15 g glucose per tube	None
Dex4 Glucose Tablets	4 g glucose per tablet	None

Carbohydrate Loading: Effective If Done Right

Almost all athletes benefit from carbohydrate loading before long-distance events because they can then begin exercise with fully restored or even supercompensated glycogen stores. Traditionally, this loading technique consisted of three to seven days of a high-carbohydrate diet combined with one or two days of rest or a reduction in exercise volume, a method known as tapering. Your daily diet while loading should contain 8 to 10 grams of carbohydrate per kilogram of body weight, which is similar to the recommended intake for all endurance athletes. We now know that even a single day with a higher carbohydrate intake and rest or tapering can effectively maximize carbohydrate stores, so you don't need to spend a week, or even as long as three days, overconsuming carbohydrate.

> *To maximize your glycogen stores, all you is really need is one day and a combination of rest, a carbohydrate-rich diet, and excellent blood sugar control throughout the day.*

For carbohydrate loading to be effective for diabetic exercisers, your muscles must be able to take up enough glucose. The way to ensure the proper glycogen storage, and even supercompensation of stores in your muscles and liver, is to have sufficient levels of insulin when you take in carbohydrate to prevent hyperglycemia and promote glucose uptake. Consuming higher-fiber carbohydrate sources and those with a lower glycemic effect will help prevent an excessive rise in your blood sugars and will still be effective for loading. In fact, a recent study showed that poorly controlled diabetic exercisers can actually end up with higher glycogen stores when they maintain better blood sugar control by loading with less carbohydrate (50 percent of calories as carbohydrate instead of around 60 percent), so eating as much carbohydrate as the glycogen-loading scenarios recommend may be counterproductive for most diabetic athletes. For optimal liver glycogen stores, maintaining more normal blood sugars has also been shown to be the most effective strategy.

Fat: Use Some But Not as Much as Carbohydrate

Both the fat stored in your muscles (i.e., intramuscular triglycerides) and circulating around in your blood (free fatty acids) can provide some energy for muscle contractions. Although carbohydrate is the main energy source during exercise, fat is an important contributor to your fuel needs, particularly during low-intensity or slower, prolonged activities like walking the dog or taking an all-day hike. Fatty acids are stored in your adipose (fat) tissue as triglycerides and are released by hormones (mainly epinephrine) to circulate around to the active muscles. Not much of the intramuscular fat is used during activities—unless they are extremely prolonged, lasting many hours at moderate intensity—but later when you're resting they kick in some of the energy for recovery, which is largely fueled by fat from all sources. Fat is hardly used at all during high-intensity aerobic and anaerobic exercise, both of which rely on carbohydrate for ATP production.

Fat use during exercise is limited, contributing most during prolonged low-intensity activities, but fat provides most of the fuel for recovery from any physical activity.

Your blood sugar may stay more stable overnight if you eat a higher-fat bedtime snack, such as ice cream, yogurt, or soymilk, on days when you've been particularly active. Fat is metabolized much more slowly than carbohydrate and will provide an alternative energy source for your muscles five to six hours after you eat it. Eating high-fat foods for exercise (a practice called fat loading) may be detrimental to your performance, however, and it is not advised. Also, keep in mind that any fat that you eat before and during exercise isn't digested and ready for use for many hours, and the fat consumed may slow the absorption of any carbohydrate that you eat.

The current dietary guidelines recommend a fat intake of 20 to 35 percent of daily calories. Many diabetic exercisers may consume more than 35 percent as fat, which is fine as long as they take into account the type of fat. You should aim to minimize your intake of saturated fats (mostly solid at room temperature, found in cheese, margarine, meats, and more), trans fatty acids (bad partially hydrogenated fats added to foods by manufacturers, now listed on food labels), tropical oils (coconut, palm, and palm kernel oils), and interesterified fats (the new trans fat substitute added by food manufacturers). All these fats can raise the levels of the bad type of cholesterol (LDL) in your blood and raise your risk for heart disease and stroke. If you choose to have a moderate fat intake after prolonged exercise to prevent later-onset lows, pick better fats like those found in nuts, peanut butter, olive oil, fish, flaxseed, and dark chocolate, or at least choose lower-fat varieties of dairy and other foods (e.g., fat-reduced ice cream, yogurt, and cheese).

Protein: Important for Recovery and Muscle Repair

During most exercise, protein contributes less than 5 percent of the total energy, although it may rise to 10 to 15 percent during a prolonged event, such as a marathon or Ironman triathlon. Regardless, protein is never a key energy source for exercise, but it is critical for other reasons. Taking in enough protein in your diet allows your muscles to be repaired following strenuous exercise and promotes the synthesis of hormones, enzymes, and other body tissues formed from amino acids, the building blocks of protein. About half of the 20 amino acids (shown in table 4.2) are considered essential in your diet, meaning that you have to consume them or your body will suffer from protein malnutrition, which causes the breakdown of muscles and organs over time. Your body can make the rest of the amino acids by itself, but you need to have enough of all of them—essential and nonessential—to synthesize protein during recovery from exercise, which is a vital process if you want to experience any increase in the strength, aerobic capacity, or size of your muscles.

The current recommended intake of protein is 10 to 35 percent of total daily calories. Athletes who train regularly likely should consume somewhere in that range, as long as they are minimally consuming at least 1.2 to 1.8 grams of protein

Table 4.2   Amino Acids

Essential amino acids	Nonessential amino acids
Histidine	Alanine
Isoleucine	Arginine
Leucine	Asparagine
Lysine	Aspartic acid
Methionine	Cysteine
Phenylalanine	Glutamic acid
Threonine	Glutamine
Tryptophan	Glycine
Valine	Proline
Serine	Tyrosine

Note: Essential amino acids are defined as those that cannot be manufactured in your body and must be included in your diet.

per kilogram of body weight (e.g., 84 to 126 grams of protein for a 70-kilogram exerciser). Typically, an ounce (28 grams) of chicken, cheese, or meat contains about 7 grams of protein. Taking in more protein and slightly less carbohydrate postexercise may also help keep blood sugars stable after exercise and facilitate the uptake of both into your muscles.

Because protein is not a major energy source during exercise, you really don't need to worry about consuming any right before or during an activity. Research has

RESOURCES FOR ACTIVE PEOPLE WITH DIABETES
Insulindependence.org

Insulindependence, Inc. is a worldwide project aimed at changing diabetic lives through adventure travel, educational outreach, and Web-based community support. A nonprofit organization incorporated in California, Insulindependence, Inc. operates through a global network of outdoor enthusiasts who work together to promote healthy, proactive lifestyles to diabetic people who lack financial resources, positive role models, or adequate guidance in professional health care. This group believes that extreme forms of activity actually precede stability in blood sugar levels, a trend attributable to the cycle of inspiration that begins with the decision to push beyond the limits of convention.

Cofounded by President Peter Nerothin and run by Vice-Presidents Nate Heintzman and J.R. Roever, this organization offers online networking, international teen and adult expeditions, team training for selected endurance events (Ironman Wisconsin in 2008, for example), online educational resources, and public speaking. For more information about their upcoming events and more, visit www.insulindependence.org or e-mail Peter Nerothin at peter@insulindependence.org.

shown, however, that taking in some protein along with carbohydrate right after hard or long workouts may help your body replenish its stores of muscle and liver glycogen more effectively. Although the benefits of postexercise protein have not been studied in diabetic athletes, taking in a small amount of protein along with your carbohydrate (in a ratio of 1:4) after an activity may help prevent low blood sugars later. Protein takes three to four hours to metabolize after you eat it—more time than carbohydrate but less than fat—and a small portion of it is converted into glucose, which can raise (or prevent drops in) your blood sugars when it finally does show up in your bloodstream. For that reason, you may also want to have some in your bedtime snack (along with fat and carbohydrate) when you're trying to prevent nighttime lows after a day of strenuous or prolonged activity.

NUTRITIONAL SUPPLEMENTS: HELPFUL OR HYPE?

The list of advertised nutritional supplements that claim to enhance athletic ability is staggering. Most "proof" of these claims comes from studies done by the manufacturer of the product or from testimonials by people, often celebrities, who use the products. Thus, the problem for most athletes is determining which nutritional claims to believe.

Probably the best ergogenic aid for most diabetic athletes is simply keeping blood sugars normal during exercise. Your performance can suffer from early fatigue (caused by hypoglycemia) or sluggishness (a common result of elevated blood sugars). You need to regulate your carbohydrate tightly during exercise to prevent either of these problems. Refer to table 4.3 for nutritional supplements that may potentially benefit diabetic athletes and table 4.4 for potentially harmful ones.

Table 4.3 Supplements of Potential Benefit to Diabetic Athletes

Nutritional supplement	Potential beneficial effect
Antioxidants	Reduction of oxidative damage to cell membranes induced by exercise and hyperglycemia
Caffeine	Increased release of fatty acids, better hormonal response to hypoglycemia during exercise
Carbohydrate, glucose intake	Intake of appropriate amounts of carbohydrate before, during, and after exercise to prevent exercise-induced hypoglycemia
Chromium, vanadium, and zinc	Improvement in insulin sensitivity (especially in type 2 diabetes)
Glycerol	Hyperhydration and prevention of dehydration with exercise and hyperglycemia
Sports drinks[1]	Prevention of hypoglycemia (if the drink contains glucose fructose), as well as dehydration and electrolyte imbalance during prolonged exercise, especially in the heat
Water, fluid replacement	Prevention of dehydration, especially because of hyperglycemia or exercise in the heat when perspiration is greater

[1] Sports drinks can also cause hyperglycemia if carbohydrate intake exceeds the necessary amount during exercise.

Table 4.4 Supplements of Potential Harm to Diabetic Athletes

Nutritional supplement	Potential harmful effect
Amino acid supplements	Amino acid imbalance in the body, added stress on kidneys because of excess nitrogen excretion
Caffeine	Potential for greater water loss and dehydration, especially during exercise in the heat
Carbohydrate loading[1]	Hyperglycemia before, during, or after exercise, as well as reduction in insulin sensitivity; hypoglycemia if consumed before exercise and too much insulin is taken for carbohydrate
Creatine[2]	Added stress on the kidneys, especially if kidney disease is present, because of excess urinary excretion of creatinine
Fat loading	Slower carbohydrate absorption rates during exercise if consumed before or during activity, increased insulin resistance, ketone production, and obesity in the long term
Protein supplements	Added stress on kidneys because of excess nitrogen excretion, especially with nephropathy

[1] Carbohydrate loading can also be beneficial to ensure proper replacement of muscle and liver glycogen levels before and after exercise. Adequate insulin must be available to prevent hyperglycemia and facilitate glucose uptake into muscle.

[2] Creatine will create the greatest kidney stress during the initial loading period (five to seven days). During the ensuing maintenance period of supplementation, added stress on the kidneys may be minimal if their function is normal.

Amino Acid Supplements: Do You Need Them?

Have you ever heard that you have to take amino acid or protein supplements to bulk up? As discussed, amino acids are the building blocks of proteins, and you have to consume enough of the essential ones (refer back to table 4.2) to build and repair your muscles and other body proteins. You can buy almost every amino acid individually as a supplement, and many more are offered in combinations (e.g., branched-chain amino acids). Athletes have tried supplementing with practically all the amino acids to produce a performance-enhancing or strength-boosting effect. The latest rage is whey protein, derived from milk protein, because it has a high concentration of three essential branched-chain amino acids (leucine, isoleucine, and valine), considered by many bodybuilders and strength athletes to be the ultimate amino acids for muscle growth and repair.

The biggest myth about amino acid supplements, and protein in general, is that you have to load up on them to gain muscle mass. The protein requirement for strength-training athletes may be about twice as high as normal (1.6 to 1.8 grams of protein per kilogram of body weight daily instead of the usual 0.8 grams, where 1 kilogram equals 2.2 pounds), but most people in the United States already consume more than these higher amounts of protein in their diets. To gain 1 pound (.45 kilogram) of muscle mass a week (a realistic amount), a strength-training athlete needs only an additional 14 grams of quality protein per day, easily attainable in less than two glasses of milk or 2 ounces (57 grams) of lean meat, chicken, fish, or cheese. The recommendation for endurance-training athletes is even less at 1.2 to 1.6 grams of protein per kilogram of body weight daily.

Taking specific supplemental amino acids may cause an imbalance in your system—an overabundance of some and a relative deficit of others. What's more, you can still gain unwanted weight or have high blood sugars if you take in excess calories as amino acid supplements, which are stored simply as excess body fat or converted into blood glucose. These supplements are also expensive. Diabetic exercisers may also need to be concerned about the potential effects of excess protein consumption on the kidneys. Excess nitrogen found in all amino acids has to be converted into a waste product called urea, which then has to be excreted by your kidneys or sweat glands. When you take supplemental protein or amino acids, your kidneys have to work overtime getting rid of it. If they're healthy, excreting it is not an issue, but it can additionally strain kidneys that have any damage from long-term diabetes. The bottom line is that taking amino acid supplements is generally a waste of money and can potentially put additional strain on ailing kidneys. If you are determined to increase your intake of essential amino acids, consider simply increasing your intake of healthy foods high in protein such as egg whites, nonfat milk, legumes (beans), and lean meats and poultry.

Glycerol: Possible Benefits to Hydration

Athletes have supplemented with glycerol (also called glycerin), a simple compound that forms the backbone of triglycerides (storage fat). Glycerol is also commonly added to protein bars to help make them moist and to sweeten them, although it doesn't cause a significant blood sugar response when taken as part of protein bar and is eliminated from your body mostly unused. Glycerol has the capacity to attract water molecules, which leads to a hyperhydration effect, so its potential performance-enhancing effect, if it has one, comes through increasing water retention and how much blood you have. The recommended dose is one gram of glycerol per kilogram of body weight, diluted in other fluids, and consumed one and a half to two and a half hours before exercise.

As you know, dehydration can have a detrimental effect on performance in endurance activities because it can lead to early fatigue and serious heat stress disorders; if you start with more fluid in your blood from consuming glycerol, you can sweat more before becoming dehydrated. Diabetic athletes may be more prone to dehydration if their blood sugars are higher than normal. Of course, drinking plenty of water and other fluids during exercise (but not too much) is still vitally important even if you use glycerol, especially during prolonged exercise in the heat and humidity.

Vitamins: Do You Need to Supplement a Healthy Diet?

Many athletes take supplemental vitamins and minerals; maybe you're one of them. In some cases, there may be either sports-related or diabetes-related reasons to supplement with certain vitamins and minerals. Many athletes supplement their diets with specific vitamins like antioxidants and vitamin B_{12}, hoping to improve performance or enhance recovery. Diabetes itself can affect vitamin and mineral status, but that doesn't always mean that you need a supplement. The ones that you should consider for supplementation are discussed in this section.

Multivitamin and Mineral Supplements

Recent research suggests that taking these supplements may be advisable for anyone with diabetes. A wide range of vitamins and minerals affect glucose metabolism and insulin function, yet people with diabetes routinely don't get enough of them, especially when on calorie-restricted diets. Choose supplements with adequate amounts of the B vitamins, antioxidants (like vitamins C and E and alpha-lipoic acid), magnesium, chromium, vanadium, and lutein. Also, select supplements that don't have fillers, such as sugar, artificial colors and flavors, or common allergens (e.g., gluten, wheat, dairy, yeast, and corn). One supplement made specifically for people with diabetes, Alpha Betic, is high in all these micronutrients and doesn't have the fillers. When choosing a general supplement, however, beware of taking in too much copper or iron because these minerals can lower insulin action.

Antioxidants

Exercise increases the production of oxygen free radicals like superoxide, a chemical substance with a lone, unpaired electron that can damage cell membranes and DNA. By exercising you enhance your vitamin-based, antioxidant enzyme systems that naturally squelch most of these potentially damaging compounds. The vitamins with antioxidant qualities are C, E, and beta-carotene (a precursor to vitamin A). Other potential antioxidants are CoQ_{10} (ubiquinone) and the mineral selenium. Cocktails of all five combined are often sold as supplements. Another powerful antioxidant compound found in foods is alpha-lipoic acid, which may help prevent and treat nerve-related problems (common to diabetes) and protect against other oxidative damage.

Antioxidant supplements are believed to help limit the cellular damage that may occur from free radicals produced during exercise, or in the case of diabetes, from poor blood sugar control, as depicted in figure 4.1. Although such supplementation doesn't enhance sport performance, it may play a role in protecting your muscles from cellular damage during strenuous training and protecting the rest of your body from radical-generated complications.

Besides its antioxidant effect, vitamin C helps form the collagen that makes up connective tissues, ligaments, and tendons. It also aids in the absorption of iron from the gut and in the formation of adrenaline. Some people take large doses of vitamin C in an attempt to prevent the common cold and other viral infections. Although doses up to 1,000 milligrams of this vitamin appear to be safe, 200 milligrams per day is likely enough, which can easily be obtained if your diet contains plenty of fruits and veggies like citrus fruits, green leafy vegetables, broccoli, peppers, strawberries, and potatoes.

Vitamin E, another antioxidant, helps maintain the fluidity of red blood cells and protects cell membranes from damage through oxidation. Supplementing with 400 to 800 IU (international units) doesn't appear to be harmful and may prevent damage. In people with diabetes, vitamin E supplementation may improve blood flow to the back of the eye (retina) and creatinine clearance (an indicator of normal kidney function), but it doesn't improve glycemic control. This vitamin

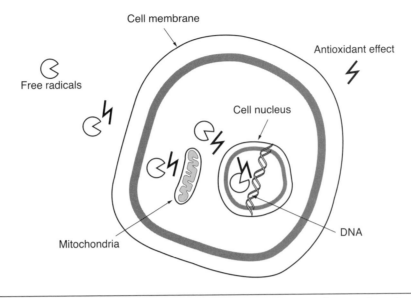

Figure 4.1 Antioxidant vitamins may help your body prevent some damage from free radical formation resulting from exercise and high blood sugars.

is recommended for athletes who are training at high altitude or in smoggy areas where oxidative stress may be greater. A fat-soluble vitamin, it is found naturally in vegetable oils, margarine, egg yolks, green leafy vegetables, wheat germ, and whole-grain products.

Supplements high in beta-carotene but low in vitamin A may also be beneficial as antioxidants. Both beta-carotene and vitamin A help maintain skin and mucous membranes, night vision, and proper bone development. Recent research indicates that diets rich in vitamin A or polyphenols (found in grapes and other foods) have protective effects against autoimmune attacks of beta cells and, therefore, have the potential to prevent type 1 diabetes, at least in diabetes-prone mice. Vitamin A is found in animal products like liver, milk, and cheese, whereas beta-carotene (its precursor) is higher in plant sources, particularly carrots, sweet potatoes, and other yellow or orange vegetables. Because your body can synthesize vitamin A as needed from beta-carotene, supplement with the latter and avoid taking large doses of vitamin A, which can be toxic.

As for CoQ_{10}, it's not an official vitamin (rather it's a lipid, or form of fat), but it's found in the mitochondria (powerhouses of the cells) and plays an important role in your cells' ability to use oxygen to make ATP. Although used as a supplemental antioxidant with the thought that it may protect the heart muscle from tissue damage because of lack of oxygen, its potential benefits remain unproven. Thus, taking it isn't advised, even though it is often included in supplements targeted at endurance athletes.

The main mineral with antioxidant qualities, selenium, can affect exercise performance if you're deficient in it, mainly by impairing your antioxidant ability during intense exercise, possibly resulting in muscle or mitochondrial damage. But you can easily obtain adequate amounts of selenium by eating grains grown in selenium-rich soil (as found in the United States and Canada), seafood, and organ meats. If you do take it as a supplement, don't exceed a daily intake of 200 micrograms, just to be on the safe side. Keep in mind, though, that selenium hasn't been proved an effective ergogenic or a preventative of diabetes-related health problems.

Finally, alpha-lipoic acid is a relative newcomer on the antioxidant supplement market, but clearly it has beneficial effects on diabetic peripheral neuropathy, as well as possibly on the memory status of people with Alzheimer's disease. If you'd rather get it naturally (albeit in a lower dose), consume more of the vegetables that contain it, such as spinach (raw or cooked), broccoli, tomatoes, potatoes, green peas, and Brussels sprouts.

Vitamin D

The only vitamin that works as a hormone is vitamin D. Its active form, calcitriol, helps your body absorb calcium and deposit it in your bones. Interestingly, it has recently been discovered that a deficiency of this vitamin may affect more than just your bone health. Low levels of vitamin D have been linked to the onset of type 1 diabetes through autoimmune mechanisms and to type 2 by increasing insulin resistance, especially when combined with low calcium intake. People commonly become more deficient in this vitamin as they age.

Close to 90 percent of the active form of vitamin D is formed through exposure to sunlight, but deficiencies today are far more widespread than they used to be because of a combination of more time spent indoors, lavish use of sunscreens (to prevent skin cancer and wrinkles), and consumption of nutrient-poor foods and drinks. Some researchers have even suggested that the use of sunscreen may be contributing to the development of skin cancers rather than preventing them. You don't need much sun exposure to make enough vitamin D in your skin—about 15 minutes on 3 days each week on your face and hands—but living in a high-latitude region and aging both reduce how much of this vitamin your skin can make with UV light exposure. You may want to consider supplementing with up to 800 IU per day (particularly if you're older) and eating more foods rich in vitamin D like fortified dairy products, nuts and seeds, and vegetable oils.

Vitamin B₁

This vitamin, also known as thiamin, was recently found to be deficient in people with both type 1 and type 2 diabetes. It has a central role in the metabolism of glucose, and it's essential for normal functioning of your nerves and for using glycogen stored in muscle during exercise. Both exercise and a high-carbohydrate intake increase the need for this vitamin, and a deficiency can lead to muscle weakness, pain in your calves, and damage to your nervous system and heart. Drinking too much alcohol can strip this vitamin from your body. Vitamin B₁ is a water-soluble vitamin widely distributed in plant and animal foods, such as whole grains, legumes, and pork, so chances are that you can take in enough by eating a balanced, healthy diet. Because researchers are not yet sure why thiamin levels are lower in people with diabetes, if your blood sugars are frequently higher than they should be, a daily supplement of up to 100 milligrams can't hurt even though the daily requirement is set at only 0.5 milligram per 1,000 calories consumed. Other B vitamins like riboflavin and biotin may also be important to people with diabetes.

Vitamin B$_{12}$

Athletes use and abuse vitamin B$_{12}$ because they believe that it enhances red blood cell production and improves oxygen-carrying capacity during endurance events. Some have also used it to try to increase their muscle mass. Although a deficiency of this vitamin can potentially impair your sport performance, it does not have an ergogenic effect if you already get enough in your diet. Vitamin B$_{12}$ is found only in animal products (meat, dairy products, and eggs); therefore, vegetarians, especially vegans who do not eat any meat or animal by-products, likely need to take B$_{12}$ supplements to prevent pernicious anemia, a form of anemia that has weakness, fatigue, and malaise as its usual symptoms. Taking supplements of this vitamin is otherwise generally not necessary or recommended, although large doses are considered harmless.

Minerals: Look to Iron and Calcium First

Minerals exert their effects on many energy-producing pathways in the body because of their involvement with metabolism and enzymes involved in ATP production. Deficiencies in a mineral like iron could certainly have a negative effect on your exercise capacity, and diabetes itself can potentially cause certain mineral deficiencies. Among the minerals that diabetic athletes may consider supplementing with are iron, calcium, magnesium, zinc, chromium, and vanadium.

Iron

An iron deficiency can affect your endurance capacity because this mineral is part of the hemoglobin molecule that carries oxygen in your red blood cells. Any reduction in hemoglobin reduces your oxygen-carrying capacity and may make your muscles feel unusually fatigued during aerobic activities. Iron deficiency is a common problem, especially in endurance athletes and premenopausal women. Dietary iron is found in both animal and plant sources, but the iron in plants (e.g., spinach, which contains the ferric form) is not absorbed as well as that found in meat, poultry, and fish (i.e., ferrous iron). You may benefit from iron supplements if you don't get enough in your diet or get your iron mainly from plant sources. Premenopausal women need about 15 milligrams daily, while men require only about 10 milligrams. Taking iron if you're not deficient won't improve your exercise capacity, though, and can reduce your insulin action, so don't supplement with iron unless you're truly deficient in it.

Calcium

Although calcium intake doesn't directly affect sport performance, adequate amounts are crucial to the long-term health of your bones and other bodily systems. Many older people experience osteoporosis (thinning of the bones), which greatly increases the risk for bone fractures. Both weight-bearing exercises and resistance training can stimulate the retention of calcium in bones, but your diet also needs to contain enough calcium. Sources of dietary calcium are dairy products, egg yolks, legumes, broccoli, cauliflower, and dark green leafy vegetables, to name a few. Supplementing with calcium (as well as foods rich in vitamin D to increase its absorption) is recommended for anyone taking in less than 1,000 to 1,200 milligrams daily (up to 1,500 milligrams when you're older). With diabetes, you should be especially diligent about getting adequate amounts of this mineral because diabetes itself can cause greater loss of bone minerals. In addition, limit your intake of phosphorus, found in colas and widely distributed in foods, which can leech calcium from your bones, and restrict intake of sodium, protein, and caffeine as well.

Magnesium

A component of more than 300 enzymes in your muscles, magnesium affects ATP use during contractions, oxygen metabolism, and your body's glucose use, as well as the health of your bones. Although supplementing is not likely to improve sport performance if you're not deficient in this mineral, having enough magnesium in your body may prevent muscle cramping and general muscle weakness, and deficiencies are more common in athletes and people with diabetes. Strenuous exercise apparently increases urinary and sweat losses that may increase your magnesium requirements by up to 20 percent.

A significant number of people routinely have magnesium intakes that may result in a deficient status, such as athletes participating in sports requiring weight control (e.g., wrestling, gymnastics). In their case, an increased intake of magnesium will have beneficial effects on exercise performance, and taking in less than 420 milligrams per day for male and 320 milligrams for female athletes may result in a deficiency. In addition, low intake of magnesium has been linked to a higher risk for developing type 2 diabetes. In people with diabetes, low magnesium levels have been linked to a higher incidence of retinopathy (diabetic eye disease) and depression, as well as poorer blood sugar control. To make sure that you're getting enough, consume plenty of foods with a higher content, including nuts, seafood, green leafy vegetables, dairy, and whole-grain products. You may also benefit from taking a magnesium supplement (not to exceed 350 milligrams daily), particularly if you are physically active, diabetic, and female.

Zinc

This mineral is involved in wound healing, growth, protein synthesis, and immune function. It is also a component of more than 300 enzymes, some of which involve ATP production using the lactic acid system. Low-calorie diets or excessive sweating may contribute to loss of zinc, and having diabetes may make you more prone to deficiencies from excessive urinary loss of this mineral with hyperglycemia. One study of people with type 1 diabetes found that zinc supplementation of twice the recommended daily intake corrected zinc deficiency and improved the activity of one antioxidant enzyme. In people with type 2 diabetes, zinc supplements may reduce insulin resistance in muscle. Zinc supplements haven't conclusively been found to enhance muscular strength or athletic performance, however, and the intake of large doses may interfere with normal intestinal absorption of other essential minerals like iron and copper, impair immune function (instead of improving it), and raise levels of bad LDL cholesterol while decreasing the good HDL. Thus, it's best not to supplement with doses above what's recommended, which is 8 milligrams (females) or 11 milligrams (males) per day. Better yet, simply consume an adequate amount by eating organ meats, poultry, seafood (especially oysters), dairy products, asparagus, spinach, and whole-grain products.

Chromium

Believed to enhance insulin sensitivity, chromium may improve your blood sugar, storage of glycogen, and performance during endurance exercise. People with type 2 diabetes have taken large doses of chromium to attempt to improve insulin action, and athletes have used it to try to increase lean body mass and reduce body fat. No well-designed studies have shown chromium supplementation to have a significant effect on muscle and fat mass, muscular strength, or muscular endurance, however, and chromium supplementation won't make you lose weight. In fact, taken in excess, this mineral may accumulate in cells and cause damage to DNA.

Supplementing with chromium is recommended only if you consume a high-carbohydrate diet, exercise strenuously, or have inadequate intake. The combination of chromium picolinate and biotin (a B vitamin found in organ meats, egg yolks, legumes, and green leafy vegetables) may improve blood sugar control and cholesterol levels in people with either type 1 or type 2 diabetes. The best approach is to get adequate chromium through food sources, including organ meats, oysters, cheese, whole-grain products, nuts, asparagus, and beer. If you take supplements, try not to exceed 200 micrograms a day until the safety of taking larger doses is certain.

Vanadium

A nonessential mineral, vanadium (vanadyl sulfate) has been tried as an ergogenic aid by athletes. Supplementation with vanadyl salts can improve glucose metabolism in adults with type 2 diabetes by exerting an insulin-like effect on glucose and protein use in the body. Although vanadium may help control blood glucose, it doesn't have any effect on an athlete's body composition or sport performance. Vanadium is found in shellfish, grain products, parsley, mushrooms, and black pepper, but you should limit your supplemental intake to no more than 1.8 milligrams per day because in high doses it can be toxic to your liver and kidneys.

Caffeine: Going Beyond the Morning Cup of Coffee

Do you need to have that cup of steaming java in the morning to start your day off right (or just to feel awake)? If you do, you're not alone, and you're probably drinking it more for the caffeine than any other reason. Caffeine is a stimulant found naturally in coffee, tea, cocoa, and chocolate that directly stimulates the central nervous system and increases arousal. At the same time, it increases your body's release of adrenaline, which can mobilize fat and provide an alternative fuel to working muscles.

Caffeine also stimulates the release of calcium in contracting muscles, allowing greater force production and muscular strength, which is probably its most important effect as far as athletes are concerned. It potentially increases performance in almost any event or physical activity that you choose to do, long or short, intense or easy. Most athletes use caffeine in an attempt to improve how well they perform and feel, but apparently they do so in the dark. A recent study showed that most athletes believe that caffeine will benefit them and they seek it out before sports participation, but few have any idea how much of it they're consuming in various drinks and other caffeinated substances. For your reference, here are the numbers:

A 6-ounce (180-milliliter) cup of brewed coffee contains 100 to 150 milligrams.

A cup of tea contains 50 milligrams.

A 12-ounce (360-milliliter) can of caffeinated soda contains 40 to 55 milligrams.

A cup of hot cocoa or decaffeinated coffee contains 5 milligrams.

A regular No Doz tablet contains 100 milligrams.

A Vivarin tablet contains 200 milligrams.

Currently, all doses of caffeine are legal in sports, although it has a history of being alternately banned, limited, and legalized by the International Olympic Committee. Its turbulent status may have something to do with the fact that it's one of the few supplements that can improve your performance, even in running times for various distance events from 1 mile (1.6 kilometers) up to marathons and in power events. You may be able to increase the effectiveness of caffeine by abstaining from it for two to three days before your sporting event and then consuming it right before you start. A short period of withdrawal actually causes you to be less habituated to its effects (although you may have to suffer through withdrawal symptoms like headaches and irritability). Another recently discovered benefit of caffeine is that it may enhance your body's hormonal release in response to a bout of low blood sugar and enhances your brain's ability to respond to adrenaline that improves its function.

A potential downside of caffeine, though, is that it can exert a diuretic effect, meaning that when you consume caffeinated beverages, you could lose more of your body water by having to urinate more than when drinking noncaffeinated drinks. Hyperglycemia increases water loss as well. So you'll need to be especially cautious about maintaining proper hydration when ingesting caffeine, especially if you exercise in a hot environment where you'll be sweating more or when your blood sugars are already elevated. The good news is that any caffeine that you consume right before or while exercising has a minimal diuretic effect, so you don't have to worry about becoming dehydrated from using it then. Another concern is that caffeine may increase your insulin resistance, but it's also likely that any such effect will be minimized during exercise. When caffeine comes naturally in coffee, it appears to have less effect on insulin action than straight caffeine does (perhaps because of the other compounds found in coffee), but the latest research shows that drinking coffee may still raise your blood sugars slightly (if you're not exercising).

Creatine: The Power Supplement, but for Diabetes?

Creatine is an amine present in animal products but also formed in the liver and kidneys from other amino acids in your body. Normally, your daily dietary intake of creatine is one gram, and another gram is synthesized by your body to reach the two-gram amount that you need. Creatine is present in all muscle cells both in its free form and as creatine phosphate (CP), a main component of the phosphagen energy system (refer to chapter 2). Many athletes have tried creatine monohydrate powder supplements to increase their performance in power sports. Oral supplementation increases free creatine and CP stores in muscles. It adds body weight as well because excess water is retained in muscle with the extra creatine.

Loading up with 20 to 30 grams of creatine monohydrate in four equal doses over the course of a day for five to seven days may improve your performance in explosive sports, primarily those that involve high-intensity, short-term, and repetitive exercise bouts with brief recovery periods. After taking it, you may be able to train at a higher level, which could lead to an increase in your muscle mass and gains in strength and power. The initial creatine-loading phase is typically followed by a maintenance dose of 2 to 5 grams per day. Other athletes have tried supplementing with 3 grams per day for four weeks without a loading phase, and doing so works equally well. Most athletes then cycle off loading for a while before starting again. Loading up on creatine doesn't work for endurance activities, however, and may even be detrimental for distance running because of weight gain. Also, consuming large amounts of caffeine when you're loading on creatine may interfere with the effects of creatine to a certain extent, so you may want to avoid taking in both. Also, drink plenty of fluids because creatine supplementation can have a dehydrating effect.

To date, there are no known long-term detrimental effects from creatine supplements, although the excess has to be removed by your kidneys as creatinine. The effect on diabetic kidneys has not been studied, so athletes with diabetes should be cautious in supplementing with it. Your intake should not exceed 20 grams per day for a period of five days (loading phase), and the subsequent intake should be no more than 3 grams per day for maintenance. If you have any evidence of kidney disease, you are best advised not to load up on creatine at all because of the additional stress it can place on your kidneys.

Ginseng: A Recovery Hoax?

Ginseng is derived from plants and sold in different forms: Chinese or Korean, American, Japanese, and Russian or Siberian. This herb is believed to stimulate the hypothalamus, which stimulates the release of various endocrine hormones from the pituitary gland. It is marketed to athletes for its purported ability to speed recovery from exercise by enhancing the resynthesis of muscle glycogen and protein stores and its beneficial effect on hemoglobin levels and oxygen transport. Unfortunately, well-controlled research has not been able to prove these effects in athletes. Consuming American and possibly Korean red ginseng before a glucose load may decrease your blood glucose response, though, as shown by a number of studies that have now investigated the antidiabetic effect of these forms of ginseng. Other forms may have variable effects on blood pressure (raising and lowering it), so supplementing with ginseng is generally not recommended for diabetic exercisers. If you do decide to use them, be aware that there is no quality control for commercial ginseng products, so you never really know how much (if any) that you're getting in the supplements.

*A*thlete *P*rofile

Name: Nikki Wallis

Hometown: Llanberis, Wales, United Kingdom

Diabetes history: Type 1 diabetes diagnosed in 1994 (at age 23)

Sport or activity: Mountaineering, rock climbing, alpine climbing, skiing, and general fitness training

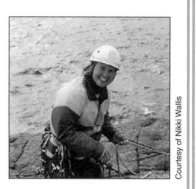

Greatest athletic achievement: Participation in an all-Italian expedition to Broad Peak in the Greater Karakorum, Pakistan (my first to high altitude), where I reached Camp 2 solo with fixed ropes, and winning the DESA Athletic Achievement Award (2005)

Current insulin and medication regimen: I currently use an AccuChek Spirit insulin pump with Humalog. My average hourly rate is 0.4 to 0.5 unit, which peaks to 0.7 to 0.8 unit in the early hours of the morning (4:00–6:00 a.m.) and late afternoon (5:00–7:00 p.m.). I increase my basal by 25 percent for stressful situations (e.g., public speaking). If I am not exercising for long periods, my insulin requirements almost double, but if I lower my carbohydrate intake, my basal requirements go down. My usual CHO-to-insulin ratio is 1.2 units per 10 grams.

Training tips: Learn to think like your pancreas. Learn to do trial and error responsibly with your diabetes (food, medications, and exercise) to become the greatest master of your condition but change only one factor at a time to see the effect. Always, for the rest of your life with diabetes, positively challenge what you have and what you are given with what you want and where you want to be in sport. Get in touch with other people who are already doing what you want to do and find out how they do it. Learn what questions you need to ask your health care professionals but also learn your own diabetes profile. Sometimes, take some time out from intensive diabetes management. Don't be impatient. Learn about "insulin on board" issues to minimize your risk of overcorrecting for highs. Last, but not least, never forget to test your blood sugar levels!

Typical daily and weekly training and diabetes regimen:

▶ *Monday:* 5-mile (8-kilometer) tempo run, for which I typically lower my basal rate by 25 to 30 percent starting one to two hours beforehand; supplement with 10 grams of carbohydrates every 45 minutes.

▶ *Tuesday:* Climbing-wall strength training; for strength workouts, I make no changes because my blood glucose levels rarely drop during them.

▶ *Wednesday:* Rest day.

▶ *Thursday:* 8-mile (13-kilometer) run, rock climbing; for climbing, I don't usually need to change my basal rates, but I reduce any boluses for food by about 30 percent.

▶ *Friday:* 3-mile (5-kilometer) run, strength training, and gym work; my shorter runs are usually more intense, so I have to reduce my basal rate by 50 percent one to two hours beforehand.

▶ *Saturday:* Mountain walking (all day at work), for which I reduce my basal rates by 30 to 40 percent and take about 65 percent of my usual boluses for carbohydrate.

▶ *Sunday:* Mountain walking (all day at work).

Other hobbies and interests: I have trained mountain and urban search and rescue dogs, including my own, as a handler with Search and Rescue Dog Association (Wales). I am an active member of the Llanberis Mountain Rescue Team and work as a ranger for Snowdonia National Park. I am founder of Mountains for Active Diabetics (www.mountain-mad.org), now the international source of practical advice and information on managing diabetes during remote adventure travel, alpine climbing, and rock climbing. In addition, I run an outdoor training company called Active Diabetes (www.active-diabetes.co.uk) that provides training and outdoor hill instruction for people with diabetes. I am qualified by the UK Mountain Leader Training Board.

Good diabetes and exercise story: In MADiDEA 2007, held in Montana, Doug Bursnall, Mauro Sormani, David Panofsky, Jeff Mazer, Lisa Seaman, Herbert Hausmann, and I took a three-day backcountry hike to Mount Cowan, where I was introduced to the wilderness delights of huckleberries and whortleberries. We had all taken turns buying and carrying food for different stages of our trip. Jeff and I had forgotten a dessert, so I promised a "Montana Mountain Special" to be made of munchy bars, crushed trail mix, and as many berries as I could find during our descent, topped with grated chocolate and coconut flakes, a mountain mad diabetic's delight. Intriguingly, this story is not directly linked with this dessert.

Instead, a few days later, I was walking up to Hyalite Peak with John Schroeder and his son, Chris, and we stopped frequently to eat huckleberries and whortleberries along the way. Anyway, I later did a blood glucose test, and it read 22 mmol/L (about 400 mg/dl). No way! I had had breakfast as normal, had been walking as usual, and had reduced my basal by 30 percent. The Guardian CGMS monitor that I was wearing was not showing any warnings of such high sugar levels, and I felt fine as well! Chris then reminded me about the whortleberries we had eaten. After washing my fingers in a nearby stream and retesting, I was much relieved to find that it had simply been whortleberry sugar on my fingertips. Luckily, I had not bolused with insulin based on my initial glucose reading. It just goes to show that when we get more techno gizmos, sometimes we can forget the basics even when we're experienced with diabetes.

CHAPTER 5

Exercise and Blood Glucose Monitoring Guidelines

In the earlier days of diabetes treatment, before blood glucose meters existed, physicians often advised their patients using insulin not to engage in any physical activity. Without a doubt, being active can increase your risk for low blood sugars both during and after an activity, especially if you are an insulin user, and being active can even cause hyperglycemia. But you can exercise safely and effectively by following a few basic guidelines and safety precautions, such as the current published recommendation pertaining to exercise that is discussed in this chapter, although many diabetic athletes make small adjustments that aren't listed in the overall guidelines.

Many reports indicate that the increasing incidence of type 2 diabetes is associated with a declining level of physical activity and weight gain. If you have type 2 diabetes, you may be able to control your blood sugars with diet and exercise alone or along with oral and other diabetic medications like insulin. Regardless of your regimen, exercise can be a vital component in the prevention and management of your diabetes. You can lower your insulin resistance with regular physical activity, and the potential health benefits are enormous. But being aware of your health complications and the effect that physical activity may have on them is important. This topic is also addressed in the following sections.

CURRENT EXERCISE AND DIABETES GUIDELINES FOR INSULIN USERS

The American Diabetes Association (ADA) publishes clinical recommendations for exercise for people with type 1 diabetes (and other insulin users). Because of the possibility of worsening your metabolic control during exercise (resulting in either hyperglycemia or hypoglycemia), the guidelines address the areas of metabolic control, blood glucose monitoring, and food intake for physical activity. See table 5.1 for a summary of these guidelines.

Table 5.1 Exercise Guidelines for Athletes With Type 1 Diabetes and Other Insulin Users

Metabolic control before exercise
• Avoid exercising if fasting glucose levels are >250 mg/dl (13.9 mmol/L) and ketosis is present, and use caution if glucose levels are >300 mg/dl (16.7 mmol/L) and no ketosis is present.
• Ingest carbohydrates if glucose levels are <100 mg/dl (5.6 mmol/L).
Blood glucose monitoring before and after exercise
• Identify when changes in insulin or food intake are necessary.
• Learn the glycemic response to different exercise conditions.
Food intake
• Consume carbohydrate as needed to avoid hypoglycemia.
• Keep carbohydrate-based foods readily available during and after exercise.

Metabolic Control Before Exercise

The first guideline states that you should avoid exercising if your blood glucose levels are more than 250 mg/dl, or 13.9 mmol/L, and you have ketones, which are by-products of your body's attempt to use fat as a fuel when glucose is not getting into your cells. Building up too many ketones in your blood makes it more acidic, which can cause a potentially fatal coma. If your glucose levels are more than 300 mg/dl (16.7 mmol/L) without any urinary ketones, then you are advised to use caution.

Not everyone follows this recommendation. Some diabetic athletes have never experienced ketosis or just never check their urine for ketones because their sugars are never that high for long. Most find that exercising reduces their blood sugars or that a small dose of rapid-acting insulin before an activity brings them right back down to normal. If you have insulin in your system and are only high because you miscalculated with your last insulin dose, then extended aerobic exercise is likely to lower your blood sugars, regardless of its intensity. A common practice of athletes is to administer 0.5 to 2 units of rapid-acting insulin before exercise and wait 10 to 15 minutes before beginning. As discussed in chapter 3, the main danger of this is that you may overestimate your insulin needs, so err on the side of caution if you try this correction technique. Underestimating how much insulin you need is far better than ending up with severe low blood sugar from taking too much before your workout. If you have ketones from being sick, having an infection, or running high for too long, don't exercise until you get your blood sugars under better control. When you have ketones and high sugars, doing any exercise can cause your blood glucose to increase even more and put you into DKA (diabetic ketoacidosis), which is serious enough to be potentially life threatening.

The second metabolic control before exercise guideline says, "Ingest added carbohydrates if glucose levels are less than 100 mg/dl (5.6 mmol/L)." However, when you're on a temporary basal rate on your pump or have low levels of circulating insulin for other reasons, you may not need to eat anything. Your blood sugars are affected by how long you plan to exercise, what type of exercise you are doing, how intense it is, and even how hot or cold it is. Most athletes eat something before prolonged, less intense activities, but not necessarily before weight training, sprinting, or other hard, shorter workouts. The time of day also makes a difference, because doing early morning exercise may not drop your sugars as later-day activities do. Depending on all these factors, your personal cutoff level to eat carbohydrate preexercise may be 75 mg/dl (4.2 mmol/L) instead of 100 (5.6 mmol/L), or whatever you find works best for you. If you're wearing a pump, you may just choose to suspend it completely instead of eating anything.

Blood Glucose Monitoring for Type 1 Diabetics

Two other guidelines address blood glucose monitoring practices. The first guideline recommends that exercisers "identify when changes in insulin or food intake are necessary." Most insulin users agree that glucose monitoring is essential in establishing a pattern and making changes, although it still involves a lot of trial and error. Many athletes minimally check their blood sugars before and after exercise, and sometimes during. You'll likely need to do more testing for new and unusual exercise than for established routines. Blood glucose meters nowadays are inexpensive (although the strips to use in them aren't), they're a joy to use, and you can choose one with the features that you like (even special colors). An added bonus is that it takes only five seconds to find out what your blood sugars are. Most insulin users test anywhere from 4 to 15 times a day. Others are now wearing continuous glucose monitors so that they get a glucose reading every five minutes all day long.

The second guideline states that diabetic exercisers should learn the glycemic response to different exercise conditions. Establishing patterns, even with a blood glucose meter, is still an inexact science because of the multitude of variables that can affect your response at any given time. The variables are too numerous for you to guess perfectly every time, but general trends are predictable for most activities. Establishing a trend usually involves a lot of trial and error because everyone is unique. Learn your own responses by checking your blood sugar levels before, during, and after exercise. Ideally, a somewhat predictable pattern will emerge to help you anticipate your responses to future bouts of similar exercise.

Food Intake

The last two guidelines for insulin users address carbohydrate intake. The first states that exercisers should "consume carbohydrate as needed to avoid hypoglycemia." You can find diabetic athletes' favorite rapidly absorbed carbohydrate sources to prevent and treat hypoglycemia in chapter 4, but to reiterate, they include regular soda, sports drinks, sports bars, glucose gels, juice, hard candy, glucose tablets, dried fruits, skim milk, bread, carbohydrate bars, and others. If you want to lose (or maintain) weight and don't want to have to eat extra calories to prevent lows, you need to minimize your circulating insulin levels as well as you can during all activities.

The second recommendation states that carbohydrate-based foods should be readily available during and after exercise. If you're an insulin user and have ever been caught out doing something without having anything with you to treat hypoglycemia, you're not likely to forget again! The recommendations no longer tell people how many carbohydrate grams to consume, which is a good thing because the amount varies on a case-by-case basis. When I ask athletes how much they consume to prevent lows, they usually answer, "It depends." You have to rely on testing your blood sugars and trying different amounts of carbohydrate a few times to figure out what works for you.

Continuous Glucose Monitoring

Some continuous glucose monitors recently received approval from the FDA. They're still invasive, requiring you to place a probe under your skin. These monitors are not a closed-loop system either, meaning that you still have to check the blood glucose readings and make regimen adjustments yourself, but getting readings every 5 minutes 24 hours a day can be extremely useful to people who are trying to learn their patterns and keep their blood glucose in good control.

The continuous glucose-monitoring (CGM) models currently available as of the publication of this book are shown in table 5.2. Insurance reimbursement is hit or miss (as of 2008), depending on the insurance provider and the person's overall diabetes care needs. These models vary in price, with start-up costs varying for the models. You also have to continue to buy supplies to use them, particularly the sensors themselves, which can be quite pricey without insurance coverage (although better reimbursement is likely in the near future). They all have user-set high and low alarms, insertion devices, associated computer software to manage data, and fairly similar accuracy, but only the Abbott monitor has a built-in FreeStyle glucose meter, one of the meters made by them.

The CGM systems recently approved for use in the United States are admittedly first-generation products, meaning that they're likely to improve when newer versions come out, just as each new model of blood glucose meter and insulin pump came with enhanced technology. Athletes have had varying experiences with them so far. In general, though, most athletes have found that the trending aspect can be helpful during exercise, although the actual readings lag behind by at least 15 minutes. This lag may result in your ending up symptomatically low before the device detects it because of how rapidly your blood sugars can change during hard exercise. Many exercisers have also experienced technical failures with the newer versions of these monitors during physical activity, but the CGM systems are still likely to be the wave of the future when it comes to managing blood sugars effectively, especially with exercise.

EXERCISE GUIDELINES FOR TYPE 2 DIABETES

Exercise guidelines for people with type 2 diabetes differ somewhat from those for insulin users. The majority of type 2 exercisers rely on a combination of diet, exercise, and medications to control their blood sugars and overcome insulin resistance.

Table 5.2 Continuous Glucose Monitoring Systems

	Abbott Freestyle Navigator	Medtronic MiniMed ParadigmReal-Time System	Medtronic MiniMed Guardian RT	DexCom STS
FDA-approved sensor life	5 days	3 days	3 days	7 days
Glucose results displayed on insulin pump?	No	Yes, using Paradigm 522 and 722 pumps, CGM on pump screen	No	No
Length of sensor probe and insertion angle	6 mm, 90°	13 mm, 45°	13 mm, 45°	13 mm, 45°
Start-up initialization	10 hours	2 hours	2 hours	2 hours
Calibration	Calibrate at 10, 12, 24, and 72 hours, with no more calibrations for the final 2 days of the 5-day wear	At 2 hours, again within 6 hours, and then every 12 hours	At 2 hours, again within 6 hours, and then every 12 hours	Must calibrate with Lifescan One Touch Ultra, twice to start and then at least once every 12 hours
Frequency of readings	Every minute	Every 5 minutes	Every 5 minutes	Every 5 minutes
Display of directional trends?	Yes, directional and rate-of-change arrows; 2-, 4-, 6-, 12-, or 24-hour glucose graph; can go back 28 days	Yes, arrows display how fast, in what direction, and 3- and 24-hour graphs	No, must manually scroll; can upload data to software for analysis	Yes, displays 1-, 3-, or 9-hour glucose graphs
Waterproof transmitter?	Yes	Yes, up to 8 feet (2.4 meters) deep for 30 minutes	Yes, up to 8 feet (2.4 meters) deep for 30 minutes	No, but shower patch makes watertight
Monitor to transmitter range	10 feet (3 meters) (but possibly more)	6 feet (1.8 meters)	6 feet (1.8 meters)	5 feet (1.5 meters)
Sensor storage	4 months at room temperature	6 months refrigerated, 1 week at room temperature	6 months refrigerated, 1 week at room temperature	4 months at room temperature
Transmitter batteries	Watch battery; replace monthly	Nonreplaceable; 9-month life	Nonreplaceable; 12-month life	Nonreplaceable; 6-month warranty
Monitor batteries	Two AAA batteries; replace every 3 months	No separate monitor; results displayed on pump	Two AAA batteries; alerts when replacement needed	Must recharge the battery every 5 days; charge time 3 hours

Athletes with type 2 diabetes may need a preexercise evaluation by a physician to ensure that being more active will not worsen any existing health problems given that their diabetes may have gone undetected for longer. They will also benefit from frequent blood glucose monitoring to determine the effects of exercise, although they are much less likely either to have lows or to develop DKA.

Preexercise Medical Evaluation

If you have type 2 diabetes and want to start a moderate or vigorous exercise program, you should probably have a checkup to detect any macrovascular or microvascular complications, such as heart disease or nerve problems, that may get worse with exercise. For example, if you have lost sensation in your feet, you may benefit from limiting weight-bearing exercises (like walking or jogging) and focusing on non-weight-bearing activities like cycling or aquatic activities. If you have central nerve damage (i.e., autonomic neuropathy), your exercise capacity may be limited and risk of a silent heart attack (one that you're not aware of) may be greater. Some people develop orthostatic hypotension, which means that their blood pressure drops when they stand up; if you have similar symptoms, you'll need to be more careful about your hydration levels and what types of activities you choose to do.

If you have had diabetes for five or more years, you may want to consider having an exercise stress test to screen for reduced blood flow during exercise because of blockages in your coronary arteries or arrhythmias (abnormal heart rhythms) elicited by exercise. If cleared by your physician, you can safely participate in any activity. If you have complications, you can usually exercise safely if you take special precautions (discussed later in this chapter).

Blood Glucose Monitoring for Type 2 Diabetics

Even if you don't get low blood sugars during exercise, monitoring your blood sugars frequently is still advisable, especially beforehand and afterward. Doing so can be motivational, especially when you see your blood sugars go down from an activity. Depending on your medications, you may have to make some changes to keep your blood glucose levels optimal. For instance, if you use certain oral medications (discussed in chapter 3), you may have higher risk for developing hypoglycemia. Luckily, type 2 athletes are not prone to developing DKA even when their blood sugars run high, but knowing your starting blood sugar level is still important so that you can prevent lows and dehydration from physical activity.

EXERCISE PRECAUTIONS FOR ALL DIABETIC ATHLETES

If you're in good control of your blood sugars and don't have any serious diabetic complications, then exercise away to your heart's content. Keep certain precautions in mind, though, particularly ones related to hypoglycemia during and following the activity, hyperglycemia, and dehydration. If you have any complications, you may also need to take extra care. The following sections contain the recommended precautionary measures.

Prevention of Hypoglycemia or Hyperglycemia With Exercise

Hypoglycemia can occur during or after exercise, but you can often prevent it with changes in insulin, meds, and food intake. Following either repeated bouts of high-intensity or long-duration exercise, eat some carbohydrate within 30 minutes to 2 hours after exercise. You'll be more insulin sensitive then, so your body will need less insulin to take up blood glucose into your muscles to reform glycogen.

Glycogen is restored at a rate of only 5 to 7 percent per hour. The rate is slightly faster when stores are low, but it slows down as they start to fill up. Insulin action starts to wane, too, as your muscles restore their glycogen stores. On a positive note, the sooner your glycogen is replaced, the less likely you are to develop late-onset hypoglycemia, which can occur up to 24 to 48 hours following exercise. Monitor your blood glucose levels at 1-hour intervals after exercise to make adjustments to prevent lows or highs. A low carbohydrate intake after exercise or carbohydrate eaten without adequate insulin (albeit less than normal) may compromise or delay your body's glycogen restoration.

Although less of a problem for most type 2 athletes, low blood sugars can still occur with exercise if you are taking certain oral medications or insulin injections. The ones with the highest risk are Diabinese, DiaBeta, and Micronase, which have a longer duration (refer to the discussion in chapter 3). If you begin exercise with blood sugars in a normal or near-normal range, especially if you use any of these

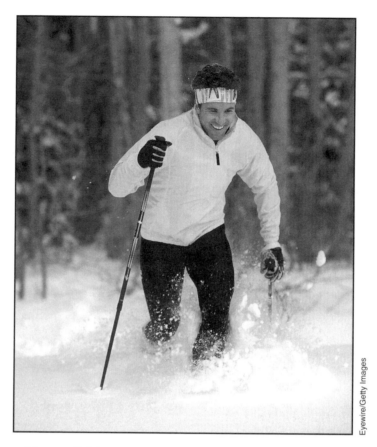

Following repeated bouts of high-intensity or long-duration exercise, like cross-country skiing, eat some carbohydrate within 30 minutes to 2 hours after exercise.

meds, then you may need to eat some extra carbohydrate to prevent lows. When your blood sugars are already elevated when you start (in the range of 150 to 300 mg/dl or above, or 8.3 to 16.7 mmol/L), you are less likely to experience lows or need to eat anything. If you use insulin, simply follow the recommendations based on your insulin regimen. If you begin regular exercise training, talk to your doctor about possibly reducing the dosages of your oral meds, Byetta, or insulin, especially if you start to have more frequent lows associated with your workouts.

Prevention of Dehydration and Overhydration

If your sugars have been running high, you may be prone to dehydration because of water losses in your urine (polyuria). Likewise, if you have the type of neuropathy (autonomic) that makes you dizzy when you stand up, you may be more likely to become dehydrated during exercise and not realize it. Normally, thirst centers in the brain are not activated until you have already lost 1 to 2 percent of your body water, and autonomic neuropathy can make you even less likely to realize that you're thirsty until it's too late. Make certain that you hydrate adequately before exercise and drink fluids early and frequently to compensate for sweat losses during exercise, especially when it is hot. Drinking cool, plain water is fine for moderate exercise lasting up to an hour. For longer workouts, use sports drinks or diluted fruit juices to replace both water and carbohydrate. Keep drinking more after an activity because it takes up to a day to restore fluids lost through sweat and ventilation. You'll find more hydration tips in table 5.3.

An equally valid concern is overhydration, or drinking too much fluid. In some cases, taking in too much fluid is worse than dehydrating, as discussed in the last chapter. One rule of thumb is that you should not weigh more after exercise than you did when you started; if you do, you probably consumed too much fluid. Whenever you start to feel thirsty, swig a mouthful (about 1 ounce, or 30 milliliters), and drink that amount every 10 to 15 minutes or so. If you don't sense when you're getting thirsty, just start drinking about 15 minutes into your exercise session. If you've already had plenty to drink and need some more carbohydrate, try glucose tablets or a gel instead.

Table 5.3   Hydration Tips for Exercise

- Drink cool, plain water during and following exercise, especially during warmer weather, and take frequent breaks to have a chance to cool down, preferably out of the heat and direct sunlight.

- Don't force yourself to drink more than the amount of fluid that satisfies your thirst. Otherwise, water intoxication may result.

- To know how much fluid to replace after exercise, weigh yourself before and after a prolonged activity and replace only as much weight as you have lost (1 liter of water weighs 1 kilogram, or 2.2 pounds).

- If you prefer fluids with some flavor, try flavored waters, sports drinks that have no added carbohydrate or calories (such as Champion Lyte), or Crystal Light (with a pinch of salt if you want it to taste more like a sports drink).

- Drink regular sports drinks (containing glucose) only when you need some carbohydrate to prevent or treat hypoglycemia during physical activities.

Exercising Safely with Complications

If you have any diabetes-related health problems, you likely can still exercise safely, but you may need to take special precautions to do so. Microvascular complications include nerve damage, eye problems, or failing kidneys, and the large-vessel ones (macrovascular) involve heart or peripheral vascular disease and hypertension.

Peripheral Neuropathy

If you have some peripheral loss of sensation from nerve damage (i.e., neuropathy), you have greater risk of injuring your feet from exercising because nerve damage can blunt signals of pain or discomfort from high impact, friction, or pressure from your shoes and socks. The ADA recommends that you use silicone gel or air midsoles in shoes, as well as polyester or blend (cotton and polyester) socks on your feet to prevent blisters and keep them dry to minimize exercise-related trauma. Picking the right shoes to wear is also essential for preventing problems; they should fit snugly without excessively squeezing or constricting your feet. A recent study found that more than 60 percent of people with diabetes wear shoes that don't fit them well. Wearing supportive, cushioning, well-fitting shoes is vitally important to the health of your feet and lower-leg joints, especially when exercising. You can find tips for picking appropriate shoes in chapter 7.

If you've lost sensation in your feet, consider switching to non-weight-bearing exercises, which are recommended to improve tone, balance, and awareness of your lower extremities. Recommended exercises include swimming, pool walking, water aerobics, stationary bicycling, rowing, arm ergometer work, upper-body exercises, tai chi, seated exercises, and other non-weight-bearing activities. Range-of-motion exercises can also help prevent contracture of your lower limbs. You may want to avoid activities like prolonged walking, jogging, treadmill exercise, and step exercises that can cause blisters or foot trauma that you may not be able to detect. Daily monitoring before and after exercise for blisters and other potential damage is critical to catching and treating problems early.

Exercise cannot reverse peripheral neuropathy, but it can slow its progression and prevent further loss of fitness resulting from being inactive. Even if you aren't aware of having lost much sensation, if you develop a diabetic foot ulcer on the plantar (bottom) surface or sides of your feet, you probably have this condition. Have a doctor look at any changes on the skin of your feet right away to avoid the possibility of gangrene and possible amputation of your toes or part of your foot.

Autonomic Neuropathy

Central, or autonomic system, nerve damage puts you at high risk for having some problems during exercise, including having a silent heart attack. If you ever suddenly start to feel extremely fatigued or have other unexplained symptoms, stop exercising and get checked out by a doctor if the symptoms persist more than a couple of minutes. With this type of neuropathy, you can also develop low blood pressure more easily when you change positions, such as going from sitting to standing, which could cause you to become dizzy or faint. You may also have difficulty maintaining your normal body temperature and staying hydrated, so you should avoid exercising outdoors in extreme heat or cold.

This condition can also affect how quickly you digest your food. With gastroparesis (a delayed emptying of food from your stomach caused by autonomic neuropathy), if you try to treat a low by eating carbohydrate during exercise, raising your blood sugars may take longer. You may also experience lows followed by high blood sugar levels during exercise and afterward because of delayed digestion. To stay on top of things, you'll need to monitor your blood sugars closely. In addition, use the RPE scale (discussed in chapter 1) to monitor your exercise intensity because autonomic neuropathy can cause your exercise heart rate to be lower than expected.

Proliferative Retinopathy

This complication results from the formation of weak, abnormal blood vessels in the back of your eyes (retina) that can break, tear, or bleed into the vitreous fluid, filling your eye with blood and obscuring your vision (although sometimes only temporarily). In general, exercise does not accelerate the proliferative process. You may need to take certain precautions, however, depending on whether you have background retinopathy or a more advanced and active stage of retinopathy. With moderate or greater proliferation, you should avoid activities that dramatically increase your blood pressure, such as heavy weight lifting, power lifting, or heavy Valsalva (breath-holding) maneuvers. For more severe retinopathy or active hemorrhaging, avoid activities that cause a large increase in your blood pressure or involve pounding and jarring, including boxing, heavy competitive sports like basketball or football, weightlifting, jogging, high-impact aerobics, racket sports, and strenuous trumpet playing; they all increase the risk that you will have a retinal tear, retinal detachment, or vitreous hemorrhage. You can, however do exercises like swimming, walking, low-impact aerobics, stationary cycling, and other endurance exercises at a low to moderate level as long as your eyes are not actively bleeding. Exercising while you're experiencing a retinal hemorrhage will likely cause the release of extra blood into your eye and further block your vision, so wait until the hemorrhage has stopped and then see your eye doctor before doing any intense exercise.

Nephropathy

If you're in the early stages of kidney disease, exercise may increase rates of albumin (protein) excretion in urine. But there is no evidence that regular endurance activity speeds progression of this disease. In fact, exercise apparently increases protein excretion in diabetic people without kidney disease (through exercise-induced proteinuria), so for accurate results on your kidney function tests, don't exercise while doing a 24-hour urine collection to assess microalbumin and protein in your urine. If you have more severe kidney disease, your exercise capacity may be limited, which is why intense or excessive exercise is usually not recommended, but light to moderate exercise will not further damage your kidneys. If you're on dialysis, you can even exercise on a stationary cycle during your treatments with no ill effects. Don't exercise, however, if your hematocrit, calcium, or blood phosphorus levels are unstable because of the need for dialysis. If you have had renal transplant surgery, wait 6 to 8 weeks until your new kidneys are stable and free of rejection before you start exercising again.

Heart Disease

Exercise benefits you and lowers your risk of heart disease by favorably altering elevated blood fats (cholesterol, triglycerides, HDL, and LDL) and coagulation defects as well as lowering your insulin levels. The most consistent effect of regular exercise is a decrease in circulating blood fat (triglycerides). Keep in mind, though, that simply having diabetes still puts you at higher risk for cardiovascular complications. If you have central nerve damage, be especially vigilant for any changes during exercise that may indicate decreased blood flow to your heart (such as extreme fatigue), because you may not get the usual symptoms like chest discomfort. Your risk is greater if you have had diabetes longer than 10 years and if you have any other risk factors, evidence of microvascular changes, peripheral vascular disease, or nerve damage to your central nervous system. In these cases,

*A*thlete *P*rofile

Name: Robert L. Stewart, DPM

Hometown: Virginia Beach, Virginia, USA

Diabetes history: Type 1 diabetes diagnosed in 1959 (at age 47)

Sport or activity: Field events at the Senior Games and Olympics, fitness activities, walking, table tennis, golf

Greatest athletic achievement: Set world record for age group (95 to 99 years old) in shot put (22 feet, 3 inches, or 6.78 meters) and long jump (6 feet, 9.5 inches, or 2.07 meters) in 2007 at the Senior Olympics; won gold medal in javelin, high jump, and discus throw as well, but did not set world records

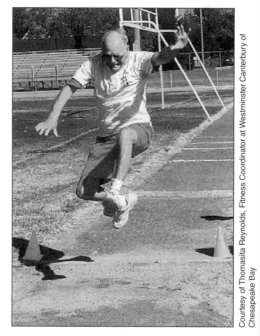

Courtesy of Thomasita Reynolds, Fitness Coordinator at Westminster Canterbury of Chesapeake Bay

Current insulin and medication regimen: Humalog and Lantus. I really like Lantus. I've had diabetes for almost 50 years, and it is pretty brittle, so my doctor has me checking my blood sugars seven to eight times a day and making adjustments to my rapid-acting insulin.

Training tips: I really don't train much for my field events. I just maintain my good health by exercising regularly, managing my diabetes, and eating a strict diet, which includes eating two tablespoons of ground, organic flax and other supplements every morning. My son always tells me that if I actually practiced the techniques for these events, I'd do even better. I guess he's right, but I just like to get out there and do as many events as I can.

Typical daily and weekly training regimen:

▸ *Monday:* formal exercise class that includes weights, running in place, and stretching (offered in the fitness area of my retirement community, Westminster-Canterbury)

▸ *Tuesday:* walking on the beach

▸ *Wednesday:* formal exercise class, square dancing

▸ *Thursday:* walking on the beach

▸ **Friday:** formal exercise class

▸ *Saturday:* walking on the beach

▸ *Sunday:* walking on the beach, line dancing

Other hobbies and interests: I was a practicing podiatrist for almost 60 years, mostly in Winston-Salem, North Carolina, and it was always gratifying to help my patients with their foot problems. My wife and I moved to Virginia Beach 14 years ago. She used to be a master's swimmer, and she set a backstroke record at the age of 60. We raised our kids to always be active, too.

My wife passed away in 2000, but I still live in the retirement community where we moved in Virginia Beach. We have a lot of activities offered where I live, and I partake of all of them. We had a golf croquet tournament not long ago that went on for two days straight, and I won all eight of my games, which was the talk of the place for a while. I used to do a lot of cycling, and I played a lot of tennis before I lost the sight in my left eye. I'm also a poet, and I write poems for all of our family occasions; I even wrote one for my recent 95th birthday in May 2007.

Good diabetes and exercise story: Probably the best story is when I set the world record in my age group in the long jump. I never did field events when I was younger, not even in college, because I was always working and never had the time for sports. I admit that being as old as I am gets rid of a lot of my competition in any event, but when you're breaking world records, that means you're competing against every single person who ever tried to do what you did at your age, and that puts you into some great competition.

You get six tries at the long jump, and my fourth one broke the world record. They have to bring out the official measuring tape when it looks like a new record, so I waited while they confirmed it. On my sixth and final try, I broke my own world record, setting a new one that beat the old one by more than a foot! Again, the measuring tape came out while I waited. It was exciting!

you should undergo a graded exercise test under a doctor's supervision before you embark on a moderate- or high-intensity exercise program. An exercise stress test will detect any significant coronary artery blockage or abnormal heart rhythms that exercise may exacerbate.

If you know that you have cardiovascular problems, at least initially do your exercise in a medically supervised environment where you can be monitored easily. Start an exercise program with low-intensity aerobic exercise and progress slowly. Periodically have an exercise stress test done to test for ischemia (reduced blood flow) so that you don't exercise harder than would be good for you. (Believe me; you really do want to prevent cardiovascular events or abnormal heart rhythms.) You also may need to avoid heavy weight training because of the excessive strain that it places on your heart and blood vessels. One of the best ways to prevent a second heart attack is to exercise regularly, so following these guidelines to do it safely will benefit your heart and your overall health.

Hypertension

Regular exercise can lower your body fat levels and reduce insulin resistance as well, resulting in modest decreases in both systolic (the higher blood pressure reading) and diastolic (the lower number) blood pressure. If you have hypertension, you must be careful to avoid certain high-intensity or resistance exercises, which may cause your blood pressure to rise to dangerously high levels. These activities may include heavy weight training; near-maximal exercise of any type; activities that require intense, sustained muscular contractions in the upper body, such as water skiing or wind surfing; and exercises that require you to hold your breath (Valsalva maneuver), like power lifting.

If you have elevations in your blood pressure, moderate-intensity aerobic exercise is generally recommended for you. If you want to do resistance work, focus on doing low-weight, high-repetition training, which usually causes less dramatic increases in blood pressure than heavy lifting does. Avoid doing near-maximal efforts, isometric exercises, and breath holding because all these activities can cause extreme increases in your blood pressure.

> *Despite the potential risks associated with exercise, the benefits to people with diabetes generally far outweigh the risks.*

Think of your diabetes as a reminder to take better care of yourself, to eat right, and to exercise daily. Find a way to exercise as much as you can because doing so can only help improve your diabetes control and prevent long-term health problems. Usually, exercise benefits you far more than it can hurt, but take precautions where necessary, especially if you have any complications, and use your common sense. You can safely participate in less strenuous forms of exercise, even with almost any complication. Learn to manage your blood sugars effectively during any type of physical activity by following the basic guidelines discussed in this chapter and by monitoring your body's response.

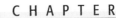

Thinking and Acting
Like an Athlete

Athletes come in all shapes and sizes. In my opinion, an athlete is anyone who exercises regularly. You don't have to be continually competing in athletic events to qualify, and even if you just exercise recreationally, you may be dealing with some of the same issues that elite athletes do when it comes to being emotionally and mentally fit for activity.

This chapter addresses how to know whether you're really an athlete (likely, you are), how to keep your mental stress under control (particularly when you are competing in events), how to relax more effectively, how to use your mind to enhance your physical performance, how to keep your motivation for exercise strong, and how to deal emotionally with getting an athletic injury. You'll also read an inspiring story about a diabetic athlete who finished his first full-length triathlon dead last but still came out a winner.

ARE YOU REALLY AN ATHLETE?

A diabetic marathoner from Pennsylvania, Bill King says that being active and seeing yourself as an athlete is more about your spirit than your athletic capability. "I'm an athlete," he says, "because when I look in a mirror, I see myself as one. If you have an active lifestyle, you will immediately gain self-esteem." He runs marathons and trains four to five days a week, so he qualifies as a true athlete, but even if you train less, you can still benefit from seeing yourself that way. Use your vision of yourself as an athlete to stay motivated to be active every day of your long and healthy life.

Kerry White agrees with Bill King's approach. She is a female diabetic athlete who in her 30s won the solo female division of the Race Across America (RAAM), a grueling cycling road race that goes from the West Coast to the East Coast of the United States. After recently winning a 2006 DESA Athletic Achievement Award, she said in her acceptance speech, "As I aspire to uphold the role of an athlete mentor, I can attest to the fact that the quality of being a great athlete is not really athleticism. My various experiences as a road cycling team member and individual mountain bike and Nordic athlete in ultraendurance events have brought to me the realization that athleticism without integrity, honesty, and the ability to share the euphoria of exercise with others is nothing. The importance of being not just an athlete but also always maintaining a positive outlook for what you are doing and treating those who support you in your endeavors with the ultimate respect and integrity is paramount. Without those who support, the athlete is nothing."

Even if you've done nothing noteworthy or remarkable athletically—except for exercising with diabetes, of course—you can consider yourself an athlete. Joyce Meyers, an exerciser with type 2 diabetes from Chicago, Illinois, is a perfect example. She says that being an exerciser at all is her greatest accomplishment. "After a period of time of exercising, you begin feeling better, which is self-fulfilling. When you feel better, you go exercise even when you don't really want to." Joyce has some other words of wisdom as well for any reluctant exercisers out there. "Treat exercise like you would diet: one step at a time and keep working at increasing it. Add a walk and a healthy shared meal with a friend after exercise as reinforcement to good behavior. Work these aspects into your life so that you miss them when they are not there. Don't expect miracles overnight, though, and don't expect to necessarily become the perfect hourglass figure. Just exercise for sake of exercising, feeling good, and having lower blood sugars."

BEING COMPETITIVE WITH YOURSELF, OTHERS, AND DIABETES

Simply having diabetes can instill in you a determination and willpower to fight the odds and survive—the exact qualities that many elite athletes have and what it takes for them to reach the top of their sport. Thus, your desire and drive for control over your diabetes parallels the desire to be a world-class athlete, and the two go hand in hand. Why can't you accomplish what others may tell you is impossible because of having diabetes?

Perhaps in some perverse way, diabetes makes all of us say to ourselves, "I'm not normal because I have diabetes, so why should I strive to be only an average person?" Many diabetic athletes are driven by the desire to prove that they can do it (whatever their unique "it" is) and that diabetes is not going to stop them. Take Al Lewis, a resident of Vancouver, British Columbia, for example. He has been a competitive master's swimmer and all-around athlete despite having diabetes for 70 years (since the age of 4). Even now, he believes that being competitive is important. "I'm even more competitive with diabetes than I am with other swimmers," he says. "It's all about being successful with diabetes." For him, exercise has been a big part of his success, the element to which he attributes most of his longevity with diabetes.

Andy Bell from Columbia, Missouri, concurs. "There is nothing that I don't do. I exercise daily, play sports, and compete in submission wrestling tournaments." He also realizes the effect that having diabetes has had on his life, though, and on his desire to compete. "I love that I have competed in two Brazilian jujitsu tournaments—a sport that I have only been doing for a couple of years now. I feel like these have been my greatest accomplishments as a diabetic athlete." He explains where the diabetes part comes in: "For me, it goes way back to the time of my diagnosis. At 14, I had already led a life of an athletic child, playing competitive soccer since I was 6, along with a lot of other sports. Getting diabetes struck me down. I lost the undeniable confidence, more like cockiness, that I had always had as a nondiabetic athlete. My self-esteem was shot, and I stopped competing in leagues and organized recreation because I didn't feel like I could do that stuff anymore. It has been a very slow recovery process, one taken on by me, and me alone. Now, I actually can embrace having this disease and fight it. Learning how to do martial arts and jujitsu actually has been literally fighting for my life. I have found that I am still that athletic, competitive little squirt that I was before my diagnosis. Not only do I have more confidence but I am now a better athlete than most people I know."

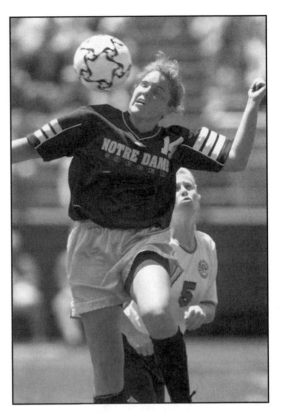

Battling diabetes can instill in you a determination and willpower to fight the odds and survive—the exact qualities that many elite athletes have.

RESOURCES FOR ACTIVE PEOPLE WITH DIABETES
HypoActive (Australia)

HypoActive, a group based in Melbourne, Victoria, in Australia, promotes an active lifestyle for people with type 1 diabetes. The group formed to provide information, ongoing support, and inspiration to people participating in exercise challenges, who can learn from other people with diabetes in the process. HypoActive has a strong commitment to assist in empowering all type 1 diabetic exercisers, and each year they provide opportunities to participate in a number of select endurance challenges, lobby for more research into the effects of exercise on type 1 diabetes, and encourage others to exercise more often. The group meets monthly in Melbourne, but has key links throughout Australia and New Zealand.

Founded by President Monique Hanley, this group features online articles about diabetic athletes' latest endeavors, along with educational articles and links to research about diabetes and exercise. For more information, visit their Web site at www.hypoactive.org, or e-mail Monique Hanley at monique@hypoactive.org or Vice-President Spike Beecroft at spike@hypoactive.org.

*A*thlete *P*rofile

Name: Monique Hanley

Hometown: Melbourne, Australia (originally Yarragon)

Diabetes history: Type 1 diabetes diagnosed in 1998 (at age 19)

Sport or activity: Cycling, including track and criteriums, and a bit of road racing

Greatest athletic achievements: Winning the Race Across America (RAAM 2007) as part of Team Type 1; finishing third in the women's 3,000-meter individual pursuit at the Australian National Track Championships (2007)

Current insulin and medication regimen: Insulin pump (currently OmniPod)

Training tips: One thing I have learned the hard way is to acquire trend data before heading out on a training ride. A single glucose test is not enough to know what direction you are headed.

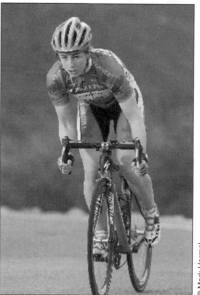
© Mark Harmel

Typical daily and weekly training and diabetes regimen: I really have no typical week of training. All year round I use different training phases and focuses, depending on the schedule and event plan. The following is a typical transition week of training, four weeks out from the RAAM event. (I also was working less then.)

▶ *Monday:* Two-hour ride at low intensity at 5:30 a.m.; I use a 50 percent reduced basal on my pump, and I eat a 25-gram bar in the first half hour and final hour of the ride (the first bar may or may not require insulin, depending on morning blood glucose). Then I ride to work and home again (35 minutes each way at low intensity) with no adjustments.

▶ *Tuesday:* Time trial resistance or cycling time trial consisting of three 10-minute efforts done as hard as possible behind a motor bike (motor pacing), with 15 minutes of recovery between efforts. Adjustments include 50 percent basal reduction but no food. Same transportation to work.

▶ *Wednesday:* Ride to work and two-hour afternoon workout at medium- to high-level intensity, with a similar basal reduction and 25 grams of carbohydrate per hour with no insulin.

▶ *Thursday:* Same morning ride as Monday, followed by my usual ride to work. In the afternoon, I repeat my Tuesday track motor pacing.

▶ *Friday:* I usually motor pace on the road for two hours, but when it's raining I instead do a general track session in the evening, group pursuit work (shorter, 4-minute efforts with 15 minutes of recovery, variable gearing), and normal transportation to work.

▶ *Saturday:* Low-intensity road cycling for four and a half hours, for which I reduce my basal insulin 50 percent and eat 25 grams of carbohydrate per hour without any additional insulin.

▶ *Sunday:* One-hour low-intensity road ride with no changes in insulin.

Other hobbies and interests: I am the president of a group called HypoActive, which promotes an active lifestyle for anyone with type 1 diabetes, based in Melbourne, Australia. I enjoy taking photos and occasionally dabble in sports journalism, but I don't have much time for these things!

Good diabetes and exercise story: There is nothing better than nailing a race with a good performance, aided and abetted by great blood sugar levels. Unfortunately, in cycling, your diabetes control may be great and the race doesn't turn out as planned, or vice versa. One example of when it all came together perfectly, though, was at our State Track Titles in 2007. My season goal was to perform well at this weekend event and earn selection to represent my State of Victoria at the National Track Championships, not an easy feat. There was a huge amount of pressure on me to realize my goal and perform my best over this weekend, and I also needed to slash seven seconds off my personal best for the individual pursuit.

My event was scheduled for a Saturday morning in January in the midst of a hot (and unusually humid) Australian summer. Nerves always push my blood sugars up from all the rush of adrenaline, so I entered the scratch race on the Friday night purely to soak up some of the anticipation and level myself out for the following morning. The race went well for me, and I picked up a bronze medal. The next morning my blood sugars were rock solid in the 90s (around 5 mmol/L). I followed my warm-up plan to a tee, stopping to check frequently and drinking a sports drink for rehydration and blood sugar maintenance. My sugars stayed rock steady—perfect. All I had left to do was to ride the ride of my life.

Unbelievably, the race went well, really well. I stuck to the race schedule and managed to catch the other pursuit rider midrace, which was a great feeling. The final four laps hurt terribly, but this was pursuit racing—it's never easy! Still, the last two laps just hurt so much. I finally crossed the finish line and looked up to see my time—3:49. I had qualified for a spot in the state team! The pain in the legs only hit me as I slowed down, and I crawled off the bike and sat on the ground for a long time, unable to move. It turned out that the reason was that we had accidentally ridden a much harder gear than intended. But my head was so focused on what I needed to do that I charged on, only fading slightly in the final laps. Accompanying me the whole way were some great numbers showing up on my glucose meter—a great partnership! I just wish all my races (and blood sugars) worked out like that!

EFFECT OF MENTAL STRESS ON DIABETES CONTROL AND HEALTH

We often underestimate how significantly our minds can affect our bodies. For example, you can undergo the hormonal elevations that occur during intense training simply by experiencing mental stress or anxiety, which also releases adrenaline, cortisol, and other hormones that raise your blood sugar levels. Feeling upset or anxious additionally stresses your immune system, resulting in elevated levels of cortisol and blood sugars and a reduction in your ability to fight off colds and other illnesses.

Being physically active, on the other hand, has a positive effect on your mood, stress levels, and self-image, all of which positively influence your diabetes control when they are enhanced. The good news is that you can train and control your nervous system response to mental stress by doing physical and other types of training. Moreover, you achieve optimal athletic performance only when you train both your body and your mind.

Endorphins Lower Mental and Physical Stress

One of the purported mental benefits of exercise is the release of brain hormones called endorphins. These mood-enhancing, feel-good hormones bind to the natural receptors of your brain and are responsible for the runner's high, a feeling of euphoria that you may get after you have been exercising for a while. You may also recognize it as your second wind, when you start feeling good enough during a workout to keep on exercising. Some people are positively addicted to this release of endorphins and need to get their daily dose. Endorphins may improve your body's insulin action, thereby reversing or decreasing insulin resistance. In fact, endorphin release may be a major mechanism in the enhanced insulin action attributed to moderate aerobic training. In that case, go for maximal endorphins on a daily basis. As a side benefit, you will be less depressed and anxious and enjoy a greatly improved mood and likely better physical health.

Training the Mind and the Body

Although each workout causes some physical damage to your muscles, you ultimately end up stronger, faster, and better, and your body responds by releasing fewer stress hormones during workouts. Similarly, when you practice using relaxation techniques to control your stress levels, your mind learns to reduce your body's sympathetic stimulation as well. The more consistently you practice relaxation, the easier it is to avoid eliciting a strong stress response when "life happens" the next time. During recovery, your parasympathetic nervous system keeps your heart rate low and digestion high, so it's no wonder that a warm shower, a big meal, and a long nap after a workout make you feel more relaxed. You're in an anabolic (building and repairing) state then, and your glycogen is being restored while your muscles are being repaired and strengthened.

Relaxation Techniques to Help Control Your Stress

Sport psychologists recommend relaxation to enhance performance in athletic events. Relaxation techniques can help you control the stress of competition as well as the stress coming from other avenues of your life. To relax, you can sit quietly and focus your mind. You can even use relaxation techniques while exercising. For example, punch the air with your fists to release your anger or anxiety and consciously relax the tense muscles in your body. Use your imagination to visualize more blood flowing to all the parts of your body that need it (like your heart, muscles, and diabetic feet). Some studies have shown that people can enhance blood flow to their feet simply by visualizing it, verifying that a strong mind–body connection really exists. Also, take deep and steady breaths and release them slowly, particularly during your warm-up and cool-down periods when you're not working as hard. Whenever you start to feel winded during a workout, take deeper breaths to bring more oxygen into your lungs and body.

Yoga for Peak Performance

Other techniques include stretching and yoga, which calm your mind and enhance parasympathetic activity, the branch of your nervous system that lowers your heart rate, breathing, and stress responses. If practiced in its true spirit, yoga can balance your body and mind, which enhances both athletic performance and mental well-being, by counterbalancing the effects of your sympathetic nervous system. Vigorous styles of yoga that are a workout in themselves are not as good for relaxing and maximizing the benefits of your parasympathetic activity; go for the kinder, gentler type for maximal relaxation. If you're mentally stressed, practicing such techniques can help train your mind and body to reduce its sympathetic drive, thus enhancing the quality of the often-limited time that you have for recovery. Additionally, working your joints and muscles with yoga or stretching to maintain and increase your range of motion around joints helps prevent injuries. Thus, whether your goal is injury prevention or simply to be a better athlete, staying flexible can enhance your performance.

ENHANCING PERFORMANCE WITH YOUR MIND

Visualization techniques get many athletes to the pinnacle of their respective sports. Moreover, they may improve mental awareness and sense of well-being. Whether you call it guided imagery, mental rehearsal, meditation, or visualization, you can practice the technique by creating a mental image of what you want to happen or feel during an athletic event. Imagine a scene, complete with images of either your previous best performance or how you want to do the next time, and then become one, so to speak, with that desire. Try to imagine all the details, both physical and mental. Include visual images, physical sensations, and auditory cues (such as the cheering of onlookers). Call up these images repeatedly, just as you repeatedly do physical training. Believe it or not, with mental rehearsal you can train your mind and body to respond in the way that you're imagining and to perform the skill or event that you're visualizing more effectively.

Visualization can improve both physical and emotional responses. Imagining a positive outcome can build experience and confidence in your ability to perform when the time comes and the stress is greater. By reducing your response to the emotional stress of the event, visualization may help you keep your blood sugars under better control. Competition is tough, and diabetic athletes have one extra (often overwhelming) variable to deal with that nondiabetic participants don't. In this case, effective visualization might be one way to gain back the advantage.

A Diabetic Athlete's Ironman Experience
(What It's Like to Finish Dead Last, but Alive)

The true spirit of all diabetic athletes is exemplified by the story of Jay Handy of Springfield, Illinois, (founder and president of the Diabetes Sports and Wellness Foundation, www.dswf.org), when he completed his first full-length triathlon, the 2003 Ironman Wisconsin. He trained for months and did everything right, but it was only his mental visualization and sheer determination that ultimately got him through the race. Needless to say, things did not go as planned for him that day. The weather was unseasonably hot, which always means trouble for any athlete, diabetic or not. His 2.4-mile (3.9-kilometer) swim went better than he had expected, given that he's normally a marathoner and a distance cyclist. As he recalls, "A quick glance at my watch indicated I was out of the water 20 minutes faster than I had planned. It was the fastest I had ever swum in my life! This was going to be a great day, I remember thinking. Already ahead of schedule by 20 minutes and feeling great!"

The story continues during the 112-mile (180-kilometer) bike course that followed the swim: "I had rigged up a homemade contraption to hold my OneTouch Ultra Meter onto the bike itself, so I could check my blood sugars without slowing down. My blood sugars were all perfect. Everything was perfect. All the hours of planning were paying off. I was so happy. By then it did occur to me that the air temperature was rising. 'No problem,' I thought as I methodically counted my electrolyte pills and salt tablets inside their plastic bag. Every 30 minutes, I would take one salt tablet and two electrolyte pills. 'Perfect,' I thought. 'I have just enough for the remaining five and a half hours I need to finish the bike race.'" Later on in the cycle portion, friends and family kept his emotions high. "All sorts of people I knew had come out to cheer me on," he recalls. "They would yell as I passed, and I would raise my arm in a fist or give thumbs up. It was a mutual exchange of excitement. I felt like the luckiest person in the world, and I just hoped that I wasn't going to disappoint them."

Here's where his race began to go downhill (figuratively, not literally). "By mile 80 (kilometer 130) the temperature was 90 degrees Fahrenheit (32 degrees Celsius), it was extremely humid, and for the first time I started to feel slight cramps in my legs. It was time to take another salt tablet and my self-prescribed electrolyte pills. I reached back toward my right jersey pocket where I kept them. It was empty, so I checked my center pocket. Not there. The left pocket? Only my emergency diabetic supplies were there. My heart sank, and my mind went completely blank for at least a mile. I also knew that, according to the rules of the event, there would be no tablets at the aid stations and that no one could give me any now that the race was in progress. I looked down at a strip of paper I had taped to my handlebar. It was from an e-mail that Julie R. had sent me two days earlier. It read, 'May God give you the strength and endurance to finish.' I thought to myself, 'I may need those two elements more than ever in my life on this day.'"

"Ten miles (16 kilometers) later, I started up the first of three tough climbs. I saw someone walking up the climb and thought that looked smart. I stopped, thinking I would simply jump off and begin walking. Instead, I fell over with locked legs due to cramped quads. It was excruciating, and I screamed into the treetops. I could see other bikers slowly ascending past me, none making eye contact for fear they might catch what I had."

"Finally, one cyclist stopped and asked what he could do for me. I said, 'Kick. Kick me. Kick me behind my knees.' He did, and it broke the clenching spasm. As I lay down in a fetal position in the dust, I had an overwhelming desire to shut my eyes and go right to sleep, but instead I forced myself to get up. I lifted my bike and started to walk like a stick man, unable to bend my knees. At the top of the hill, I slowly got onto the bike and began to spin my pedals with very little resistance." During the remainder of the bike course, Jay's quads cramped up twice more, but he finished it with a minute to spare to make the time cutoff to start the final 26.2-mile (42.2-kilometer) run portion of the event. "I was slightly delirious, but made it into the transition area. I saw several bodies on the ground moaning and in various stages of exhaustion."

After the final transition, Jay recalls, "I came out in my running gear—including my 'Running on Insulin' shirt—walking like a stick man. My legs kept locking at the knees. My wife Kim and my two daughters, Schuyler and Grace, were there. I could hear Grace begin to cry, and Kim said to me that I did not have to do this. I told her my legs would hopefully loosen up because different muscles are used for biking and running. A man held up two cups of water, and asked, 'Are you OK?' I said that I was and walked out of the chute onto the course. The crowds were cheering, not for me but for the finishers heading in the opposite direction, and I was just beginning the marathon. I had never felt so alone amongst so many people."

He recalls that the first mile of the marathon course seemed to take forever. "How am I ever going to do this?" he wondered. "My next thought was, 'Let's break it down; 1 mile done, only 25.2 to go.' But that thinking did not help at all because the distance left was just too daunting. Instead, I focused on taking each step and pushing through the pain. My friend Mark called my cell phone when I passed mile 2. He was already at mile 13 (kilometer 21) or so, and he suggested that I might want to consider doing just the half-marathon and quitting then. Later, Mark admitted that he thought I was about through at mile 2 when we spoke."

"By mile 6 (kilometer 10), my legs did loosen up some. I thought maybe I could run a little, just to speed things up. I tried a light jog for 100 feet (30 meters), but that was a major mistake. My legs stiffened right up. I knew the only way to propel myself forward was by speed walking, and I felt every step." At that point, he only had about 20 miles (32 kilometers) to go to finish. "With about 1.5 miles (2.4 kilometers) before the halfway mark, which is also at the finish line because there is a turnaround there, I called my wife. I told her I didn't think I could go on because the pain was too great. I told her I was sorry; after all she had done to support me, that I wasn't going to finish. I wanted to cry, but there were no tears. She said I had a lot to be proud of, it was fine, and I need not apologize. She said she'd meet me at my finish."

When Jay got there, all his supporters were there cheering the end of his race (albeit cut short). "When I hit State Street, I knew I had only seven blocks to finalize the decision to quit. I started to think again of the e-mail Julie had sent me about having the strength and endurance to finish. I thought of all the people who made an effort to see me through the race and of their encouragement. Finally, I thought of the diabetic children. I couldn't DNF (did not finish) this race. Yet, I also couldn't fathom going back out there again and doing another 13.1-mile (21.1-kilometer) loop. When I came up Pinckney Street, three blocks from my decision point to either exit or loop around, I saw Hans, a friend of mine who is a former Olympic athlete. He had a certain look in his eye, one that was different from all the other spectators. All he said was, 'Jay, you can do this.' I looked to my right and there was my whole family and a host of others rooting for me. I heard the roar of the crowd; they all thought I was finishing, as did the official there. Ten feet (three meters) before the turnaround, I looked at my wife, raised my arm, and whirled my hand in a circle to indicate I was going back out. There was no way I could walk off. I had to keep going."

During the last 13.1 miles (21.1 kilometers), several people came along on bikes and met up with Jay to encourage him and keep him company, although he was still on his own, walking in the dark for most of that final distance. He recalls the finish vividly: "I was finally approaching the one and a half blocks to where the finishing arch was still in place. I came around the corner and into the glow of spotlights, along with the roar of cheers from hundreds of people. There were still people there for me—for me! The announcer said, 'And the final finisher is number 1076, Jay Handy, a type 1 diabetic!' The crowd's roar was unbelievable. There were 50 yards (46 meters) left to the finish, but I had to run it. It seemed as though the pain had lifted, at least for a moment. I came across the line with my arms up and smiling. It was 12:07 a.m. Moments later, the medical team asked if I was OK. Other than the terrible pain in my cramped legs, I felt pretty good."

"Two volunteers came up, and one handed me a T-shirt," Jay recalls. "The other said, 'He needs his medal.' I protested, saying, 'No, no, I didn't earn one. It's after midnight, and I barely missed the time cutoff.' She looked to an official, who answered for her, saying, 'Yes, you do. You completed the distance. Therefore, you are finisher and an Ironman.' The volunteer then draped the medal over my head and down around my neck. I had finished—dead last, but still alive—and with a medal after all! Success." Jay, you did all diabetic athletes proud!

(As an aside, you should know that the temperature that day reached 93 degrees Fahrenheit, or 34 degrees Celsius, and a quarter of the competitors sought medical attention during the event. Also, 276 athletes dropped out of the race, the highest in the competition's long history, compared with just 39 the year before under better conditions. Jay's diabetes management was excellent throughout the race; his problems that day were the same as those of any athlete with a functioning pancreas. He has completed many more Ironman competitions since his first one with great success.)

STAYING MOTIVATED TO EXERCISE

Even elite athletes have days when they're not as motivated to exercise as they are on other days. You know those days—the ones when you have trouble putting on your exercise gear, let alone finishing your planned workout. For the sake of your diabetes control, though, don't use one or two bad days as an excuse to discontinue an otherwise important exercise or training routine. See table 6.1 instead for some motivating behaviors and ideas for regular exercisers and anyone else who may not always feel motivated to work out.

As for other tricks that you can use, start with reminding yourself that regular exercise can lessen the potential effect of most of your cardiovascular risk factors, including elevated cholesterol levels, insulin resistance, obesity, and hypertension. Even just walking regularly can lengthen your life, and if you keep your blood sugars in control with the help of physical activity, you may be able to prevent or delay almost all the potential long-term complications of diabetes.

To motivate yourself to exercise, you also need to control your feelings of depression. When you are depressed, the last thing you may want to do is exercise. The funny thing about physical activity, though, is that it reduces your feelings of depression and anxiety. If you can simply get yourself up and going, you may feel your depression lifting by itself.

Table 6.1 Tips for Keeping Your Motivation for Daily Physical Activity

- Get yourself an exercise buddy (or even a dog that needs to be walked).
- Use sticker charts or other motivational tools to track your progress.
- Schedule structured exercise into your day on your calendar or to-do list.
- Break your larger goals into smaller, realistic stepping-stones (e.g., daily and weekly physical activity goals).
- Reward yourself for meeting your goals with noncaloric treats or outings.
- Plan to do physical activities that you really enjoy as often as possible.
- Wear a pedometer (at least occasionally) as a reminder to take more daily steps.
- Have a backup plan that includes alternative activities in case of inclement weather or other barriers to your planned exercise.
- Distract yourself while you exercise by reading a book or magazine, watching TV, listening to music or a book on tape, or talking with a friend.
- Don't start out exercising too intensely or you're likely to become discouraged or injured.
- If you get out of your normal routine and are having trouble getting restarted, simply take small steps in that direction.

Removing potential barriers to exercise can help as well—excuses such as exercise being inconvenient or taking too much time. If you stop thinking of exercise only as planned activities and instead simply try to move more, you'll be more active all day long without feeling as if you have to come up with big blocks of time to fit it in. Most people expend the majority of their calories each day during unstructured activities rather than during a formal exercise session. Doing something during the day is always better than doing nothing, particularly when it comes to keeping your insulin action higher and your diabetes better controlled.

Finally, keep in mind that having diabetes is the best reason to be physically active, maybe the only one that you need. For you diehard competitive athletes, see more tips in table 6.2 about how to build your self-confidence and stay motivated to compete and improve your athletic performance.

RECOVERING FROM INJURY—EMOTIONALLY SPEAKING

Maybe an injury has left you unable to do your usual workouts. Taking some time to let your body repair itself (as discussed in the following chapter) is fine, but having a physical injury that keeps you from your normal routine can be emotionally devastating, especially for diabetic athletes who have to deal with changes in their physical state when their exercise routines are altered. Physical activity may normally be your social outlet, your stress reducer, or a significant source of meaning and purpose in your life—even some of your identity. Athletes who lose their

Table 6.2   Keys to Building Self-Confidence and Motivation

- Manage mental stress and disappointment effectively.

- Stop all negative self-talk.

- Increase your ability to maintain and regain concentration.

- Mentally prepare well for competition.

- Improve communication with teammates and coaches.

- Set, reset, and manage your individual and team goals.

- Notice, avoid, and recover from competition burnout.

- Regain your mental fitness after an injury.

guiding light, so to speak, may have a negative reaction to injury that can lead to depression and lack of motivation.

An injury may not be life threatening or even permanent, but because your injury likely resulted in a loss of some kind, you may still find yourself going through the stages that people go through when a loved one dies. These stages—denial, anger, bargaining, depression, and finally acceptance—can be traveled in any order and sometimes repeated. Usually you have to reach the last stage, acceptance, to deal effectively with any physical injury (or diabetic complication).

In times like those, assemble a group of people around you who can provide support, including physical therapists, health care practitioners, coaches, trainers, family and friends, counselors or therapists, and good doctors (especially if you need to have surgery to repair the damage). Next, set realistic goals for your recovery process, including the time that it will take and the necessary steps. To minimize the fitness that you will lose during your recovery, try to come up with alternative activities. For many running injuries, athletes spend time in the pool either running or swimming. Finally, think positively and set yourself on a road to faster recovery. As for the physical aspects of recovering from an athletic injury, those are discussed fully in the following chapter.

CHAPTER 7

Preventing and Treating Athletic Injuries

If you exercise regularly, eventually you're likely to experience some kind of an athletic injury, regardless of whether you have diabetes. Having diabetes, however, increases the likelihood of developing certain joint problems like frozen shoulders and trigger fingers, so the more you know about how to handle and prevent joint and other injuries—both acute and overuse ones—before they develop, the better off you'll be. You will also benefit from knowing some tricks for preventing and treating delayed-onset muscle soreness and overuse syndrome discussed in this chapter.

IDENTIFYING ACUTE AND OVERUSE INJURIES

Acute injuries are sudden, sharp, traumatic injuries that occur immediately (or within hours) and cause pain, most often resulting from obvious causes like an impact, fall, sprain, or collision or even through carelessness (e.g., dropping a dumbbell on your foot). Some common examples are ankle sprains, shoulder dislocations, and hamstring muscle strains. Diabetes is not usually a contributing cause unless you fall and injure yourself because of having gait abnormalities related to diabetic neuropathy. In any case, if you experience sudden-onset joint pain, swelling, reduced range of motion, weakness, numbness, or tingling, your injury should be treated sooner rather than later.

> *Never ignore acute pain in your knee, ankle, elbow, or wrist joints, which is most likely related to ligament (connections between bones) or tendon (muscle to bone) damage.*

If a specific point on a bone, muscle, or joint is painful (which you can check by pressing your finger into it), you may have a significant injury, especially if pushing on the mirror image spot on the other side of your body doesn't hurt. As for swelling, it's usually obvious. Almost all sports injuries, such as twisting an ankle, cause the affected areas to swell, which results in pain, stiffness, or a clicking sound as

107

the ligaments that connect bones to other bones across joints snap over one another (they may have been pushed into a new position by the swelling). Any significant swelling will cause you to lose mobility around that joint (reduced range of motion). Weakness when comparing one side of your body to the other is also a sign, along with numbness or tingling that may be related to compression of a nerve.

On the other hand, longer-term injuries often result from excessive or repetitive training that causes an overuse injury or syndrome. These injuries are nagging and persistently uncomfortable. For instance, rotator cuff tendinitis in your shoulder tends to feel worse at night after you lie down, when you often experience a dull ache in the affected shoulder. Common examples include tennis elbow (lateral epicondylitis), swimmer's shoulder (rotator cuff tendinitis and impingement), Little League elbow, runner's knee, jumper's knee (infrapatellar tendinitis), Achilles tendinitis, shin splints, and plantar fasciitis. In most sports and activities, overuse injuries are the most common and challenging to diagnose and treat, and they often worsen over time if neglected.

IMMEDIATE AND CHRONIC TREATMENT OF INJURIES

Treatment of acute injuries is best handled with RICE—rest, ice, compression, and elevation. You never want to heat an acute injury because heat increases circulation to the area and causes it to swell, which is what you're trying to limit with the ice, compression, and elevation.

Follow these steps for immediate treatment of an acute injury:

- Immediately stop whatever activity you're doing.
- Wrap the injured area in a compression (ace) bandage.
- Apply ice (using a bag of crushed ice or even a bag of frozen vegetables) for 15 minutes, let the area warm back up, and reapply two or three times total, as tolerated.
- Elevate your injured joint to reduce swelling; if it's your ankle, try to get it up higher than the level of your heart.
- See a physician for proper diagnosis and treatment of any serious injury.

Reducing Inflammation With Meds

Taking anti-inflammatory medications, otherwise known as nonsteroidal, anti-inflammatory drugs (NSAIDs), many of which are available in drugstores without a prescription, is often helpful. Aspirin, ibuprofen (sold as Advil or Nuprin in the United States), and naproxen (e.g., Aleve) all fight inflammation and reduce pain, but acetaminophen (commonly sold as Tylenol) limits only pain. Your doctor may also prescribe anti-inflammatory medications like Relafan, Celebrex, Daypro, and Naprosyn.

Follow RICE to treat both acute and overuse injuries (after workouts that aggravate the latter), and consider treating them with NSAIDs.

If an affected area becomes inflamed enough that you can't control it with rest and NSAIDs or prescription pain medications, or if it's painful for several weeks without any improvement, you may want to look into having a cortisone injection to relieve pain and joint tenderness. Keep in mind that although the injections are localized, they can affect your whole body, and most cortisone preparations increase insulin resistance. For instance, Kenalog, a common steroid, may increase your blood sugars into the range of 300 to 400 milligrams per deciliter (16.7 to 22.2 millimolar), while others like Depomedrol may cause fewer problems, raising them only into the 200s (11 to 16 mmol/L) until the steroid wears off after a few weeks. Whether you take insulin or other medications, you may need to increase your doses temporarily to cover these glycemic effects.

Using Cold Therapies

Ice therapy is arguably the best immediate treatment for acute injuries because it reduces swelling and pain by causing blood vessels in the iced area to constrict; this vasoconstriction limits fluid influx into the area. When using this therapy, you should apply ice to the affected area for 10 to 15 minutes at a time, several times a day, and for up to 3 days. If you treat a chronic injury with ice, use it following (but not before) activities to prevent or reduce inflammation. The easiest method is to use an ice pack that conforms to the shape of the area that you're icing down, but you can also use a bag of frozen veggies (like peas), ice frozen in a paper cup (you peel down the edge of the cup as the ice melts), or a bag of ice wrapped in a thin towel for comfort.

When Should You Heat Your Injuries?

Most athletes know to apply ice to an acute injury like a sprained ankle but aren't so sure about when to use heat. If anything is hurting you (either an acute or chronic injury) after a workout, use ice. Heat is better for chronic injuries or injuries without inflammation and swelling, such as sore joints, stiffness, or nagging pain. Using heat therapy before exercise may even increase the elasticity of your joints' connective tissues, stimulate blood flow, or relax tight muscles and spasms. Apply heat for 15 to 20 minutes at a time, and use enough layers between your skin and the heating source to prevent burns, particularly if you are heating an area in which you have lost some of your sensation (e.g., neuropathic feet) and would be unlikely to realize if it is too hot. Moist heat is best, so try using a hot wet towel. You can also use special athletic hot packs or heating pads, but never leave them on for more than 20 minutes at a time or while asleep. Heated whirlpools and spas are also effective, but avoid using them if you have open sores or ulcers on your feet or lower legs.

OVERUSE INJURIES: WHICH ARE MOST COMMON AND WHO GETS THEM?

By definition, an overuse injury is caused by excessive use of a particular joint. Overuse injuries are more common in people with diabetes because of structural changes in their joints caused by long-term elevation in blood glucose levels. But regardless of the contributing cause, all overuse injuries are treated the same way. Moreover, their onset can usually be linked to changes in athletic endeavors or techniques. For example, if you have been running 3 miles (5 kilometers) several days a week at a moderate pace and then you suddenly begin running 5 miles (8 kilometers) six days a week at a faster pace than before, you're setting yourself up for an injury. You should make only gradual increases in your training duration, frequency, or intensity so that your body will have time to adapt. Exercise is all about causing damage to your muscles to stimulate their rebuilding to become stronger, faster, or more aerobic—a result that can occur only if you allow adequate time for recovery and recuperation of both muscles and joints.

> *All athletes have a higher chance of getting an overuse injury at some point by overstressing muscles, joints, and bones with repetitive or damaging movements, particularly by rapidly increasing their training.*

Some people are prone to developing overuse injuries, but their development is more often related to anatomical, biomechanical, or other considerations. For instance, imbalances between your strength and flexibility around certain joints (e.g., quads versus hamstring strength) can predispose you to hamstring pulls. Uneven body alignment, such as knock-knees, bowed legs, unequal leg lengths, and flat or high-arched feet, can also contribute. Even having old injuries leads to a greater likelihood of overuse injuries, along with factors like the type of running shoes you use, the terrain (hilly, flat, or uneven), and whether you work out on hard surfaces like concrete roads or floors or softer ones like grass, dirt or gravel trails, asphalt, and cushioned floors.

Many overuse injuries involve inflammation of an area, or redness, soreness, and swelling, designated as "itis" at the end of its name. Tendinitis is inflammation of tendons, which attach muscles to bones; it is a common overuse injury that results from a tendon rubbing repeatedly against a bony structure, ligament, or another tendon or from being impinged. Tennis elbow is a type of tendinitis on the outside of the elbow common in tennis players as well as rowers, carpenters, gardeners, golfers, and other exercisers who repeatedly bend their arms forcefully. Swimmers often develop tendinitis and other impingement syndromes in the rotator cuff (shoulder) because of the overhead movement required by the sport. In sports that involve running and jumping, tendinitis often occurs in the knee, foot, and Achilles (heel) tendons. The more common athletic overuse injuries, symptoms, and treatments are listed in table 7.1.

Anyone with diabetes is prone to developing overuse injuries with a slower onset that can limit movement around joints. Common injuries are shoulder adhesive capsulitis ("frozen shoulder"), carpal tunnel syndrome (wrist pain), metatarsal

Table 7.1   Common Athletic Overuse Injuries, Symptoms, and Treatment

Injury	Area affected	Symptoms	Treatment and prevention
Carpal tunnel syndrome	Wrist	Pain, weakness, or numbness in hand and wrist; loss of grip strength	Rest, ice, NSAIDs, surgery if longer than six months
Tennis elbow	Outside of the elbow	Painful to touch or bump, pain when shaking hands or turning a doorknob	Rest, ice, NSAIDs, use of a strap around the upper forearm, using a two-handed backhand, exercises
Rotator cuff tendinitis	Shoulder	Pain when lifting arms, combing hair	Rest, ice, NSAIDs, stretching and strengthening exercises
Chondromalacia patella	Knee	Knee pain made worse by bending the knees, doing full squats, or sitting for long periods with bent knees	Rest, ice, NSAIDs, strengthening the inner quads with weight training
Iliotibial band friction (ITBF) syndrome	Knee	Pain along the outside part of the knee or lower thigh	Rest, ice, gentle stretching (IT band and gluteal muscles), running on both sides of the road, wearing proper shoes
Shin splints	Front of lower legs, along the tibia bone	Generalized pain along the bones of lower leg	Rest, ice, NSAIDs, slow progression of training program, avoiding running on hard surfaces
Plantar fasciitis	Heel, bottom of foot	Heel pain during first steps each morning and following periods of inactivity	Rest, ice, NSAIDs, stretching and massaging the plantar fascia, exercises
Achilles tendinitis	Heel and calves	Pain in the heels and tight calf muscles	Rest, ice, NSAIDs, frequent stretching of the calves and thighs, limited wearing of high-heeled shoes

fractures (of the foot bones), and neuropathy-related joint disorders (e.g., Charcot foot) in people with peripheral neuropathy. Trigger fingers, which result in curled fingers because of shortening of ligaments, usually require cortisone injections or surgery to repair them. People who have had diabetes for a long time are additionally prone to nerve compression syndromes at the elbow and wrist that may be

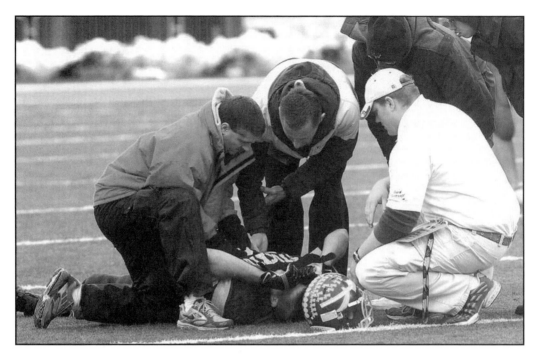

Ignoring minor overuse injuries can lead to more serious injuries, so make sure to rest or cut back on the intensity of exercise to give your body a chance to heal.

aggravated by repetitive activities, prolonged gripping, or direct nerve compression during weight training, cycling, and other activities. In most cases, good control of your blood sugars can reduce your risk for developing these injuries.

Preventing Overuse Injuries

If your nagging aches and pains are only minor, simply cutting back on how hard, how often, and how long you do the activities that irritate your joints may bring relief from your symptoms. In other words, give your joints a rest! One way to prevent problems in the first place is to adopt a hard–easy workout schedule in which you alternate and vary your workouts by the day to avoid stressing your joints in the same way with every workout. If your problems are being caused by anatomical concerns, fix what you can (such as getting orthotics to correct leg-length discrepancies) and then consider doing other activities that don't cause as much risk of injury, such as working out on an elliptical trainer a few days a week instead of always running outdoors on concrete or asphalt. In addition, working with a coach or teacher or taking lessons can help you improve your training and technique. Make sure to do a proper warm-up and cool-down, ice down inflamed joints after workouts, and use NSAIDs to control inflammation and pain.

You may also benefit from cross-training. To use this approach, you do other activities to maintain overall fitness levels while your injured area recovers. For example, if you have lower-leg pain, you can still work out your upper body by doing activities that allow your legs to rest and recuperate. Try alternating weight-bearing activities like walking or running with non-weight-bearing ones, such as swimming, upper-body work, and stationary cycling so that you don't injure another part of your body.

> *After you resume your normal activities, work to strengthen the muscles around the previously injured joint to prevent recurrence, especially following tendinitis.*

Strengthening the muscles around an affected joint, after the pain is gone, is critical to preventing the return of the problem. For example, following a shoulder joint injury like rotator cuff tendinitis and impingement, focus on doing resistance work using all sections of the deltoid muscle in particular, along with exercises for the biceps, triceps, pectoral muscles, upper-back muscles, and neck muscles. In table 7.2 you'll find some other suggestions for preventing injuries.

Table 7.2   General Tips for Exercising Safely and Avoiding Injuries

• Never bounce during stretches because doing so can cause injuries, although dynamic stretching is fine (movement stretches).
• If you haven't exercised in a while, start slowly and progress cautiously to avoid delayed-onset muscle soreness (DOMS) or an acute injury.
• Warm up with stretches and easy aerobic work before you begin to exercise vigorously.
• Choose an exercise that suits your condition; for example, swimming might be suitable if you are recovering from an ankle or knee injury.
• Vary your exercise program occasionally or try out new activities; doing so emphasizes different muscle groups and increases your overall fitness.
• Cross-train to reduce the risk of injury by varying muscle and joint usage.
• Wear appropriate shoes and socks, and check your feet after you exercise.
• Avoid going back to your normal activities until your symptoms have almost completely gone away.
• For best results don't forget to warm up and cool down.

Choosing the Proper Footwear

Wearing proper shoes is critical to preventing many lower-extremity and foot problems. The best type of shoes to wear varies by activity. Walkers and runners generally need some cushioning, whereas tennis players require footwear with greater stability for side-to-side movements. For most activities, though, you will benefit by picking your shoes based on whether you rotate on your feet toward the arch of your foot or toward the outside edge.

To determine how you step, look at the wear pattern on your shoes. For example, exercisers who overpronate (rotate their feet too far to the inside), have flat feet, or carry a lot of extra body weight wear out the insides of their soles first. If you have this problem, motion-control shoes may help. Generally heavy but durable, they are rigid, control-orientated running shoes that have firm midsoles designed to limit overpronation; they also come in varieties with more cushioning. If your shoes do not compensate for overpronation, you may place extra stress on your knees, hips, and ankles that can result in injuries. Conversely, supinators usually have high arches and more rigid feet and thus wear out the soles of their shoes on the outside edge. If you're a supinator, you will generally do better in highly cushioned shoes with plenty of flexibility to encourage foot motion. If you have normal arches, you'll want to aim for shoes with moderate control, such as those with a two-density midsole. If you're unsure which type of arches your feet have, wet your feet and make a footprint to see how much of the arch region of your foot shows.

Recognizing and Treating Overtraining Syndrome

Overtraining syndrome frequently occurs in athletes who are training for competition or a specific event without allowing adequate time for rest and recuperation. Becoming more fit and improving your performance is a balancing act between training and recovering from it. You're not stronger or faster right after your workout, but rather after your body has repaired the damage that you did to it with the exercise. Overloading your body excessively without enough recovery time can result in both physical and psychological symptoms.

The symptoms of overtraining are not hard to recognize when you know what to look for. They include chronic tiredness, lethargy, soreness and aches, chronic pain in your muscles and joints, an unexpected drop in your performance, insomnia, an increased number of colds and upper-respiratory tract infections, mild depression, and general malaise.

> *To determine whether you have overtraining syndrome, measure your resting heart rate first thing in the morning. If it is increasing over time, you're likely overtraining.*

Getting sick more frequently means that excessive training is compromising your immune function, and because overtraining results in elevated levels of cortisol, you may have more problems controlling your blood sugars as well. If you start feeling chronically tired, drained, and lacking in energy, cut back on your training schedule a bit and see whether that helps; if you're overtraining, it will. Cross-training (or doing different activities) can also help if you're overworking certain muscles or joints, and it may help you maintain or improve your psychological outlook. Total recovery can take several weeks. Proper nutrition and stress reduction are important to the recovery process.

Arms and Shoulders

The most common problems affecting the arms and shoulders are carpal tunnel syndrome (wrist), tennis elbow (lateral epicondylitis), rotator cuff tendinitis in the shoulder, and frozen shoulder (i.e., adhesive capsulitis). Most, but not all, involve tendinitis, which occurs more commonly in people with diabetes because of glycation of collagen structures in joints that limits their mobility and results in minor swelling and inflammation of tendons. Others involve impingement syndromes or inflammation of other joint-related structures.

Carpal Tunnel Syndrome

Carpal tunnel syndrome results from a squeezing of the median nerve, which runs from your forearm down into the palm of your hand. That nerve controls sensations to your thumb and most fingers, as well as impulses to some small muscles in the hand that allow the fingers and thumb to move. The carpal tunnel is a narrow passageway that contains ligaments, tendons, and the median nerve. When the area becomes inflamed from overuse, the nerve is compressed, resulting in pain, weakness, or numbness in your hand and wrist that can radiate up your arm.

Symptoms often first appear in one or both hands during the night because sleeping with flexed wrists aggravates the condition. Your grip strength will suffer. Forming a fist, grasping small objects, or doing other things with your hands may become more difficult. Carpal tunnel syndrome is more common in the dominant hand and more common in women because their carpal tunnel area is smaller. Contributing factors include trauma or injury to your wrist that causes swelling, mechanical problems in your wrist joint, repeated use of vibrating hand tools, and fluid retention during pregnancy or menopause, among others. Carpal tunnel problems can be treated by wearing a wrist brace (to prevent wrist flexion), by icing the area, by taking NSAIDs, and sometimes by having surgery when pain lasts longer than six months. Stretching and strengthening exercises can help prevent its recurrence.

Tennis Elbow

Technically known as lateral epicondylitis, this overuse injury is literally a pain in your elbow, mainly where your forearm muscles attach to the bony prominence on the outside (the epicondyle). Some of the symptoms are pain that radiates from the outside of your elbow into your forearm and wrist (especially if you touch or bump that area) or that occurs when you extend your wrist, a weak grip (not good for your tennis game!), and discomfort in that area when you shake hands or turn a doorknob. Repeatedly contracting the forearm muscles can cause it, as can playing tennis and using poor technique with your backhand stroke; if you use a two-handed backstroke, you're much less likely to develop tennis elbow. But it's not just tennis that you have to worry about. You can get tennis elbow from repeatedly twisting a screwdriver, hammering, painting, raking, weaving, playing string instruments, and more. The typical treatments apply, including rest, ice, and use of NSAIDs to reduce pain and inflammation. Many athletes find that wearing an adjustable strap or brace around the top of the forearm helps keep the pain from coming back again. You'll also want to do stretches and strengthening exercises after the pain is gone as a preventive measure.

Athletic Shoulder Issues

Shoulders can experience a variety of problems resulting from athletic pursuits, such as rotator cuff tendinitis, bursitis, and impingement syndrome. These conditions have similar symptoms and often occur together. For instance, if the rotator cuff and bursas are irritated, inflamed, and swollen, they may become impinged, or squeezed, between the head of the humerus (the long upper-arm bone) and the acromion process (a bony structure in the shoulder). Repeated motion involving the arms over many years may also irritate the tendons, muscles, ligaments, and surrounding tissue.

In tendinitis of the shoulder, the rotator cuff and biceps tendons can become inflamed, usually as a result of being pinched by surrounding structures. When the rotator cuff tendon becomes inflamed and thickens, it may become trapped under the acromion process. If squeezing occurs, impingement syndrome results. Tendinitis and impingement syndrome are often accompanied by inflammation of the bursa sacs that protect the shoulder, or bursitis. Sports that involve overuse of the shoulder and occupations that require frequent overhead movements are other potential causes of irritation to these structures and may lead to inflammation and impingement.

Slow onset of pain in the upper shoulder or upper arm and difficulty sleeping on that shoulder are symptoms, as is pain when you try to lift your arm away from your body in particular directions or overhead. Treatment normally includes rest, ice, and anti-inflammatory meds, but it can also involve physical therapy, gentle stretching, and exercises to strengthen the muscles surrounding your shoulder joint. If you don't experience improvement in 6 to 12 months, your physician may recommend arthroscopic surgery to repair damage and relieve pressure on the tendons and bursas.

Frozen Shoulder, or Adhesive Capsulitis

This condition usually results from inflammation, scarring, thickening, and shrinkage of the capsule that surrounds your shoulder joint. Any injury to your shoulder can lead to frozen shoulder, including tendinitis, bursitis, or rotator cuff problems. Unlike those overuse injuries, however, frozen shoulder usually limits the ability to move your shoulder in all directions, not just specific ones.

Frozen shoulder usually involves three stages. Initially, the pain increases with movement and is usually worse at night, much like you get with rotator cuff tendinitis. But you will likely experience a progressive loss of motion around your shoulder joint in all directions, with increasing pain for 2 to 9 months. Stage 2 involves diminishing pain and more comfortable movement of your arm, but the tradeoff is more limited range of motion (ROM) for 4 to 12 months. Finally, in the last stage, most people experience gradual restoration of motion over the next 12 to 42 months, although some may need surgery to restore more normal ROM.

Treating a frozen shoulder often involves a combination of anti-inflammatory medications, cortisone injection, and physical therapy. If you don't treat it aggressively, a frozen shoulder can be permanent. Physical therapy is often the key and includes treatments like ultrasound, electrical stimulation, icing, and ROM and strengthening exercises. Months of physical therapy may be required for full recovery, depending on the severity of the scarring of the tissues around your shoulder. You should also try not to reinjure your shoulder during its rehabilitation by avoiding sudden, jerking motions or heavy lifting.

One Diabetic Athlete's Account of Frozen Shoulder

Delaine Wright of Hopkinton, Rhode Island, recalls her experience with getting frozen shoulders: "In truth, with my first frozen shoulder, I had no idea what was going on. It came on gradually, and by the time I realized what was happening, I couldn't put my hands in my back pockets, struggled with bra clasps, and eventually couldn't put a coat on without cringing (and even at times bursting into tears) from the pain. I couldn't lie down flat at night because of it, and for more than a year, I slept sitting straight up in bed propped up on five or more pillows because it felt better when I was nearly upright. I felt 80 years old! My husband and I had a few laughs over it, but sometimes even the shaking of a laugh hurt.

My ROM was so bad that with my arms out straight, I couldn't raise my hand any higher than just below my shoulder. But the worst part was the pain. I tried everything: physical therapy (the most painful thing), chiropractic manipulation (which I don't suggest), and more. The only thing that got me past the most painful point was a cortisone injection that included an analgesic like novocaine, and I had to have two of those a couple of months apart. During that time I kept up with the physical therapy—active and passive stretches—especially the gravity-assisted ones, lightweight one-arm hangs, and others. I found valerian root and heating helpful at night to sleep, and I regularly got a massage. I also used flax seed (oil and ground) and still do to assist in decreasing inflammation because I think it helps. I experienced about a four-month painful freezing stage, followed by eventual regression and slow return of my ROM, but the whole process took about a year.

Just as I was getting over the one shoulder, the other started. The second time wasn't as bad, although whether that was because I knew what to expect and immediately did what worked for me the first time (the analgesic and cortisone injections, stretching, but no formal physical therapy) or because the second shoulder was a milder case, I'm not sure. Although I have never fully returned to my pre–frozen shoulder ROM and am definitely stiff, at least the pain is gone. Regular yoga practice helps, along with my trapeze and aerial exercise. I've just accepted that there are some things that I will never be able to do anymore even though I'm not that old. I can't externally rotate my shoulders like most people can—I can barely accomplish a backbend because I can't get my arms in that rotated, over-the-head position, and I can't exactly manage some of the Ashtanga yoga arm wraps and such—but I suppose that's OK. I accept my body and its limitations.

I was always looking for the 'why' of my frozen shoulders, but I never found it. I had never had a shoulder injury, and my blood sugars were and had always been in good control. The whole experience certainly allowed me to appreciate the complexity of the shoulder. The good news is that it does go away eventually (with some intervention), but I'll never take my shoulders for granted again."

Knees and Shins

Knees are a critical joint for movement. They are made up of a conglomeration of tendons, ligaments, meniscal padding (cartilage), a joint capsule, a sliding kneecap (patella), synovial fluid, and more. Your athletic knees can get all sorts of aches and pains, including chondromalacia patella, iliotibial band friction syndrome (IBFS), ligament and meniscal tears, and shin pain, to name a few. The origin of each is different, although most of the treatments of these injuries are similar.

Chondromalacia Patella

Also known as patellofemoral syndrome, this overuse injury is the most common cause of chronic knee pain. It results from poor alignment of the kneecap (patella) as it slides back and forth over the lower end of the femur, or thighbone, whenever you bend your knee. If you have this, your patella tracks abnormally during bending, sliding toward the lateral (outside) edge of the femur instead of straight. You may feel some discomfort in your inner knee area related to the resulting inflammation that is made worse by activities like running, jumping, climbing or descending stairs, and prolonged sitting with bent knees (like in airplane seats). If you're experiencing pain, you'll want to avoid activities that irritate it and use ice and NSAID therapy. One thing that can help is selectively strengthening the inner part of your quadriceps (front of thigh) muscles with resistance training. In addition, you should avoid doing full squats (bending your knees to a 90-degree angle), particularly when you're using weights; do quarter squats instead.

If you have "runner's knee" and are unsure of the cause of the pain, you can start by assuming that it is this overuse injury and treat it as such. Treatments include rest, icing your knee, doing quarter squats to strengthen the quadriceps muscles, stretching your iliotibial band, replacing your running shoes every 350 to 500 miles (550 to 800 kilometers), and possibly getting orthotics for your shoes.

Iliotibial Band Friction Syndrome

Iliotibial band friction syndrome, also known as ITBFS, is an overuse injury that causes an ache or burning sensation on the lateral (outside) portion of your knee during physical activity. ITBFS is common among runners and cyclists. The iliotibial (IT) band consists of tough fibers that run the length of the outside of your thigh, attaching to your buttock muscles (gluteal muscles) and tensor fasciae latae (TFL, or hip abductor muscle) at the top, crossing the knee, and attaching to the tibia, or shinbone, at the lower end. Its primary function is to act as a stabilizer when you move around, whether walking, running, or cycling. Running on a sloped surface (such as always running on one side of the road) can aggravate the IT band because doing so tilts your pelvis, as can excessive pronation of your foot, leg length discrepancy, lateral pelvic tilt, bowed legs, and tight gluteal or quadriceps muscles. Apparently friction occurs as or just after your foot hits the ground when you're running; downhill running reduces the knee flexion angle and can aggravate ITBFS, whereas sprinting and fast running increase it and are less harmful. Treatment includes rest, ice, correcting your training errors, wearing good shoes and orthotics, and gentle stretching, particularly of the iliotibial band itself and gluteal muscles.

To stretch out your IT band, cross your right leg over your left while standing and extend your left arm against a wall or another stable object. Push your right hip in the opposite direction while leaning your weight to your left toward the wall. Your right foot should remain stable, but allow your left knee to flex. If you're doing it correctly, you'll feel the stretch in your right hip and down the outside of that leg.

Ligament and Meniscal Tears

Although usually more of an acute injury, tears in either the ligaments supporting the knee or the cartilage (meniscus) cushion there require prolonged treatment and often surgery. Ligaments are more easily injured in sports that require starting and stopping rapidly or quick directional changes, such as basketball. The anterior cruciate ligament (ACL) and the medial collateral ligament (MCL) are the most often injured, but the posterior cruciate (PCL) and lateral collateral (LCL) ligaments can also be affected. During an acute injury, you will often hear a loud popping noise that may or may not be accompanied by pain. An MRI scan is usually required to confirm these tears, and nowadays arthroscopic surgery, which is minimally invasive, is used to treat partial tears.

If you tear the cartilage in your knee, you have usually torn a meniscus, which is a small, C-shaped piece of cartilage that serves as a cushion between the thigh (femur) and tibia (shin) bones on both sides of your knee; the lateral meniscus is the outside one, the medial one is on the inside. You can tear your menisci alone or along with one of the ligaments (most often the ACL) as a result of twisting or pivoting with your foot planted, by decelerating, or by a sudden impact. Manual tests can determine whether it's torn, but often the tear must be confirmed (and treated) arthroscopically.

Shin Splints

Although not a specific diagnosis, shin splints result from generalized pain that occurs in the front of the lower leg along the tibia (the shinbone). This injury has a number of different potential causes, but it is most likely a cumulative stress injury that occurs from overtraining or excessive running on hard surfaces, resulting in inflammation in those areas or stress fractures in the tibia or fibula (lower leg bones). Your bones can heal themselves over time, but if you don't rest them after a crack starts to appear, they can fracture. If you're a beginning runner, you have higher risk for developing shin splints and stress fractures because you are probably not accustomed to the high impact of running.

How can you tell whether you have shin splints? Watch out for pain on the medial (inside) part of your lower leg that gets worse with running or other weight-bearing exercise (especially when done on hard surfaces). Other symptoms are an aching pain that lingers after exercise, as well as increased pain with activity such as running, jumping, hill climbing, or downhill running. Taking all your jogs along the edge of the ocean on the packed sand running barefoot is a sure way to get this overuse injury! Generally, icing your shins after workouts, taking NSAIDs, and resting are effective ways to treat it. Return to your activities gradually, using pain as your guide. Get new, well-cushioned shoes with adequate support to lower your risk. Also, make sure to stretch properly, warm up effectively, train moderately, progress your workout schedule conservatively, and avoid running or jumping on hard surfaces or for long distances on tilted or slanted surfaces. If the pain doesn't subside using these treatments or if you have a single point of intense pain, consider seeing a podiatrist with expertise in lower extremities and diabetes to pinpoint the exact cause.

*A*thlete *P*rofile

Name: Sean Busby

Hometown: Mission Viejo, California, USA

Diabetes history: Type 1 diabetes diagnosed in 2003 (at age 19)–first misdiagnosed with type 2 before losing 30 pounds (14 kilograms) in two weeks and finally being put on insulin

Sport or activity: Professional snowboarder

Greatest athletic achievement: Within months of my correct diagnosis, I was able to get back on the pro tour to compete and regain my West Coast championship title. I was also featured on the cover of *Diabetes Focus* and *Inner Strength* magazines.

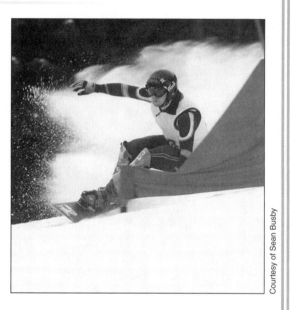

Courtesy of Sean Busby

Current insulin and medication regimen: Either insulin pump or Lantus and NovoLog regimen

Training tips: Test, test, and test! Testing my blood sugars has been the key to my success in understanding how my body is acting in certain environments, including different climates, various humidity levels, competition stress and excitement, time zone changes, complex training schedules, and different altitudes. When I travel around the world for competitions, I test my blood sugar every two hours throughout the night and record everything, including corrections that I made for high or low blood sugars. Two days before my competition I can then look at my log, see how my body is acting in the new environment, and make appropriate corrections to get the most out of my sleep and be prepared to compete. I still check at least once through the night, even before the race (usually at 2:00 a.m.).

Typical daily and weekly training and diabetes regimen:

► **Monday:** Up early. I usually eat a healthy complex carbohydrate and reduce my basal. After breakfast I attend gate training from 8:30 a.m. to 1:00 p.m. I try to keep my blood sugars around 140 to 150 (7.8 to 8.3 mmol/L). If over 180 (10 mmol/L), I give myself insulin and take a break until they go back down. After training I eat a lunch with some protein and some carbohydrate, take a quick siesta, and then go on to the mountain for a light afternoon recovery ride.

► **Tuesday:** Day off for recovery; no training, but I usually participate in a light hike, run, or gym workout. I may also go free ride the mountain with some of my friends, take the snowmobiles out, or explore the backcountry.

► **Wednesday:** Same routine as Monday.

▸ *Thursday:* Meet at our training-center gym from 10:00 a.m. to noon. I reduce my basal because of strenuous core, leg, or upper-body exercises. Back on the hill training from 2:00 p.m. until about 6:30 under the lights to work on fundamentals and different skills. For this I may not reduce my basal because we will be having many discussion and video analysis breaks.

▸ *Friday:* Same routine as Monday and Wednesday.

▸ *Saturday:* Day off snow—very light workouts only!

▸ *Sunday:* Same routine as Monday, Wednesday, and Friday.

Other hobbies and interests: I love snowmobiling and winter mountaineering—snowboard touring in the backcountry. Backcountry riding provides the thrill of being out in the wilderness away from ski resorts and an escape from civilization.

Good diabetes and exercise story: While I was trying to win back my West Coast championship title, my insulin ran out. I had brought an extra insulin cartridge with me that day but had accidentally left it down in the lodge. In first place and with one run left in the event, I began to develop the early stages of DKA, and the stress was making my sugars shoot even higher. Also, the high altitude was making me severely dehydrated. In the starting gate of my final run, I felt as though I was going to pass out, so I asked the start judge to hold the race so I could do an emergency rehydration. The event coordinators and judges put a 10-minute hold on the event to allow me to rehydrate and evaluate my situation. I was questioning whether I should disqualify myself from the event and my potential first-place medal or finish the final run and possibly hold on to first place. I knew that I had to get down the mountain either way, so I decided to get back in the gate and go for it. If I were to pull out of the course because of my sugars, I would know that I had at least tried to finish it. Also, I asked that a ski patrol crew be placed at the bottom. My final run quickly became one of my most challenging snowboard runs and races. I knew that my body could tolerate a little more stress but wasn't sure exactly how much more. As I raced, I reminded myself on every turn to turn quickly across the multiple fall lines throughout the course—usually effortless for me—but I could tell that my cognitive thinking was becoming slower. As I crossed the finish line, I nearly collapsed. Ski patrol then quickly rushed me down to my insulin by snowmobile. I later found out that I had gotten first place and went to stand on the podium. It was a rad feeling. That day I not only won and regained my West Coast title but also beat the hardest competitor I have ever faced—diabetes!

Feet and Ankles

Because of the amount of stress placed on your feet and ankles, they are also a common site of overuse injuries, including plantar fasciitis, chronic sprains, Achilles tendon problems, blisters, calluses, and ulcers. For people with diabetes, particularly if they lose some of the feeling in their feet, blisters, calluses, and ulcers can lead to larger problems, possibly even gangrene and the need for amputation. In some cases, foot deformities (e.g., Charcot foot) are more likely to develop following a sprain and continued walking when you have neuropathy; at such times, a foot cast may be necessary for appropriate healing to take place. In addition, people with any type of diabetes have greater risk of fractures of the metatarsals (long bones in the feet), likely because of some loss of calcium and other minerals associated with long-term diabetes. In athletes without neuropathy, though, plantar fasciitis is the biggest concern, followed by problems with the Achilles tendon.

Plantar Fasciitis

An inflammatory overuse injury, plantar fasciitis is the most common cause of heel pain. It is usually recognizable by your first steps in the morning being painful. Your feet are extended when you sleep (in a position called plantar flexion), which allows the fascia that makes up the underside of your foot to shorten. Pain also occurs at the start of activity and generally goes away with use, but it returns after a long rest when you restart being active. Plantar fasciitis is common in runners and in those who gain weight quickly because the plantar fascia runs the length of the inside of your arch, and it is stretched to flatten your arch slightly each time your heel hits the ground. The plantar fascia isn't very flexible, so repetitive stretching from impact can result in small tears in the fascia, which then become inflamed.

You're more likely to get this injury if you have very flat feet or high arches, excessive pronation (tipping your ankle inward to flatten your arches), a tight Achilles tendon, obesity, or sudden weight gain. It can also result from a rapid increase in your workout intensity or duration, wearing shoes with poor cushioning, a change in your usual running or walking surface, or having to stand upright for excessively long periods. A type 2 diabetic athlete from Mesa, Arizona, found out the hard way that you can also develop this problem from not wearing shoes at all. Her fitness routine includes doing "Dance, Dance Revolution" (a video game on Playstation and Wii), which she did in her socks until she developed plantar fasciitis. After taking two months off from it, she now does the game wearing proper athletic shoes.

If you find yourself with plantar fasciitis, taking NSAIDs can help control the inflammation and resulting discomfort. In addition, take some time off from the activities that are most irritating to that area, including walking barefoot on hard surfaces. It may also help to stretch the plantar fascia and massage that area by rolling your foot over a 3- to 4-inch (8- to 10-centimeter) diameter tube like a rolling pin, soup can, or tennis ball. You can also try taping your heel and arch and using medial, longitudinal arch supports and good shoes.

A new stretching technique may reduce pain when performed several times a day. To do it, you need to cross one leg over the other, pull your toes toward your shin for a count of 10, and repeat 10 times. To prevent recurrence, try doing strengthening exercises, such as scrunching up a hand towel with your toes or pulling a towel weighted with a soup can across the floor. After exercising, ice your heel where it is most sore for 15 to 20 minutes to relieve pain.

Achilles Tendinitis

This type of tendinitis is caused by inflammation, irritation, and swelling of the Achilles tendon, which is the one that connects the two calf muscles, the gastrocnemius and the soleus, to your heel bone (the calcaneus). You use these muscles for pushing off your foot or going up on your toes and, of course, for walking and running. As an overuse injury, it occurs most commonly in walkers, runners, and basketball and volleyball players because of the large amount of stress that jumping puts on this tendon. As you age, you can also experience Achilles problems from arthritis, which can cause extra bony growths on the heel (i.e., spurs) that inflame the tendon. Having an inflammation in this area also increases your risk for experiencing rupturing of your Achilles tendon, correctable only with surgery.

Usual treatments include rest, ice, NSAIDs, exercises, and occasionally a cast, boot, or brace worn to keep it from moving and becoming more inflamed before the swelling goes down. To prevent Achilles tendinitis, progress slowly when starting an exercise program after being inactive for a while and make sure to stretch your calves and thigh muscles properly. Another point of caution is relevant if you've been wearing high-heeled shoes and switch to flats. Your Achilles tendon and lower leg muscles adapt to a shortened position because the high-heeled shoes prevent your heel from stretching down to ground level; putting on flat shoes to exercise causes your tendon to stretch farther than it's accustomed to, which can cause it to become inflamed. If you wear high heels regularly, stretch every morning and night to keep this tendon a more normal length to prevent problems.

Muscle Cramps: Are They Preventable?

If you experience painful, involuntary contractions of your muscles, you're having a muscle cramp. They can occur in any muscle but are most common in the legs, feet, and muscles that cross two joints, such as your calf muscle (the gastrocnemius, which crosses your knee and your ankle joints), quadriceps and hamstrings (the front and back of your thighs), and your feet. Not all of them are that painful; they range in intensity from a slight twitch to severe cramping that makes the muscle feel rock hard and that can last from a few seconds to several minutes. They can also ease up and then recramp several times before disappearing.

Although the exact cause of muscle cramps remains unknown, they're likely related to poor flexibility, muscle fatigue, or doing new activities. Athletes are more likely to get cramps in the preseason when they are less conditioned and more subject to fatigue. Cramps often develop near the end of intense or prolonged exercise, or the night after. Of course, if you're exercising in the heat, cramps can also be related to dehydration and depletion of electrolytes (sodium, potassium, magnesium, and calcium) lost through sweating. When these nutrients fall to certain levels, you're more like to experience cramping.

Cramps usually go away on their own without treatment, but there are effective ways to deal with them. For starters, stop the activity that is causing your muscles to cramp (if you can). Then, gently stretch and massage the cramping muscle, holding your joint in a stretched position until the cramp stops. To prevent cramps, increase your fitness level and avoid becoming excessively fatigued during an activity. Warm up before you start intense workouts and stretch regularly when you're done exercising, focusing on your calves, hamstrings, and quads.

Treating and Preventing Muscle Soreness

Feeling stiff or tight after training is neither uncommon nor cause for alarm. Stretch out all your muscles and joints after workouts. If you find yourself slightly sore the day after exercise, low-level exercise, light stretching, and gentle massage can help. But if you are still rather sore a day or two later and you feel stiff and weak, you are likely experiencing delayed-onset muscle soreness (DOMS), which peaks 24 to 72 hours after an activity. You may even be so stiff and sore that you find it difficult to walk downstairs or fully straighten out your joints.

Although unpleasant, DOMS is different from an acute injury and requires no special treatment. DOMS is a common occurrence, particularly if you are just beginning an exercise program or changing to a new or unusual activity. The cause is likely minute tears in your muscles and connective tissues. As these damaged areas become inflamed and swollen, your nerves are sensitized and you feel the pain. Two or three days may pass before you reach the maximum point of pain, and a week or more may be required to resolve completely. Mild activity, stretching, gentle massage, hydrotherapy (such as getting into a hot tub), and NSAIDs can all help relieve discomfort, but they don't speed up the healing process—the best healer is simply time. The good news is that your body responds with "stress" proteins that it builds into the repaired muscles, almost eliminating the possibility that you will reach that level of soreness in the same muscles for six to eight weeks afterward, even if you overdo it again.

The amount of tearing (and resulting soreness) depends on the activity, the intensity of your workout, and the duration of the workout. Any unaccustomed movement can lead to DOMS, but eccentric muscle contractions (when the muscles are contracting while lengthening) cause the most soreness. Examples of eccentric muscle contractions include going downstairs, running downhill, lowering weights, and doing the downward (gravity-assisted) part of squats and push-ups. As far as

---

RESOURCES FOR ACTIVE PEOPLE WITH DIABETES

Mountains for Active Diabetics (UK)

Mountains for Active Diabetics (MAD) is an international association of mountain sports enthusiasts, many of whom have diabetes, who are interested in the challenges of managing diabetes in the outdoors, particularly at extremes of altitude, temperature, and exertion. The philosophy of the association is that "with careful planning, it can be done." By way of example, many MAD members have summitted the world's highest peaks, crossed endless expanses of desert and snow, run ultramarathons, bicycled all over the world, and climbed vast walls of Himalayan rock and ice. Their stated mission is to help people with diabetes "reach their personal summits."

Founded by Nikki Wallis (UK) in 2000, MAD encourages sharing of practical diabetes issues through electronic access to some of the world's most experienced diabetic mountaineers. The organization also organizes the annual MADiDEA event, an active three-day, mountain-based meeting with exciting topical evening lectures. The iDEA half was started by American diabetic mountaineer David Panofsky, along with Todd Clare and Catalunyan Ernest Blade, culminating in the International Diabetic Expedition to Aconcagua in 2000 (www.idea200.org). You can find more information about the organization on their Web site, www.diabetic.friendsinhighplaces.org, or by e-mailing webmaster@friendsinhighplaces.org.

diabetes goes, the bad part about DOMS is that you won't be able to restore glycogen in affected muscles until they're fully repaired, which can lead you to be insulin resistant and cause your blood sugars to be harder to manage. In addition, certain muscle pain or soreness can be a sign of a serious injury, so if the soreness doesn't get better within a week, consult your physician.

ARTHRITIS

Although exercise is good for you, too much exercise may increase your risk of joint injuries and osteoarthritis, the most common form of arthritis. Trauma to, or overuse of, the joints can cause osteoarthritis. If you've ever had an injury to one of your joints, you are more prone to developing arthritis there. But it's unclear whether long-distance running causes knee and hip joints to deteriorate. Some endurance athletes have been tested and found to have an increase in arthritis-related changes, but they don't necessarily have more symptoms. The latest studies suggest that long-distance running doesn't increase the risk of osteoarthritis of the knees and hips if you're healthy, and it might even have a protective effect against joint degeneration. Diabetes does not increase your risk for arthritis, although hip fractures may be more common among those with diabetes, particularly those who do not regularly participate in weight-bearing exercise that helps stimulate and strengthen the hips and lower-limb bones.

If you have already developed some arthritis in your joints, don't despair; you can still exercise safely. A recent study found that being regularly active may reduce the pain in your affected joint or joints and that stopping activities may cause you to revert to your preexercise pain level. But your activities shouldn't cause pain in your joints while you're exercising. Obviously, activities of higher intensity or longer duration have greater potential to cause pain, so use pain as your guide to know how much to do. Also, avoid sports with high risk of joint trauma, such as contact sports and others with frequent directional changes like racquetball.

INJURIES AND THE OLDER ATHLETE

No one likes to think or talk about it, but everyone has to face the fact that getting older by itself causes changes in physical performance. For instance, the world record in the clean-and-jerk power lift is 20 percent lower in men and 40 percent lower in women in athletes over 50 years of age. Even if you continue to compete in athletic events past your mid-20s, after that you'll be past your peak for most sports and at greater risk for getting acute and overuse injuries.

From your mid-20s on, you'll experience a slow decline in your maximal heart rate, aerobic capacity, lung function, and nerve function (unrelated to diabetes). Although being active lowers your risk for colds, certain cancers, heart disease, and other illnesses, these other physiological changes can't be entirely prevented. The result is that you'll have lower overall strength and endurance as you get older. You're likely to experience selective loss of the fast-twitch muscle fibers used for power and speed, although using those fibers will prevent you from losing them as quickly. In addition, loss of calcium and other minerals from bones accelerates with age, particularly in postmenopausal women, but weight-bearing and resistance exercise can slow and reverse those losses to some extent. Although your body's maximal ability to use oxygen during exercise typically declines 1.5 percent per year, highly trained older athletes show a slower, though steady, rate of decline of only 0.5 percent annually. Moreover, training will keep your breathing muscles stronger and fitter.

Although runners of any age who exercise moderately tend to be physically better off than less active people their age, extensive training for marathons, ultramarathons, and triathlons can increase the risk of injury. Doing that level of training may cause your joints to wear out more quickly than they will if you do more moderate amounts of activity. Many older athletes spend up to a month each year unable to exercise because of injuries. With injury prevention in mind, include an adequate warm-up period with stretching exercises to lower your risk.

Older athletes face some general physical problems that make specific injuries more common. For instance, your joints become less flexible with age, and changes in your body's connective tissues combined with arthritis mean that your knees, hips, and other joints must bear greater stress during exercise than your muscles do. Such changes make running a particularly damaging activity for your joints over time. Stretching regularly can help slow the loss of flexibility but can't prevent it completely, so at some point most runners have to choose alternative activities like walking or working out on lower-impact conditioning machines. Diabetes itself can cause you to lose flexibility faster, particularly if it is not well controlled.

For various sports, you may have to make other adjustments as you age to prevent injuries. For instance, swimmers are more likely to experience rotator cuff tears and should avoid excessive use of hand paddles (which increase stress on the shoulders) and swim fins (which aggravate knee problems), and they should increase swimming distances gradually. Older cyclists are more likely to suffer from compressive or inflammatory syndromes involving nerves in the upper body. These problems are largely preventable by reducing training. Older cyclists should also use the correct seat height, wear padded gloves, use a padded seat (like a gel pad), wear padded cycling shorts, and avoid resting on their hands on the handlebars. Older golfers can develop shoulder problems; neck, lower-back, and wrist pain; and golf or tennis elbow. If you golf, warm up properly, stretch, and do strengthening exercises, especially for your back muscles.

You should now realize that despite the risk of injuries, both acute and overuse, that comes with being physically active, your joints, muscles, bones, and body as a whole will be better off if you stay fit and active. You can prevent overuse injuries by varying your training and treat any injuries that you do get by following the guidelines given in this chapter.

Guidelines
for
Specific Activities

CHAPTER 8

Fitness Activities

Being physically fit is the way to go! Whether you participate in aerobic dance classes, learn martial arts, pump up with weights, or push your limits on the stair stepper, you are not alone. We all want an athletic, toned, fit look, and most of us know we have to sweat some to get it. Besides, being physically fit has many health benefits, especially when you have diabetes (if you've forgotten what they are, go back and read up on them in chapter 1). As I always say, having diabetes should be your excuse to exercise regularly, not a misguided reason for being a sedentary couch potato!

The activities included in this section run the gamut from low-intensity activities (e.g., yoga) to intense, brief ones like heavy weight training and kickboxing to endurance-based race walking and stationary cycling. Most of these activities, however, are endurance activities that use the aerobic (oxygen) system. You can participate in most fitness endeavors in a health club or fitness gym, although others like walking can be done inside on a treadmill or outdoors. Stretching and yoga can be done in a class or on your own just about anywhere.

All the remaining chapters in this book, including this one, give general guidelines for maintaining control over your blood sugars during and after the included activities (in this case, fitness ones), separated out by diabetes regimen (insulin pump, basal-bolus, or noninsulin and oral medication users). Then for each activity, you'll find specific recommendations and examples of some diabetic athletes' individualized changes in insulin, diet, or both.

Examples from type 2 diabetic and type 1.5 (LADA) athletes who use no medications or only oral ones, or who inject Byetta, are given throughout part II as well. You'll find them listed under either diet changes alone or combined regimen changes.

GENERAL RECOMMENDATIONS FOR FITNESS ACTIVITIES

Fitness activities vary widely with respect to the energy systems and fuels that your body uses while you're doing them. For example, aerobic dance is mainly an endurance activity, but it may also contain elements of muscular toning, strengthening, and stretching. Some martial arts may involve only short, intense movements. Conditioning machines like stationary cycles or rowers can provide aerobic and anaerobic conditioning, depending on how hard and how long you use them. For a review of the various energy systems and fuels, refer to chapter 2.

Regular participation in fitness activities can cause you to lose fat weight, gain muscle mass, and improve your blood sugar control. Your insulin sensitivity is likely to improve, resulting in a need for lower doses of insulin or other medications. The actions of different types of insulin and oral meds are covered in chapter 3, as well as what you need to know about them when exercising. Although you may be proficient in regulating your insulin doses on your own or with some input from your diabetes care providers, you should adjust prescribed doses of other meds under the direction of your physician.

GENERAL ADJUSTMENTS BY DIABETES REGIMEN

How you adjust your medications and food intake for any activity will vary with which diabetes regimen you use, which type of exercise you do, and how long and intensely you exercise. In general, the guidelines in this section simply let you know whether you will likely have to change your medications, worry about eating more carbohydrate, or do both.

If you use any brand of an insulin pump, the first section that follows is for you. Other insulin users (nonpumpers) should read the second section on basal-bolus regimens instead (unless, of course, you're interested in finding out more about what pump users need to do). Even if you still use an intermediate-acting insulin instead of a basal one, the guidelines still apply; just think of that insulin as being a basal one except around the time that it peaks, when it acts more like a short-acting one that needs to be adjusted further in advance (e.g., the breakfast dose for after-lunch exercise). If you don't use insulin, go right to the third section, "Noninsulin and Oral Medication Users," for advice that applies to you.

Insulin Pump Users

If you reduce your basal insulin doses by 25 to 100 percent during most of these activities, you'll likely prevent your blood sugars from going too low. Remember, a nondiabetic exerciser's body reduces the amount of insulin that is available during the activity, thus keeping his or her muscles from taking up too much blood glucose. With an insulin pump, you can lower your basal insulin easily by reducing the rate before and during exercise or by disconnecting it altogether. Depending on what the activity is and how much you lower your basal insulin, you may still need to eat some extra carbohydrate. If you exercise right after you eat, you may need to lower your meal bolus by 10 to 50 percent, as well as reduce your basal rate and eat extra carbohydrate. Of course, what you do varies with the activity, its duration, and its intensity. You'll likely need 10 to 30 grams of carbohydrate per hour if you don't have lower insulin levels. Depending on what you do, you may also need to keep your basal insulin rates lower overnight. But for most weight training or stretching activities you may need to make only minimal changes.

Basal-Bolus Regimens

For most fitness activities (except really prolonged ones), you can simply lower your doses of rapid- or short-acting insulin by 10 to 50 percent if you eat within two hours of when you start to exercise, and you may need to increase your carbohydrate by 10 to 30 grams per hour, depending on how much you lowered your preactivity insulin. If you're working out more than two or three hours after your last dose of rapid-acting insulin, focus mainly on your carbohydrate intake. You may need up to 15 grams per hour if you have only basal insulin in your system, or you may get by with eating nothing at all. You may slightly lower the dose of your next injection of basal insulin following prolonged workouts, but you likely won't need to make many adjustments for weight training or stretching.

Noninsulin and Oral Medication Users

If you don't use insulin, doing most of these fitness activities is unlikely to make your blood sugars go too low. To get a better idea of how your body responds, though, test your blood sugars before and after your activities at least for the first few weeks or whenever your medications change. For prolonged activities, you may need to eat up to 15 grams of carbohydrate per hour (even nondiabetic athletes eat during prolonged workouts to help maintain their blood sugars). If you start to experience lows more often after you've been exercising regularly, talk with your physician about lowering the doses of meds that you take. If you inject Byetta and find that it is interfering with your ability to exercise, also check to see whether it's possible to reduce your dose or adjust the time of day when you take it.

Intensity, Duration, and Other Effects

The duration and intensity of your workout, the time of day that you exercise, and your starting blood sugar levels have the biggest effect on your blood sugar responses to fitness workouts. In general, longer bouts of exercise will lower your blood sugars more than short bouts will, and to compensate you may have to make more adjustments in your diabetes regimen both during and afterward. As discussed in chapter 2, intense activities may initially maintain your blood sugar levels more effectively (or even cause them to go up because of hormonal release), but you'll have a much higher risk of developing hypoglycemia later because you will have used up more muscle glycogen.

As for the time of day, any activity that you do early in the morning when your insulin resistance is higher will be less likely to cause your blood sugars to drop compared with exercising later in the day or at any time that your insulin levels are higher or more effective. Exercising right after a meal, even breakfast, will result in greater use of blood glucose, whether you take insulin or your body releases it. In addition, if you exercise after your meal-related insulin is mostly gone (two to three hours later), you'll need fewer adjustments to keep your blood sugars normal.

Lastly, your blood glucose level when you start a workout will significantly affect how much you need to eat or reduce your insulin. To avoid getting low, some athletes try to bump their sugars up to 180 milligrams per deciliter (mg/dl), or 10 millimolar (mmol/L) or higher before they ever start. But if you're too high (e.g., above 250 to 300 mg/dl, or 13.9 to 16.7 mmol/L) when you start, you may have to take some rapid-acting insulin to reduce your blood sugars.

AEROBIC CONDITIONING MACHINES

Workouts on a treadmill, stair stepper, elliptical strider, cross-trainer, stationary cycle, ski machine, or rowing machine are all aerobic in nature because they last for more than two minutes and predominantly use your aerobic system. These activities can be quite intense because they generally involve either large-muscle groups in your legs or your full-body musculature. Some, like ski and rowing machines, also involve significant upper-body work. Your regimen changes will depend primarily on the intensity and duration of your workout, as well as the time of day when you exercise. See table 8.1 for further instructions on aerobic conditioning machines.

Treadmills   As far as your blood sugars are concerned, treadmill walking or running is similar to walking, race walking, or running outdoors. The only differences arise from the environment: You'll expend more energy when you exercise outdoors in hot, cold, or windy conditions (for examples, refer to walking in this chapter, running in chapter 9, and exercise under environmental extremes in chapter 12).

Stair steppers or stair climbers   Working out on a stair stepper or stair climber is much more aerobic than sprinting up stadium steps. Although the intensity of stair climbing varies with the program that you choose (hills, manual, random, and so on), your blood sugars will respond mainly to how long you work out because the workout is never easy. If you do climbing for a relatively short time (10 to 15 minutes), you may not have to make any regimen changes. Doing it for longer will use more muscle glycogen and have more immediate and longer-lasting effects on your blood sugars.

Elliptical striders and cross-trainers   An elliptical strider is a cross between a treadmill and a stair climber, and cross-trainers emphasize more of a leg-lifting action than striders do. Although usually more intense than treadmill walking, exercising on striders and cross-trainers is less taxing on your lower-leg joints because your feet are constantly in contact with the footpads. Both generally offer an easier workout than does the stair stepper, which has more of a vertical component that requires you to lift the equivalent of your body mass.

Stationary cycles   The intensity of stationary cycling can vary widely. It can involve sprinting and intermittent increases in intensity with hill climbing, both of which provide significant stress to your anaerobic metabolism, especially the lactic acid system. Doing "spinning" on a cycle (a fast pace with lower or variable resistance) is less taxing than pedaling as hard as possible against a heavier resistance. How hard you work out will affect your blood sugars. A longer duration at a higher intensity generally lowers them more, but the time of day also plays a role; for instance, intense stationary cycling may cause your blood sugar levels to rise, particularly if you exercise in the morning. Recumbent cycles are a good alternative to regular stationary ones because the angle formed at your hip while riding a recumbent bike is more natural and is less likely to result in joint pain, so you might consider using one of these if you have a choice.

Ski machines   "Skiing" indoors on a ski machine has almost the same fitness and blood sugar benefits as cross-country skiing if you use good technique. Most people,

Table 8.1 Aerobic Conditioning Machines

Insulin: insulin pump	Insulin: basal-bolus regimen	Diet: insulin pump	Diet: basal-bolus regimen
• For shorter workouts of 20 minutes or less, reduce premeal insulin boluses by 0–20%. • Reduce your basal insulin by 25–50% during the activity or suspend it. • For longer workouts, reduce your premeal insulin boluses by 20–40%, reduce basal rate by 50–100% during exercise, or do both. • For workouts with low insulin levels, reduce only your basal rates or make no changes. • After harder or longer workouts, keep your basal rate reduced by 25–50% for 1–2 hours afterward as well.	• For shorter workouts of 20 minutes or less, reduce rapid-acting insulin doses by 0–20% if you eat within 2 hours beforehand. • For longer workouts, reduce those doses by 20–40% depending on when you work out. • For workouts with low insulin levels, you may need no insulin adjustments. • Do not change your basal insulin for these activities (especially if done regularly).	• For shorter workouts, increase carbohydrate intake by 5–15 grams for exercise. • For longer workouts, supplement with 15–25 grams of carbohydrate per hour. • You may not need any extra carbohydrate if you lower your insulin levels during your workout.	• For shorter workouts, increase your carbohydrate intake by 5–25 grams if after a meal, depending on how much you lowered your premeal insulin dose. • For longer workouts, increase your carbohydrate intake by at least 15 grams per hour. • If you only have basal insulins on board, you may not need any extra carbohydrate.

though, do not work out on a ski machine for as long as they would cross-country ski outdoors (covered in the next chapter), and they don't have to deal with the effects of a cold and sometimes windy environment. As a result, this fitness activity will generally lower your blood glucose less than skiing outdoors will for a similar length of time.

Rowers   The biggest effects of rowing come from how hard and how long you work out. Short, intense rowing will maintain your blood sugars more effectively because of a greater release of glucose-raising hormones. If you row for longer at a less intense pace, you'll have to make more adjustments to your diabetes regimen to prevent hypoglycemia. Rowing outdoors, however, may increase your body's blood glucose use because of a greater intensity elicited by temperature and wind effects (as discussed in chapter 10 covering endurance–power sports).

Athlete Examples

Although the fitness activities vary, these examples show that comparable adjustments can be made for all of them, depending on your exercise intensity, starting blood sugar levels, time of day, and circulating insulin levels.

Insulin Changes Alone

Before doing 30 minutes of exercise on an elliptical strider and 30 minutes of Pilates right after lunch, Del Mar, California, resident Marty Fedor simply lowers her normal insulin-to-carbohydrate ratio for lunch by about one-half. She keeps her carbohydrate intake and exercise routine consistent, though, which she feels is the key to maintaining blood glucose control during exercise.

Type 1 pumper Malcolm Airst (San Diego, California) compensates for an hour of hard exercise, done with his heart rate at about 80 percent of maximal on an elliptical strider, by using a temporary basal rate that is 0.1 unit per hour instead of his usual 0.75, starting about 30 minutes before exercise and lasting throughout.

For 60 minutes of hard exercise on a cross-trainer machine, Jeff Vollin from Tucson, Arizona, takes a smaller bolus ratio (1 unit of insulin per 16 grams of carbohydrate instead of 12 grams) at his preworkout breakfast and turns off the basal rate on his pump during the activity.

Diet Changes Alone

A type 1.5 diabetic exerciser taking basal Lantus insulin only, Mark Shriver of Minneapolis, Minnesota, finds that eating enough to get his starting blood sugars above 150 mg/dl (8.3 mmol/L) and then eating one gram of carbohydrate per minute during his fitness activities works for him.

For Chuck Keyserling of Rockville, Maryland, a type 2 diabetic exerciser controlled with Avandia (an insulin sensitizer) only, doing 2- to 3-hour workouts of weightlifting with interspersed sessions on an elliptical trainer may require him to eat a small snack before going to the gym. The best effect on his glucose control has come from slowly adding 5-pound (2.3-kilogram) increments to his weight training and increasing the resistance on the aerobic machines that he uses. Another type 2, Susan Rice from Black Mountain, North Carolina, finds that eating an Extend bar at night after doing her workouts at Curves helps prevent high blood sugars the next morning, whereas Claude Stone of Montpelier, Vermont, often eats a low-carbohydrate snack after his 60- to 120-minute cardio workouts at the gym.

Combined Regimen Changes

Ron DeNunzio of Lititz, Pennsylvania, sets a temporary basal rate 30 minutes before exercising, avoids taking any Symlin preexercise, and tests his blood sugars twice before starting. Before walking, biking, or doing any fitness exercises, he also eats peanut butter and crackers. He drinks some water with glucose in it during longer sessions.

A resident of Somerset, Massachusetts, Nicole Purcell may lower her basal rate on her insulin pump before, during, and after working out on an elliptical trainer, treadmill (doing slow jogging), or stationary cycle. She may also eat 15 to 20 grams of fast-acting carbohydrate with a small serving of protein preexercise without bolusing.

To work out on an elliptical trainer for a half hour three or four times a week, Kateri Routh of Chicago, Illinois, takes off her insulin pump when she works out in the afternoon and drinks a small juice box before starting. For similar morning exercise, though, she has to leave her pump on, although she lowers her basal rate by 50 percent and doesn't drink any juice.

Intensity, Duration, and Other Effects

Effect of workout intensity   Esther Pinto of Rio de Janeiro, Brazil, takes her insulin pump off during all her cardio workouts at the gym. Following her higher-intensity activities (e.g., spinning classes, strength training), she has to give a small bolus (more than the basal insulin that she missed) immediately after exercise to correct hyperglycemia. In her preexercise meals, she also reduces her carbohydrate boluses by 50 percent.

Effect of starting blood sugar levels   A San Diego (California) resident, Larry Verity always checks his blood glucose before starting a workout, usually consisting of 30 to 45 minutes of vigorous aerobic exercise in the early morning. If his blood sugars are over 180 mg/dl (10 mmol/L), then he takes half a unit of Humalog before starting. If they're less than 110 mg/dl (6.1 mmol/L), he eats 30 to 40 grams of complex carbohydrate. He also avoids taking any Symlin before working out.

Lynn Witmer of Toronto, Ontario (Canada), usually reduces her insulin basal rate by 50 percent during running, cycling, or elliptical trainer workouts, starting 15 minutes before and continuing until about 30 minutes after she finishes. But if her starting blood sugar level is below 7 mmol/L (126 mg/dl), she eats some dried fruit; for 11 mmol/L (198 mg/dl), she doesn't eat or reduce her basal rate; and when it's above 14 mmol/L (252 mg/dl), she takes a small insulin bolus as well.

Similarly, for about an hour of rowing on an ergometer, Allan Meltzer from Ottawa, Ontario, cuts back on his rapid-acting insulin dose for the last meal before he exercises, or he eats a high-carbohydrate snack to make sure that his blood sugars are high enough (about 14 mmol/L) when he starts. If his blood sugars are over that value (252 mg/dl), he has to inject 1 to 2 units of NovoRapid so that his sugars drop down during exercise as they normally do.

Effect of time of day   For K. Mathias, a type 1 athlete from Toronto, Canada, adjustments for working out for 30 minutes on varying fitness machines (stair stepper, treadmill, elliptical strider, or stationary cycle) are not necessary if she works out first thing in the morning. For the same evening exercise, she takes only half of her usual dinner bolus. Similarly, Marilyn Johnston from Swan River, Manitoba (also in Canada), finds that for 3 miles (4.8 kilometers) of treadmill walking to start her day, she often has to take a few units of NovoRapid beforehand to counter the insulin resistance that she has at that time of day (i.e., prebreakfast).

Another pumper, Jim Gehring of Bridgewater, Maine, exercises in the early morning and eats lightly if his starting blood sugars are normal. He skips all food before an hour of cycling or treadmill exercise, though, if his sugars start out above 130 mg/dl (7.2 mmol/L) because of his greater insulin resistance.

Effect of circulating insulin levels   Down in Australia, Kerry Vinall of Brisbane, Queensland, will not do her usual fitness activities within two hours of taking an insulin bolus because her blood sugars drop too rapidly during the session. Normally, she lowers the basal rate of her pump one hour ahead of exercise (to lower insulin levels), down to 20 percent of normal for stationary cycling, 25 percent for jogging, and 50 percent for weight training.

A Lantus user, Lynne Korlewitz of Crofton, Maryland, finds it easiest to maintain her blood sugars during one to two hours of early morning fitness exercise done on a treadmill, cycle, or other machine before she takes her morning dose of Humalog with breakfast. If she does cardio training alone, her blood sugars drop about 30 mg/dl (1.7 mmol/L) during the activity but decrease less or may even rise when she does resistance training as well.

AEROBIC FITNESS CLASSES (DANCE, HIP HOP, PILATES, SPINNING, AND STEP AEROBICS)

These activities are mainly aerobic in nature, with interspersed periods of greater intensity (the aerobic portions) and stretching and toning. Even if you use small weights or do repetitions like abdominal work during the classes, the workouts are still mainly aerobic because most classes last at least 45 minutes and emphasize muscular endurance over strength. Classes also vary in intensity based on how hard you push yourself and the nature of the class (e.g., high impact, low impact, step, cycling, and others).

The newer crazes in classes are Pilates and spinning. Pilates is a lower-intensity activity that focuses on flexibility, posture, balance, and core strength using a variety of techniques that incorporate breathing and spinal alignment, among other things. Spinning classes take place on specially designed stationary cycles. You pedal to motivating music (like in other fitness classes), while the class instructor talks you through a visualization of an outdoor cycling workout. You vary your pace during the class—sometimes pedaling as fast as you can against lower resistance and other times cranking up the tension and pedaling slowly from a standing position—but you should always be able to finish simply by turning the resistance down to a workload that you can handle.

For most of these aerobics classes, how hard, how long, and when you work out have a big effect on your blood sugar responses. For example, higher-intensity workouts that last an hour or more will generally reduce your blood sugars more than doing easier ones for the same amount of time. If you take classes in the early morning, such as before breakfast when your insulin resistance is higher, you'll be less likely to experience hypoglycemia than after a meal when you still have more insulin in your system. Working out more than two or three hours afterward when your insulin levels are lower is your best bet for maintaining stable blood sugars. You may still need to eat some carbohydrate, depending on where your sugars start. See table 8.2 for further instructions on aerobic fitness classes.

Athlete Examples

Aerobic fitness classes come in all sorts of types and intensities, but all of them can be modified to allow you to do them effectively.

Insulin Changes Alone

Before participating in an hour-long aerobics class (with 20 minutes each of step aerobics, kickboxing, and weightlifting), Cynthia Fritschi of Chicago, Illinois, cuts back her preactivity meal dose by about 1 unit and sets her pump at 25 percent of her normal basal rate.

Table 8.2 Aerobic Dance, Step Aerobics, and Pilates

Insulin: insulin pump	Insulin: basal-bolus regimen	Diet: insulin pump	Diet: basal-bolus regimen
• Reduce basal insulin rates by 50–100% to reduce your need for extra carbohydrate. • Consider reducing your basal rate 30–60 minutes before you start exercising, and keep it lower for 1–2 hours afterward to prevent lows (unless you want to eat). • For exercise after a meal, reduce your insulin bolus by 25–50% as well.	• Cut back your mealtime insulin dose by 25–50% for exercise following it. • For exercise before meals or early in the morning, you may not need to adjust your insulin. • You probably won't need to reduce basal insulin doses to prevent overnight hypoglycemia.	• Increase your carbohydrate intake by up to 10–20 grams per hour, depending on insulin reductions. • If you lower your insulin levels sufficiently, you may not need any extra carbohydrate.	• Consume 10–20 grams of carbohydrate per hour, depending on your reductions in rapid-acting insulin. • For exercise more than 2–3 hours after your last injection, consume extra carbohydrate right before your workout, if you need to, instead of lowering your last insulin dose (to prevent highs). • If your insulin levels are low during this activity, you may not need any extra carbohydrate.

Rachel Lanclos of Lubbock, Texas, teaches fitness classes, including step aerobics, kickboxing, yoga, and Pilates. She finds it easiest simply to remove her pump during hour-long classes.

For aerobics classes, Adelaide Lindahl, a type 1 exerciser from Bloomington, Minnesota, prefers to reduce her basal rates during the activity rather than cut back on her premeal boluses, which tends to lead to postprandial spikes. If she reduces her basal rates to 0.5 unit per hour starting an hour beforehand and during the class, she doesn't need to eat anything extra.

Diet Changes Alone

For an hour of Pilates, Michelle McCotter from Los Angeles, California, usually eats 10 to 15 grams of carbohydrate if she starts with a normal blood glucose level. If her sugars are around 120 mg/dl (6.7 mmol/L), though, she won't eat anything.

Combined Regimen Changes

A resident of West Roxbury, Massachusetts, Lulu Morrison does step aerobics four to five days per week. For this activity, she suspends her pump during the class and takes four glucose tablets before it starts if her blood sugars are less than 150 mg/dl (8.3 mmol/L). If they drop during class, she eats another two to four tablets to compensate.

Likewise, Catherine Cunningham (Lexington, Kentucky) suspends her pump during aerobics classes, of which she is the instructor. She additionally eats some protein and carbohydrate before starting classes.

For spinning classes, Karen Tank of Princeton, New Jersey, lowers her basal rate by 50 percent before starting and keeps it there until the end. She also checks her blood sugars about halfway through the hour-long class and eats carbohydrate if she starts going too low. For morning workouts, she tries to eat a breakfast higher in protein, fat, and fiber (but low in carbohydrate) so that she doesn't have to bolus much, if at all, beforehand.

Bob Paxson of Sacramento, California, teaches spinning classes. Because of how much he sweats during them, he suspends his insulin pump during a one-hour class and usually consumes about 200 calories of Cytomax during it. He has found that if he keeps his pump off longer than two hours during back-to-back classes, his blood sugars stay normal for a time but then start to rise a couple of hours later from loss of basal insulin. Consequently, for other activities like cycling outdoors, he reduces his basal rate rather than completely suspend his pump.

Intensity, Duration, and Other Effects

Effect of exercise intensity Sandy Asherman of New York City finds that doing lower-intensity Pilates affects her blood sugars differently than fast walking or using an elliptical strider does. Although she usually suspends her pump during exercise and eats 15 to 20 grams of carbohydrate before and possibly during her workout, she finds that her blood sugars stay more stable during Pilates, only decreasing about an hour afterward.

Effect of time of day Kathleen Johnson of Lake St. Louis, Missouri, finds that she exercises best in the early morning and has to make fewer adjustments then for step aerobics (as the instructor). She just doesn't eat before the class and takes no insulin boluses.

BOWLING

This activity involves extremely short bursts of activity (e.g., swinging and releasing the ball) and relies on your short-term energy (phosphagen) system. Most of the time, you do little activity between your turns. Consequently, the total energy that you use in bowling is minimal, its effect on your blood sugars is usually insignificant, and you probably won't need to adjust your regimen. But if you bowl competitively for two or three hours or more, you might need 5 to 10 grams of carbohydrate, especially if you're bowling after a meal. If you use a pump, you can lower your basal insulin by a small amount (10 to 20 percent) then.

BOXING

This activity involves short, powerful jabs and quick (anaerobic) movements, as well as constant motion of your legs during a given round. Training for boxing usually involves a combination of power and endurance moves. For recommended changes for this sport, refer to the section on kickboxing later in this chapter.

CLIMBING, INDOOR

Climbing indoors on a specially designed wall involves muscular endurance and strength to hang onto the handholds with your fingertips for extended periods without rest and to push off the wall and footholds with your legs. Your muscles are working while staying the same length (doing isometric contractions), which involves both strength and endurance of your upper-body muscles. For short climbing attempts, the intensity of this activity will likely keep your blood sugars stable, but if you climb for long periods, you may need to take in some carbohydrate to compensate, both between climbs and later to prevent lows. For some examples, read the section on rock and ice climbing (outdoors) in chapter 12.

DANCE: BALLET, MODERN, SOCIAL, BALLROOM, AND OTHERS

Dance activities often combine aerobic and anaerobic components, depending on how hard and long you dance. An extreme example is ballet, which requires power moves, such as jumping, and sustained muscular contractions when holding dance positions, along with hours of training and practice. Other types of dance are generally more aerobic in nature, but they are usually lower-level activities, necessitating fewer adjustments. Social or recreational dancing (e.g., line) may not lower your blood sugars much, but you can't be a ballerina without lowering your insulin and eating more to prevent lows. See table 8.3 for further instructions on dance.

Athlete Examples

These diabetic exercisers often make changes in their diet and insulin dosing, but the actual adjustment depends largely on the type of dancing that they do.

Table 8.3 Dance: Ballet, Modern, Social, Ballroom, and Others

Insulin: insulin pump	Insulin: basal-bolus regimen	Diet: insulin pump	Diet: basal-bolus regimen
• Reduce your basal rates by 0–20% for low-level (social or recreational) dancing. • If you're active following a meal, reduce your premeal boluses by 10–20%. • For more intense or prolonged dancing, reduce your basal rates and boluses by 20–40% during and possibly before the activity.	• For most social or recreational dance, you won't need to change your insulin much unless the activity is prolonged (more than 1 or 2 hours). • For dancing after a meal, reduce your dose of rapid-acting insulin by 10–20%. • For more intense or prolonged dance or ballet classes, cut back your rapid-acting insulin by 20–40%.	• Increase your carbohydrate intake by 0–15 grams per hour during dancing activities. • Consume an additional 0–30 grams of carbohydrate per hour for intense or prolonged dancing, depending on how much you lower your basal rates.	• Consume an extra 0–15 grams of carbohydrate per hour for dancing after a meal. • Increase your carbohydrate intake by 10–30 grams per hour for more prolonged or intense dance.

Insulin Changes Alone

Tom Somma of Virginia Beach, Virginia, notices that ballroom dancing causes big drops in his blood sugars even though it's a light activity. To compensate, he suspends his insulin pump while taking a class and tries to start out with his blood sugars around 200 mg/dl (11.1 mmol/L).

In Falmouth, Maine, Steffi Rothweiler participates in competitive Irish dancing, for which she usually sets a lower, temporary basal rate on her pump to compensate. For Irish set dancing, Andrea Limbourg of Paris, France, also lowers her basal rate when she's dancing all day in Ireland, but for helping with beginner or intermediate classes as she usually does, she doesn't need to make many changes in her regimen.

Diet Changes Alone

Jeanne Young, a type 2 diabetic resident of Mesa, Arizona, finds that doing "Dance, Dance Revolution" (DDR) on PlayStation gives her a cardiovascular workout that has helped her lose 70 pounds (32 kilograms) in a year. She exercises doing DDR after dinner, which is the meal during which she eats the most carbohydrate, to help control her postprandial glucose spike, along with taking the extended release form of metformin then. If she can't do DDR, she cycles 6 miles (9.7 kilometers) on a canal road.

Combined Regimen Changes

During swing dancing lessons, Sarah Soper (West Lafayette, Indiana) lowers her basal rate down to 65 percent of normal for an hour. For weekly jam sessions, she lowers it even more, to 45 percent for two hours. If her blood sugars are going lower before she starts, she often eats a granola bar, for which she sometimes gives a very small bolus.

A preprofessional ballerina, Jillian Wiseman of Tarzana, California, dances for three to eight hours daily, for which she makes changes in both insulin and food. She lowers her NovoLog doses (taking almost none during long days of dancing) and reduces her basal Lantus by a third to a half to compensate, along with eating more carbohydrate and protein before workouts.

Intensity, Duration, and Other Effects

Effect of exercise intensity For Jillian Wiseman, the biggest challenge is dealing with postexercise lows during the night after evening ballet practice, but she is often hyperglycemic before that when she finishes her dancing because of how hard she works. Her primary strategy for preventing such lows is to cut back dramatically on her dose of basal insulin (Lantus), which she takes in the evening, by 33 to 50 percent.

HOUSEWORK

This activity has elements of strength and endurance, depending on what specifically you're doing. Most aspects of housework minimally involve standing, and others, like sweeping or vacuuming, require you to hold out your arms from your sides for periods at a time. The best training for housecleaning and other domestic chores is to do fitness activities regularly. Doing housework for an extended period can require you to make some adjustments to prevent hypoglycemia.

Athlete Examples

Although not a sport per se, housework involves manual labor, and it can affect your blood sugars, particularly when it is intense and prolonged.

Insulin Changes Alone

When Julie Heverly of Richmond, Virginia, cleans her house two Saturdays a month for four to six hours, she has to lower her basal rate down to 50 percent of normal. Her cleaning is physically active, including going up and down steps many times, moving furniture to clean, vacuuming, and more.

A resident of Annapolis, Maryland, Shiela Bostelman finds that doing housecleaning for two hours requires her to lower her basal rate on her pump to 30 percent while doing it.

Similarly, Gayle Land of Minnetonka, Minnesota, finds that vacuuming usually takes a toll on her blood sugars, forcing her to reduce her basal rate on her pump during the activity. She also finds that playing the organ typically causes lows because of the vigorous activity of using the foot pedals and keeping her arms raised and moving over the keyboards.

Diet Changes Alone

For doing moderate housecleaning for an hour or more, Sheri Ochs of Virginia Beach, Virginia, finds that she has to eat an extra 10 to 15 grams of carbohydrate per hour to prevent lows. If she cleans more than two or three hours after her last injection of Humalog, she needs to supplement only during the second hour of cleaning, not the first.

ICE SKATING AND INLINE SKATING

These activities are mainly aerobic in nature, much along the lines of walking. The gliding effect of the skates reduces some of the energy required to cover any given distance. Ice and inline skating, if you do them at a high skill level, may involve powerful, quick movements such as jumping or spinning, which are more anaerobic.

The intensity and duration of skating will affect your blood sugar response. For instance, recreational skating requires minimal aerobic effort and, like slow walking, uses little blood sugar or muscle glycogen. Competitive skating (speed or figure, usually done on ice) is much more intense than recreational skating and will certainly require you to make some adjustments. For comparable regimen changes for competitive-level skating, refer to recommendations for ice hockey found in chapter 10. See table 8.4 for further instructions on ice skating and inline skating.

Table 8.4   Ice Skating and Inline Skating

Insulin: insulin pump	Insulin: basal-bolus regimen	Diet: insulin pump	Diet: basal-bolus regimen
• For shorter, recreational skating, reduce your basal rates by 10–20%. • For more extended skating, reduce both the basal rate (10–20%) and premeal boluses before exercise (20–40%) within 2 hours.	• Decrease your rapid-acting insulin by 20–40% for meals before exercise. • For prolonged or faster skating, reduce your insulin more or eat an additional snack.	• If you don't lower your basal rates, you may need to consume 5–15 grams of carbohydrate for shorter or easier skating. • Increase your carbohydrate intake by 10–15 grams per hour during longer bouts.	• Consume up to 15 grams of carbohydrate right before or during the activity. • If you have low insulin levels, you won't need any extra carbohydrate unless your skating is prolonged or intense.

Athlete Examples

The following example stresses how many people can make minimal adjustments for recreational skating.

Insulin Changes Alone

For inline skating, Sarah Soper from Indiana disconnects from her pump during the activity but not before giving herself about 20 percent of the basal insulin that she's going to miss up front. When she reconnects, she gives herself the other 80 percent.

KICKBOXING

Kickboxing is mostly anaerobic, involving short bursts of powerful movements. It may also involve continual movement of your legs if you're doing repeated kicks. Training for this activity involves power and endurance movements designed to increase the strength and endurance of your leg and trunk muscles. Higher-intensity, more anaerobic workouts often require you to make fewer changes than you would expect because of greater release of glucose-raising hormones. Having low insulin levels during this kind of high-intensity activity will further lower your need to adjust. If your blood sugars are higher when you finish than when you start, you may need a small amount of insulin to bring them down. See table 8.5 for further instructions on kickboxing.

Athlete Examples

This activity is most similar to intense martial arts with regard to its effects on your blood glucose levels. To compensate, you may need to make a variety of diabetic regimen adjustments.

Table 8.5 Kickboxing

Insulin: insulin pump	Insulin: basal-bolus regimen	Diet: insulin pump	Diet: basal-bolus regimen
• Take 10–30% less pre-exercise insulin depending on the workout that you're planning to do. • Lower your basal rates by 10–40% alone or along with bolus decreases. • For higher-intensity workouts, consider bolusing with 1–2 units of insulin to counter above-normal starting blood sugars, especially if kickboxing often raises your blood sugar. • For longer workouts (1–3 hours), reduce your insulin more before or during the workout.	• For kickboxing within 2 hours of eating, lower your insulin doses by 20–50%. • For higher-intensity workouts, you may need to reduce insulin doses by only 10–25%. • For longer workouts (1–3 hours), you will likely need to reduce your insulin before the workout based on when your last injection was.	• Depending on how hard you're working out, increase your carbohydrate intake by 5–15 grams per hour. • Consume less carbohydrate for shorter workouts, especially if you lowered your basal insulin. • You may need to eat more for longer workouts (1–3 hours), depending on how high your insulin levels are.	• Increase your carbohydrate intake by 5–15 grams per hour, or less if your workout is short. • For 1- to 3-hour workouts, consume 10–15 grams of carbohydrate or more per hour, depending on how low your insulin levels are and how hard you're working out.

Insulin Changes Alone

Before kickboxing workouts, Gary Scheiner of Wynnewood, Pennsylvania, cuts back on his meal bolus by 50 percent. Similarly, Kameron Hurley from Dayton, Ohio, cuts back on her dinner NovoLog injection by about 3 units before evening kickboxing.

Diet Changes Alone

Peter Thompson of Invercargill, New Zealand, who won a New Zealand middle-weight full-contact kickboxing title, usually does his kickboxing, boxing, or karate training in the evenings after dinner. Before dinner, he takes 0 to 1 unit of NovoRapid, along with Protophane (an intermediate-acting insulin). His dinner consists of mostly veggies, chicken or lean beef, and very little carbohydrate. He eats enough carbohydrate between breakfast and his afternoon tea to get him through his evening training sessions. Before particularly intense workouts, he eats a good meal of lower GI carbohydrate and protein, along with higher GI carbohydrate during the training itself.

To participate in kickboxing fitness classes, Patti Murphy Cerami of Bloomingdale, Illinois, usually has to eat some carbohydrate to prevent lows, even when kickboxing in the midafternoon. She eats about 30 grams of yellow or brown raisins with almonds mixed in.

Combined Regimen Changes

During kickboxing classes, Tom Somma disconnects his pump, but he also eats enough beforehand to make sure that his blood sugars are about 200 mg/dl (11.1 mmol/L) when he starts because this activity causes his blood sugars to decrease even with his pump off. He takes glucose tablets as needed throughout to prevent lows.

For kickboxing or boxing workouts before dinner, Alexis Pollak (La Jolla, California) needs to take 2 to 3 units of NovoLog around 4:00 p.m. to avoid ending up with high blood sugars afterward. She usually can then eat a lower-carbohydrate dinner afterward without taking any rapid-acting insulin, only Symlin and Levemir. But if her blood glucose is below 120 mg/dl (6.7 mmol/L) right before she starts, she typically eats two or three glucose tablets and tests in the middle of her workouts, using Gu packets to treat lows.

Intensity, Duration, and Other Effects

Effect of time of day   Patti Murphy Cerami chooses not to do kickboxing in the morning because doing so makes her extremely hyperglycemic because of its intensity and her body's resistance to insulin at that time of day. Instead, she works out later in the day when her insulin resistance is lower.

MARTIAL ARTS

These activities include karate, judo, taekwondo, and tai chi, which cover a wide range of exercise intensity. Most involve power moves like kicking, chopping, and punching, although disciplines like tai chi include only slow, controlled movements that are more prolonged and less intense. The intensity of the activity will have the greatest effect on your blood sugar levels. Extremely intense workouts will be more anaerobic in nature and may not cause much of a decrease during them, and in some cases your blood sugars may increase instead because of greater release of glucose-raising hormones. If you work out long and hard, however, your risk of experiencing delayed drops in blood sugar levels will be heightened by your depletion of muscle glycogen. Activities like tai chi are low in intensity and may require no adjustments. See table 8.6 for further instructions on martial arts.

Athlete Examples

These examples demonstrate the need to modify each regimen according to the type, intensity, duration, and timing of martial arts workouts.

Insulin Changes Alone

Tom Shearer of Carlsbad, California, studies kung fu. During 30- to 60-minute classes, he simply removes his insulin pump because he finds that it gets in the way.

Diet Changes Alone

A type 1.5 diabetic exerciser who takes only Actos and Janumet, Troy Strausbaugh of Lexington, Kentucky, finds that he rarely gets low during mixed martial arts

Table 8.6   Martial Arts

Insulin: insulin pump	Insulin: basal-bolus regimen	Diet: insulin pump	Diet: basal-bolus regimen
• Reduce your basal rates by 0–30% during the activity (probably 0% for tai chi). • For longer workouts (1–2 hours), cut back preexercise boluses by 10–25%. • Consider giving a bolus of 0.5–2 units after intense martial arts workouts and competitions if your blood sugar goes up.	• Reduce rapid-acting insulin doses preexercise by 0–40%. • For longer workouts (1–2 hours), reduce insulin doses before the workout by 10–50%. • Make greater changes for more vigorous activities (e.g., judo or karate) compared with lower-activity martial arts like tai chi. • Keep in mind that you may need some extra insulin (0.5–2 units) following intense martial arts competitions or workouts.	• Supplement with 0–15 grams of carbohydrate per hour as needed. • For higher-intensity workouts or martial arts competitions, you should not need extra carbohydrate unless the activity is prolonged.	• Supplement with 5–15 grams of carbohydrate per hour, depending on your insulin levels. • For higher-intensity workouts or martial arts competitions, you may need minimal carbohydrate if you have low insulin levels, unless your workout is long.

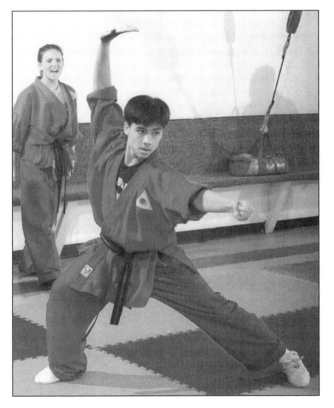

For martial arts like karate, extremely intense workouts will be more anaerobic in nature and may not cause much of a decrease in blood sugars, but if you work out long and hard, your risk of experiencing delayed drops will be heightened by your depletion of muscle glycogen.

(MMA) practices and competitions, but if he does start to feel symptomatic, he drinks a fruit smoothie with added protein.

Combined Regimen Changes

Marc Blatstein, a resident of Huntingdon Valley, Pennsylvania, practices taekwondo competitively, for which he turns down the basal rates on his pump by 10 to 20 percent an hour before he starts a workout. He also finds that he needs to drink about 4 ounces (120 milliliters) of juice before starting to prevent lows.

To compete in jujitsu practices and competitions, Andy Bell of Columbia, Missouri, tries not to take any rapid-acting insulin within two hours of when he starts, and he prefers to have his blood sugars in the upper 100 to lower 200 mg/dl (10 to 13 mmol/L) range. He finds that he does better by eating foods that take longer to digest, such as peanut butter crackers, because they help his blood sugars stay more stable. He also consumes protein-based drinks while exercising.

Intensity, Duration, and Other Effects

Effect of starting blood sugar levels   A Brazilian youth champion in jujitsu, Matehus Trigo from Rio de Janeiro, Brazil, adjusts his insulin intake based on his starting blood sugars. If he's less than 100 mg/dl (5.6 mmol/L) before a meal and his activity, he eats without taking any NovoRapid. If his sugars are 150 or higher, he takes 1 unit for every 20 grams of carbohydrate, and he eats candy if he starts to feel low during workouts.

PHYSICAL EDUCATION CLASSES AND GYM (SCHOOL BASED)

These activities can vary widely, depending on which sport or activity (e.g., basketball, soccer, running, dance, or health instruction) the PE instructor is focusing on for the day or week. Activities may be done indoors or outdoors, depending on the weather, available facilities, the nature of the sport, and more. Not all schools offer PE classes daily anymore, making their effects even more unpredictable at times. Because these classes are so variable, compensating for the activities in advance can be difficult. Your best bet may be to make sure that you have carbohydrate snacks available to eat before and during more intense activities to prevent low blood sugars.

Athlete Examples

Adjustments may need to be made on a daily basis to compensate for different activities done in PE and gym classes.

Diet Changes Alone

For Baylee Glass of Los Lunas, New Mexico, PE classes in elementary school often make her blood sugars drop, but not always. Her biggest challenge is that these activities take place at the end of her school day and in the middle of the afternoon, which makes them hard to compensate for with changes in prelunch NovoLog without causing high blood sugars before class starts. She usually just tries to eat an extra snack before PE to prevent lows, which she treats with juice, crackers, and glucose tablets when they occur.

Combined Regimen Changes

Katrina Anderson of Lancaster, Pennsylvania, takes gym classes in high school. For these, she usually cuts back on her pump boluses before exercising and eats carbohydrate. If her sugars are higher at the start of class, she takes in less carbohydrate, and if she gets low during class, she treats it with juice or Gatorade.

WALKING AND RACE WALKING

Walking is an endurance activity that uses your aerobic energy system. Your body uses fat and carbohydrate when you walk at a moderate pace, but it uses carbohydrate (both blood glucose and muscle glycogen) almost exclusively for brisk and race speeds. How long you walk will also make a difference, and you may need to alter your insulin, diet, or both for longer walks at certain times. For additional recommendations, refer to the section on hiking found in chapter 12. See table 8.7 for further instructions on walking and race walking.

General Adjustments by Diabetes Regimen

Because walking is such a common activity, an outline of some general recommendations for effective walking and hypoglycemia prevention for specific groups will be useful.

Table 8.7   Walking and Race Walking

Insulin: insulin pump	Insulin: basal-bolus regimen	Diet: insulin pump	Diet: basal-bolus regimen
• For slower or shorter walks, reduce your basal insulin minimally (0–20%). • For longer or brisker walking, cut back your basal rate during or boluses before exercise by 20–40%, or do both. • If you walk when your insulin levels are low, you may not have to make many adjustments to your insulin doses.	• For slower, shorter walks, modify your premeal insulin by 0–20%. • Reduce your insulin doses by 20–50% at meals before longer, faster walking. • Don't consider lowering your morning basal insulin doses unless your walking is going to be extremely prolonged (more than 3 hours).	• For slow-paced or short walks, you may only need 0–10 grams of carbohydrate. • For longer, more intense walks, increase carbohydrate intake by 5–15 grams per hour, depending on your insulin reductions.	• For shorter or slower walking, consume only 0–10 grams of carbohydrate. • Increase your carbohydrate intake by 10–15 grams per hour for longer, more intense walking, depending on your insulin levels during your walk.

Insulin Pump Users

If you use a pump, you have the most flexibility in controlling your insulin levels because you can suspend or reduce basal insulin when walking, giving you the most normal physiological response. If you walk at a slow or moderate pace (either walking comfortably or briskly), you may need to reduce your basal rates by only 25 percent. For more intense or extended walks, such as maintaining a race-walking pace or walking for an hour or more at a faster pace, you may lower them by 50 percent or more, along with taking smaller boluses for any snacks and meals that you have during or after walking.

Basal-Bolus Regimens

If you walk more than two or three hours after a meal, you'll have to make fewer regimen adjustments than you will if your exercise closely follows a meal. You may not need any adjustments for slow or short walks at any time, but longer or faster ones may require you to eat 15 to 30 grams of carbohydrate per hour because your muscles will be using more blood glucose as fuel. If you know that you'll be taking a substantial walk closely following a meal, you may want to lower your premeal injection of insulin by 25 to 50 percent to prevent lows.

Noninsulin and Oral Medication Users

If you take no meds, oral ones, or Byetta, walking may have very little effect on your blood sugar levels. In fact, in a recent study I conducted I found that when type 2 diabetic exercisers do 20 minutes of self-paced (slow to moderate) walking either before or after a meal, the after-meal activity keeps their blood sugars more stable, with less of a postmeal spike. If you make your own insulin, your levels of this hormone will be higher after you eat than before, and by walking then you get the double effect of exercise and insulin on your blood glucose levels. Any exercise also slows your digestion of food, which can additionally lower the glycemic effect of the foods that you eat before exercise. If you walk briskly first thing in the morning, though, your blood sugars may go up; to combat this, have a small snack before you start your exercise to cause the release of enough insulin to break the higher insulin resistance before breakfast.

Athlete Examples

The following examples illustrate a variety of changes to compensate for everything from slow strolling to race walking.

Insulin Changes Alone

A resident of Alpharetta, Georgia, Shirley Andrews plans her walks for after a meal, for which she reduces her bolus doses and her basal, letting her blood sugars climb to about 170 to 180 mg/dl (9.4 to 10 mmol/L). After 30 to 40 minutes of walking, her blood glucose level is normal again.

Emmy Parker of Atlanta, Georgia, cuts her basal rates by 50 percent during walking. Likewise, Esther Pinto from Brazil decreases hers by 50 to 70 percent for low-intensity walking on the beach.

Susan Greenback walks in her native Australia four to five times a week for about 45 minutes at a time. For this activity, she suspends her insulin pump for 30 minutes beforehand and during it.

Similarly, Christiane Engelbrecht of Brussels, Belgium, walks every day, for which she compensates by decreasing her meal bolus right before exercising. Because she usually spreads par to her bolus over several hours, she reduces the extended portion of it to compensate.

Monique Gordon, a Philadelphia, Pennsylvania, resident, lowers her basal rate by 0.1 unit per hour for walking her dog daily for about five hours total. She adjusts her carbohydrate only if she doesn't decrease her basal rate.

A type 2 diabetic race walker from Monument, Colorado, Paul Grogger uses intermediate-acting insulin only (Humulin N), which he takes in the morning and evening. For morning race-walking events, he does not take any insulin until after he finishes.

Diet Changes Alone

A type 2 diabetic speed walker, Mark Whitcombe from Orangeville, Ontario (Canada), takes only metformin, but walking, along with changing his diet to have a lower GI and eating frequent, small meals instead of large ones, has helped him lose more than 20 kilograms (45 pounds) and control his diabetes. Another type 2 exerciser, Robert Eicholz of Hollywood, California, also finds that taking a walk when his blood sugars are high brings them right back down to a more normal level.

For walking occasionally for two to three hours at a moderate pace, Sheri Ochs usually has to supplement with 5 to 15 grams of carbohydrate during the second and third hour, even when she starts walking at least three hours after her last injection of Humalog. For walking an hour or less at the same time of day, she doesn't need to make any adjustments.

For walking 2.5 miles (4 kilometers) daily, Sharon Smith of Tyler, Texas, may eat a small banana before walking to cover it. Alternatively, she reduces her Humalog by 1 unit if she plans to take her walk soon after eating.

A Georgia resident, type 2 diabetic exerciser Debra Simons finds that because she does her walking just before dinner, the meal she eats afterward is able to cover any drops in her blood sugars, although they're infrequent because she controls her diabetes with diet and exercise only.

Combined Regimen Changes

For Nordic walking (fitness walking done with specially designed poles in each hand), Sreten Dzebo of Ridderkerk, Netherlands, reduces the basal rate on his pump by 50 to 75 percent during the activity. In addition, he eats extra carbohydrate if his blood sugars are on the low side at the end of his walk.

Intensity, Duration, and Other Effects

Effect of temperature   For walking outdoors in the heat, Shirley Andrews has to lower her insulin even further because her blood sugars drop faster when it's hot outside.

WATER AEROBICS AND AQUATIC EXERCISE

Water aerobics and aquatic exercise are similar to aerobic dance except for their intensity. Workouts in the pool are not weight bearing as regular aerobic workouts are, making the water-based ones less intense for that reason alone. The good thing about water exercise is that it places less stress on your lower limb joints and feet, which can be particularly good if you have any neuropathy there. It is still aerobic in nature, with periods of greater and lesser intensity depending on how hard you want to work. Like most other aerobic activities, doing them first thing in the morning allows you to maintain your blood sugars more easily. Otherwise, lower your basal doses or cut back on premeal boluses and injections if you plan to do this activity within two hours of eating and want to prevent hypoglycemia. See table 8.8 for further instructions on water aerobics and aquatic exercise.

Athlete Examples

These examples show that both type 1 and type 2 diabetic athletes can safely engage in varying types of aquatic exercises and classes.

Diet Changes Alone

Joyce Meyers, a type 2 diabetic exerciser who uses Lantus and lives in Chicago, Illinois, tries to make sure that her blood sugars are high enough before she starts her swim aerobics to prevent lows. If she does feel one coming on, she eats a granola bar.

Similarly, Sheryl Necoche of San Diego eats a complex carbohydrate and protein before doing one hour of water aerobics and toning. Corpus Christi, Texas, resident Patricia L. Gomez started doing aquatics exercises when she injured her knee and couldn't walk for three months. For this activity, she doesn't adjust her doses of 70/30 insulin but instead snacks to prevent lows during and afterward, usually on peanut butter crackers with milk, orange juice, or Lifesavers.

Table 8.8 Water Aerobics and Aquatic Exercise

Insulin: insulin pump	Insulin: basal-bolus regimen	Diet: insulin pump	Diet: basal-bolus regimen
• Remove your pump altogether or reduce the basal rate by 25–50% during water aerobics (as long as your pump is waterproof). • For exercise following a meal, reduce both your bolus and basal rates by 15–40%.	• Decrease rapid-acting insulin by 15–40% when water aerobics follows your meal. • You shouldn't need to make changes to your basal insulin doses for this activity.	• Consume 0–15 grams of carbohydrate per hour, depending on how much you lower your insulin. • With insulin reductions, you may not need any extra carbohydrate.	• Increase your carbohydrate intake by 10–15 grams per hour. • If your insulin levels are low, you may need only 0–10 grams for water aerobics.

Combined Regimen Changes

A Jensen Beach, Florida, resident, Judy Unger does laps in the pool using Styrofoam barbells with various techniques (e.g., body row, body bicycle, and kicking) for about 25 minutes at a time. After finding that removing her pump completely led to hyperglycemia, she now keeps it on (yes, it's waterproof) and simply lowers her basal or boluses to compensate. She won't exercise with a blood glucose over 180 mg/dl (10 mmol/L), and if it's below 100 (5.5) when she is ready to start, she eats 15 to 20 grams of carbohydrate.

WEIGHT AND RESISTANCE CIRCUIT TRAINING

Weight training involves short, powerful repetitions and mainly uses your anaerobic energy sources (stored phosphagens and muscle glycogen). More often than not, weight training causes greater release of glucose-raising hormones than most aerobic activities do. Doing any intense activity, as you know by now, may require you to make minimal adjustments to prevent lows, at least during the activity, and your sugars may actually go up instead of down. Doing a prolonged weight-training session, though, can use up a lot of muscle glycogen, thus increasing your risk of later-onset hypoglycemia, even if your blood glucose rises initially.

If you do your workout with lower levels of insulin on board, such as two or more hours after eating or in the early morning, you may even need to take some insulin to bring yourself back down if you don't make your own. Many people often do weight training in combination with an aerobic workout on a stationary cycle, rowing machine, treadmill, or other type of exercise equipment to help reverse this rise. An alternative is to do circuit weight training, which usually emphasizes a greater number of repetitions with lower resistance and is slightly more aerobic in nature (meaning that it usually causes less of a rise in your blood glucose levels). See table 8.9 for further instructions on weight and resistance circuit training.

Athlete Examples

You'll see from these examples that how you choose to do your weight training affects the changes that you'll need to make to maintain control over your blood glucose levels.

Insulin Changes Alone

Guy Hornsby, a masters weightlifter from Morgantown, West Virginia, rarely has to make adjustments for his morning or afternoon training routine, although both tend to raise his blood sugars by 20 to 40 mg/dl (1.1 to 2.2 mmol/L) because of their intensity. If intense training raises his sugars more than 40 mg/dl, he gives some rapid-acting insulin to bring it down. Otherwise, he needs insulin adjustments only if he is sick or injured and can't train as he normally does. He never exercises within two hours of eating, taking Symlin, and injecting any insulin other than basal Lantus.

Table 8.9 Weight and Resistance Circuit Training

Insulin: insulin pump	Insulin: basal-bolus regimen	Diet: insulin pump	Diet: basal-bolus regimen
• Maintain your normal basal rates, reduce them slightly, or disconnect your pump during this activity, depending on your intensity and duration of lifting. • When weightlifting without doing any aerobic work, keep your basal rates the same to avoid increases in your blood sugars. • If you combine weight training with an aerobic workout, you may choose to disconnect your pump during both activities if less than an hour (any longer, though, and you may need some basal insulin). • When weightlifting after a meal, reduce your premeal bolus slightly, by 10–20%.	• You will need minimal changes to your rapid-acting insulin doses to maintain your blood sugar levels during this activity. • For weight training after a meal, prolonged training of 2 hours or more, or training combined with an aerobic workout, reduce rapid-acting insulin by 10–30%. • Doing this activity alone (with no aerobic workout) when your insulin levels are low may actually cause your blood sugars to rise, for which you may need 0.5–2 units afterward. • You will likely not need to change your basal insulin doses for this activity.	• For workouts shorter than an hour, you may not need any extra carbohydrate. • For longer training sessions of 2 hours or more, consume 0–20 grams of carbohydrate per hour.	• For shorter workouts, you may need only a small amount of carbohydrate (0–10 grams) per hour. • For prolonged training, consider an increase in carbohydrate of 5–20 grams per hour, depending on your workout intensity and circulating insulin levels.

A resident of Loughborough, England (United Kingdom), Kathryn Latham tries not to do any exercise right after meals for which she injected Humalog. If she has to work out shortly afterward, she skips her premeal insulin. She finds that weight training has a much different effect on her blood sugars than going for a run does. They're much more stable during weight-training exercises, which for her include plyometrics (e.g., jump lunges, leaps, and bounding).

Brian Worsley of Athens, Ohio, doesn't make many adjustments for weight training, but it has a prolonged effect on his blood sugars afterward. He either reduces the next dose of Humalog he takes for food or skips it to compensate.

If doing strength training alone, Susan Greenback of Australia leaves her basal rate alone during the activity. But if she's doing an exercise class at the gym that incorporates some weight training, she turns her pump off during the activity.

Janet Switzer of Millstadt, Illinois, finds that when she lifts weights with a starting blood glucose level above 110 mg/dl (6.1 mmol/L), she needs to give herself a bolus of 2 to 4 units of NovoLog. If she doesn't, her blood sugars go up from this activity.

Diet Changes Alone

For weight training two hours a week year round, Martin Desbois of Montreal, Quebec (in Canada), makes no adjustments to his insulin. But he likes to eat carbohydrate without bolusing beforehand so that his blood sugars are on the rise when he starts to exercise. That way his blood sugars remain stable during the activity.

Mike McMahon of Petersburg, Alaska, tries to start his workout with a blood glucose reading of 120 to 180 mg/dl (6.7 to 10 mmol/L). He keeps apple juice and glucose tablets close by to take as needed. Usually, he eats breakfast and waits an hour before starting his workout because he prefers to have an emptier stomach when working out. He also finds that having higher blood sugars makes him unmotivated to do his usual activity.

Combined Regimen Changes

New York City resident Ed Liebowitz decreases his basal rate by 50 percent while doing heavy weight training. In addition, he eats a Clif Builder's Bar before working out.

Bob Paxson of California generally doesn't make adjustments in his basal rate for weight training. The exception is when he's having a low blood sugar level that won't go away, even with food and glucose, in which case he may reduce his basal somewhat during the activity.

Intensity, Duration, and Other Effects

Effect of exercise intensity Scott McKinnon from Midlothian, Texas, finds that circuit weight training usually causes his blood glucose to drop. If he rests two to three minutes between sets, however, the decrease is less severe.

New York City resident Robert deBrauwere finds that heavy lifting causes his blood sugars to spike rather than decrease. To compensate, he takes a small dose of NovoLog before lifting and often immediately afterward as well.

Lorrie DiCesare of Chicago, Illinois, lowers her basal rate to 75 percent of normal during weight training, although for running she suspends it completely.

YOGA AND STRETCHING

Both of these activities are low level and require minimal muscular effort. Most stretches, especially in yoga, are static (involving no movement) and are held for a while. Because diabetes can often limit joint and muscle flexibility, doing stretching at least two or three times a week can be extremely beneficial. You shouldn't need to do anything special to compensate. Even yoga classes that last for an hour or more will use minimal amounts of blood glucose.

Athlete Examples

Doing yoga classes, particularly in a hot environment, may require more adjustments than just practicing yoga or stretching on your own.

Insulin Changes Alone

Roberta Voulon of Paris, France, usually does yoga in the morning after breakfast for about an hour. For this activity, she often reduces her prebreakfast NovoRapid by 1 unit (a 10 to 25 percent decrease in her dose).

Combined Regimen Changes

David Weingard, a resident of New York City, practices Bikram ("hot") yoga, ideally practiced in a room heated to 105 degrees Fahrenheit (40.5 degrees Celsius) with a humidity of 40 percent. He keeps his basal rates normal to compensate for his higher insulin resistance in the mornings (when he does yoga), and he ensures that he stays highly hydrated to prevent his blood glucose levels from going higher during the activity. About 50 minutes into each 90-minute yoga session, he drinks fruit water that contains 31 grams of carbohydrate, and he boluses using his normal insulin-to-carbohydrate ratio (1:15).

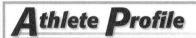

Athlete Profile

Name: Zippora Karz

Hometown: Northridge, California, USA

Diabetes history: Type 1 diabetes diagnosed in 1987 (at age 21)

Sport or activity: Professional ballerina (retired), present day repetiteur (person who stages the ballets) for the George Balanchine Trust, ballet teacher and coach

Greatest athletic achievement: Former soloist ballerina with the New York City Ballet (from age 27 until retirement in 1999); I was featured as the sugar plum fairy in *The Nutcracker,* as well as having soloist roles in Balanchine's *Apollo* and *Sleeping Beauty* and many others.

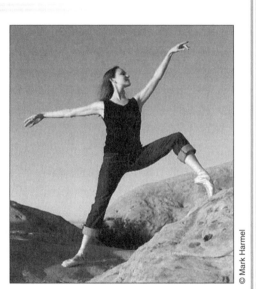

© Mark Harmel

Current insulin regimen: Levemir (for basal needs) and NovoLog

Training tips: Always check your blood sugar levels before a workout. Never assume that you know what your blood sugar levels are. Many times I thought I was low, but I was actually extremely high due to performance anxiety. I also had to learn not to overshoot before a performance because exercise increases insulin sensitivity. It was easier to eat snacks with more protein rather than a lot of carbohydrate before the performance so that I didn't need as much insulin. It's always better to be slightly on the high side than risking going too low.

One time in my early years of performing with diabetes, I felt my blood sugars dropping severely right before a key performance. My younger sister was also a member of the company then. Because of my low, she had decided to put my costume on and try to perform my role, but she didn't know it and there wasn't time to teach her, so we quickly abandoned that idea. I had taken enough glucose tablets and knew I'd be OK, but it was scary for us both. My blood sugars began to rise in time, but it was midway through my performance before I no longer felt lightheaded. From that experience, I learned never to dose with any faster-acting insulin before a performance unless I was extremely high.

If my blood sugars were ever a little above normal on my day off (Mondays, when I did just yoga), I corrected them more confidently because I wasn't going to exercise and risk going too low. The lingering effects of the exercise from the night before still had to be taken into account.

Typical daily and weekly training and diabetes regimen:

▶ **Typical training day (when dancing professionally):** My daily schedule was different each day according to which ballets were performed each night. The typical day routine was to have breakfast at 9:00 a.m., get to the theatre to stretch before class, do a technique class and warm-up from 10:30 a.m. to noon, and then rehearse until 6:00 p.m. with one hour for lunch at a different time each day. At 6:00, I would proceed to my dressing room to put on stage makeup and eat a snack. Performances lasted from 8:00 to 11:00 p.m. at the Lincoln Center, followed by dinner at 11:30 p.m. My insulin was mostly basal, and I would eat protein snacks throughout to avoid having to take much (if any) faster acting insulins that would make my blood sugars go low during the day.

▶ **Currently:** As a teacher, I work out every morning for about an hour, doing a combination of yoga, stretching, ballet, and minitrampoline. I test before, during, and after my workout. I'm better able to adjust how much strenuous movement I do, so if I feel on the low side during classes, I don't demonstrate as much and talk more. I still test throughout the day but don't have to juggle the highs and lows caused by extreme exercise and performing.

Other hobbies and interests: Long before I had diabetes, I was passionate about health, both physical and environmental. Diabetes forced me to take my interest in nutrition and ways to eat healthfully and explore it fully. I really love eating healthy foods that taste good. My childhood passions were the animals and the environment. I've recently teamed with other environmentalists and am working on ways to make a difference. Although I rode and owned horses before my professional career—and will get back to that soon—my recent joy has been rescuing Marley, a tabby cat who jumps higher than Baryshnikov. I love my time with my friends, my boyfriend, and my family.

Good diabetes and exercise story: Although every ballet was different, I usually was on stage for a time and then ran off into the wings before the next entrance. When I was in the wings waiting for the next entrance, I would do a quick blood sugar check, if there was time and if I felt low. It was much easier for me to hide the candy in my mouth when I ran back on stage if the performance was a dramatic one and not a happy one with a big smile. My forehead could look pained with my mouth shut and the sweet intact.

CHAPTER **9**

Endurance Sports

Whether you want to run a marathon, cycle across the country as fast as possible, or compete in a full Ironman triathlon, you'll be in good company. Even becoming an Olympian is entirely possible. By now, who hasn't heard of swimmer Gary Hall Jr., the fastest swimmer in U.S. history and worldwide, a 3-time Olympian, 10-time Olympic medalist (wining five gold, three silver, and two bronze by 2004), and an American record holder in 50-meter freestyle? Most of his workouts are highly aerobic with interspersed sprinting or harder intervals. The same goes for the activity of Team Type 1, the diabetic cycling team that has, hands-down, won the ultrachallenging Race Across America (RAAM) on several occasions.

Endurance sports primarily rely on your aerobic energy system. Some aspects of the sports and activities included in this chapter, however, would also qualify as endurance–power sports (discussed in the next chapter), such as sprinting 50 meters in swimming or doing all-out time trials in cycling. Whether you want to become the world's fastest swimmer or a top ultradistance runner, you'll find that diabetic exercisers have taken on all these grueling events just to prove that they can do anything that they want to do despite having diabetes. Their examples, as well as others relevant to more modest exercisers, are included in this chapter, which covers activities like cross country running and skiing, cycling, marathons, running and jogging, soccer, swimming, triathlons, and ultraendurance events and training.

GENERAL RECOMMENDATIONS FOR ENDURANCE SPORTS

Your body can use carbohydrate, fat, and protein to make ATP to fuel your muscular activity over prolonged periods, but how intense and how long your workouts are largely determine the fuel mix. For example, during less intense activities like slow swimming, your body can use more fats (triglycerides and free fatty acids in blood), along with some muscle glycogen and blood glucose. When you're working out harder, your muscles use little fat, relying mostly on carbohydrate—muscle glycogen and, to a lesser extent, blood glucose. Typically your blood sugar consists of only about five grams of carbohydrate total—the equivalent of about 20 calories' worth, or enough to run .2 mile (.3 kilometer) or less—although your liver is constantly working to replenish and maintain that amount. Depleting your muscle glycogen changes the fuels that your body may be using, causing you to slow your pace and

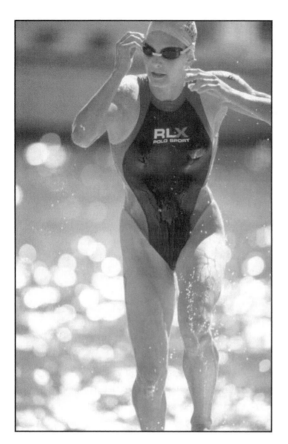

When exercising long and hard, like when competing in a triathlon, you'll need to make a combination of insulin reductions and carbohydrate increases to maintain your blood sugar levels.

rely more on fat or to start using your blood sugar at a faster rate. You can generally delay fatigue by taking in carbohydrate regularly during any prolonged activities. Doing so is especially important to prevent lows as your glycogen stores diminish.

Intense efforts use carbohydrate almost exclusively, and you can also revert back to temporarily relying more on your lactic acid system whenever you increase your pace or start using faster muscle fibers, which happens as you run and cycle up hills or sprint for the finish line. Doing prolonged events can draw on your protein stores, too: up to 10 to 15 percent of your energy comes from breaking down protein during extremely long events, although for shorter ones lasting an hour or less, it's usually 5 percent or less. For a refresher on the energy systems and fuel sources used for different types of exercise, refer to chapter 2.

When you're exercising long and hard, you'll need to make a combination of insulin reductions (shown in table 2.4), if you use it, and carbohydrate increases (table 2.3) to maintain your blood sugar levels, depending on where they start. Exercising with minimal insulin on board will help prevent lows, but for extended events you will definitely need to eat adequate amounts of carbohydrate during the activity, just as nondiabetic competitors do. Although regular training increases your body's use of fat somewhat, you will likely have to reduce your overall insulin doses, both basally and for food intake after training, because of enhancements in your insulin action. Reduce oral doses of meds only under the advice of your physician if you start to experience more frequent low blood sugars with regular training. For more information about diabetic medications and those that most increase your hypoglycemia risk, refer to chapter 3.

GENERAL ADJUSTMENTS BY DIABETES REGIMEN

You may need to supplement with 15 to 45 grams of carbohydrate every 30 to 60 minutes during prolonged activity, depending on its intensity and duration. The best way to learn how much works for you is by measuring your blood sugar responses during the exercise. You will need more carbohydrate when you exercise during an insulin peak if you do not sufficiently reduce your insulin doses, as well as extra afterward and even at bedtime to prevent a drop in your blood sugar later as your glycogen stores are being replaced over the next 24 to 48 hours.

In general, your carbohydrate requirement will not be as great during short, intense activities (see table 2.3). Although your body uses more glycogen as fuel during such activities, their intensity causes greater release of your glucose-raising hormones like adrenaline, which help maintain your blood sugars. Lowering your insulin doses will decrease your carbohydrate needs.

One last point to realize is that if you have seriously overstressed your body with an event or long-distance training, you may not be as insulin sensitive as you would expect to be for the next day or two. If you end up with delayed-onset muscle soreness, your body won't be able to replace glycogen until your muscles repair and rebuild themselves, and you may actually experience some insulin resistance while that process is going on.

Insulin Pump Users

If you are a pump user, you may lower your basal insulin during an activity by 0 to 100 percent, depending on its intensity and duration and how much carbohydrate you want to eat. In addition, you can reduce preworkout meal boluses by 10 to 75 percent if you are exercising closely after the meal. Your blood sugars will generally be easier to maintain if you don't have any rapid-acting insulin within 2 or 3 hours of starting your event or workout. Afterward, you may need to reduce your meal boluses by 25 to 50 percent, along with your basal rates (10 to 25 percent) for 2 to 6 hours, and up to 24 hours afterward to prevent later-onset and nocturnal hypoglycemia.

Basal-Bolus Regimens

For endurance activities you can reduce your preworkout doses of rapid-acting insulin by 10 to 75 percent, depending on how long and how hard you'll be work-ing, and increase your carbohydrate intake. You may also benefit from reducing your morning dose of basal insulin (if you take some then) by 10 to 30 percent before an extended activity. If you exercise when your insulin levels are lower, at least two or three hours after your last injection of rapid-acting insulin, then you will likely need fewer adjustments. Following prolonged endurance exercise, you may have to reduce your premeal insulin doses by 25 to 50 percent, lower your bedtime doses of basal insulin (10 to 30 percent) to prevent nighttime lows, and consume extra carbohydrate.

Noninsulin and Oral Medication Users

If you don't use insulin, you probably aren't any more likely to develop hypogly-cemia during a prolonged event than a nondiabetic athlete is. You'll still want to check your blood sugars to find out how your body responds. Ask your diabetes physician about lowering your doses of medications if you start seeing significant drops during or after your activities. You should still supplement with carbohydrate during extended exercise, just as nondiabetic participants do. If you use Byetta and find that it affects how you feel or perform during endurance exercise, check with your physician about possibly reducing your dose or adjusting the time of day when you take it.

Intensity, Duration, and Other Effects

Many variables can affect your blood sugar responses to an endurance activity. How hard and how long you work will definitely have a significant effect. In general, more intense activities done for a shorter time will result in a smaller drop in your blood sugars compared with prolonged, slower activities. Exercising when your insulin levels are lower—either first thing in the morning or before meals—requires substantially fewer regimen changes. Your starting blood sugar levels will affect your need for regimen changes; you'll need fewer changes when they start in a higher range. In addition, regular endurance training will likely enhance your insulin action, resulting in reduced need for insulin regardless of your type of diabetes or your medication regimen.

CROSS COUNTRY RUNNING

This competitive sport stresses endurance performance. Your body will primarily use muscle glycogen and blood glucose during it, and the harder you run, the more you'll use up. To compensate, you'll need to alter your insulin doses, carbohydrate intake, or both, depending on factors such as the time of day that you exercise, your starting blood sugar levels, and your insulin levels during your run. More intense running (such as during competitions) may temporarily raise your blood sugars, but doing it for long enough will often bring it down quickly, more so during practices than competitions because of the lesser anxiety associated with nonrace days. You'll likely need to take lower overall insulin doses during the cross country season because of the heightened insulin action you will experience from regular training, but if you are injured and have to take some time off, your insulin requirements will go up. See table 9.1 for further instructions on cross country running.

Athlete Examples

These athlete examples show that cross country running usually requires a combination of dietary and insulin adjustments to compensate.

Combined Regimen Changes

Blair Ryan of San Diego, California, is a collegiate triathlete and has run cross country and track. Before early morning races, she eats a bagel with peanut butter and covers it with a normal insulin bolus, but she aims to have her blood sugars around 180 milligrams per deciliter (mg/dl) or 10 millimolar (mmol/L), when she starts her prerace warm-ups.

During the cross country season, Joe Fiorucci of Shirley, New York, finds that he has to lower his overall Lantus insulin doses. In addition, he eats just enough food to prevent lows during practices and meets, relying on taking in Gatorade, SlimFast, or meal bars before exercising.

Svati Narula of Gaithersburg, Maryland, participates in high school cross country running. To compensate for practices, she takes her pump off while running and has a snack beforehand, such as Gatorade, half a peanut butter and jelly sandwich,

Table 9.1   Cross Country Running

Insulin: insulin pump	Insulin: basal-bolus regimen	Diet: insulin pump	Diet: basal-bolus regimen
• Reduce your basal insulin during practices or competition by 25–100%, depending on how much carbohydrate you eat. • Reduce your prepractice meal boluses by 25–50% for exercise closely following a meal. • For morning meets involving shorter and more intense runs, consider reducing precompetition boluses by 10–30%, but keep in mind that your blood sugars could go up. • Reduce your basal insulin doses during the season by 10–25%.	• For regular practices, reduce your insulin doses before exercise by 25–50% to lower the need for extra carbohydrate. • For morning meets (involving intense running), reduce your precompetition rapid-acting insulin by 10–30%; take a small amount of insulin afterward to lower your sugars, if needed. • Reduce your basal insulin doses by 10–25% during the season (compared with the off-season).	• Eat 15–30 grams of carbohydrate for every 30 minutes of running, depending on how much you reduce your insulin and where your blood sugar starts. • More intense running (competitions), especially in the morning, may require less (if any) carbohydrate because of greater release of glucose-raising hormones when insulin resistant.	• Eat an extra 15–30 grams of carbohydrate for every 30 minutes of running, depending on your blood sugars and your insulin reductions. • You will probably have to eat less for morning competitions because of greater release of glucose-raising hormones and higher insulin resistance at that time of day.

or a banana. She finds that her carbohydrate requirement before a run depends on how much insulin is in her system; if she hasn't taken any boluses for a few hours beforehand, she doesn't need to eat that much because her blood sugars stay stable during the run. During meets, her blood sugars rise more because of stress, and she has to fight the urge to eat beforehand.

Michelle Simes of Fountain Valley, California, participates in cross country running in high school. Her strategy is to make sure that her blood sugars are at least 200 mg/dl (11.1 mmol/L) before she starts a run, which she accomplishes by eating some carbohydrate. Before disconnecting from her pump for the run, she gives one-fourth of the usual basal that she'll be missing. If she's over 300 (16.7) before starting, she takes a correction bolus and waits for her blood sugars to drop before she runs.

Intensity, Duration, and Other Effects

Effect of emotional stress   On race days, Blair Ryan fights to keep her blood sugars under control before racing because the more nervous she is, the more her sugars creep up over time because of the effects of adrenaline release. She gives 1-unit boluses to bring them back down to about 160 mg/dl (8.8 mmol/L), usually 1 unit for every 80 mg/dl (4.4 mmol/L) above 180 (10). On any given day, if her adrenaline release is less, she may need to drink some fast-acting carbohydrate.

CROSS-COUNTRY SKIING

Cross-country skiing is one of the best overall aerobic exercises that you can do. Athletes who participate regularly in this activity are extremely fit aerobically. "Skiing" on a ski fitness machine (see chapter 9) can bestow similar benefits, although most people tend not to sustain the indoor activity for as long as they would ski outdoors. Changes in your diabetes regimen will depend mainly on how long you're skiing and the environmental conditions, including the temperature, windchill, and snow conditions.

The duration of your cross-country skiing is the most important factor affecting regimen changes. Skiing longer uses more muscle glycogen and increases your risk of later-onset hypoglycemia. You will likely need both to reduce your insulin and to increase your carbohydrate intake for skiing longer than an hour. Another factor is the skiing conditions on any given day. Your body will use more carbohydrate when it's cold or when you're working hard against a strong wind or stickier snow; in these cases, you'll need to adjust your diabetes regimen more to compensate. See table 9.2 for further instructions on cross-country skiing.

Athlete Examples

The following real-life examples show that you can make many combinations of regimen changes to compensate for cross-country skiing.

Diet Changes Alone

An avid type 2 diabetic exerciser, Thomas Gallagher of Madison, Wisconsin, uses cross-country skiing to control his blood sugars during the winter and cycling during the other times of the year, along with oral doses of metformin. He finds that

Table 9.2   Cross-Country Skiing

Insulin: insulin pump	Insulin: basal-bolus regimen	Diet: insulin pump	Diet: basal-bolus regimen
• For skiing an hour or less, reduce your basal rates by 50–100%, alone or in combination with a 25–40% reduction in your meal boluses before exercise. • For skiing 2 hours or more, reduce both your basal rates during the activity and your boluses pre- and possibly postexercise.	• For skiing an hour or less, reduce your rapid-acting insulin dose by 10–25% for meals before the activity. • For longer durations (2 hours or more), reduce your doses by 25–50% before and possibly following your workout. • Reduce your morning basal insulin doses (if you take them) by 20–30% for prolonged or all-day skiing.	• For skiing for short periods, increase your carbohydrate intake by 15–20 grams per hour, especially if you don't reduce your basal insulin or boluses much. • For longer durations, you may need 15–30 grams of carbohydrate per hour.	• Increasing your carbohydrate intake by 15–30 grams per hour may replace reductions in your rapid-acting insulin for shorter-duration skiing. • Consume 20–30 grams of carbohydrate per hour during longer-duration skiing and reduce your insulin doses.

this type of skiing is the best for lowering and keeping his blood sugars in check. Although some winters haven't had enough snow, he has completed 18 American Birkies (51-kilometer cross-country ski races) to date. During long skiing or cycling exercise, he drinks Heed or eats Clif Bars to keep his energy up.

Combined Regimen Changes

A world-class cross-country skier from Sormano, Italy, Mauro Sormani also participates in ski mountaineering, high-altitude mountaineering, free climbing, and more. Before skiing, he usually takes only 70 percent of his normal boluses for food and cuts back on his basal rate by the same amount. If his blood sugars ever start to go below 150 mg/dl (8.3 mmol/L) while skiing cross-country, he eats additional carbohydrate.

Before any intense exercise, Deb Martin of West Branch, Michigan, usually eats a meal without taking a bolus. For cross-country skiing, she eats at least 30 grams of carbohydrate during the first 60 to 90 minutes of this activity. She also consumes 15 grams more per hour to keep her blood sugars stable because she finds the exercise to be intense. By way of contrast, she doesn't have to eat anything to cover downhill skiing.

For cross-country skiing and other aerobic activities, Marc Konvisser of Orchard Lake, Michigan, lowers the basal rate on his pump down to 65 to 70 percent of normal if he exercises for over an hour. He also uses a half bolus for carbohydrate and drinks Gatorade.

A resident of Vail, Colorado, Kerry White participates in Nordic skiing (classic and skate), as well as backcountry touring. She has also competed in 90-kilometer Nordic ski races. For these activities, she avoids taking any Symlin or reduces her doses for meals, and she cuts back on her basal Lantus by 1 to 3 units on the morning of a race or a long workout. During exercise she uses her body's response to determine what to do with her food intake and insulin.

For Lisa Seaman of Silverthorne, Colorado, skiing includes Nordic, backcountry, and downhill. One adjustment that she makes for the first two types is to lower her basal insulin while skiing. If her blood sugars are below 150 mg/dl (8.3 mmol/L) at the start, she eats a snack as long as she plans to exercise for longer than 30 minutes. She usually checks where her sugars are after 30 to 45 minutes to see where they're headed and to prevent lows. She finds that she doesn't recognize lows as easily when she's skiing, and she knows that she comes out of her lows quicker if she treats them early with Clif Shot Bloks, Gu gels, or raisins. Another challenge with skiing is keeping her insulin warm enough. She wears an OmniPod pump and usually tucks it in beneath her clothes during this activity.

CYCLING

This activity is generally aerobic in nature, although some cycling events involve sprinting and hill climbing, both of which rely more on anaerobic energy mostly from the lactic acid system. Prolonged, hard cycling will use almost all carbohydrate, both blood glucose and muscle glycogen, and will require you to adjust more to keep your blood sugars in line.

Cycling intensity and duration, timing of exercise, and starting blood sugar levels will affect your blood sugar responses. For longer-duration cycling (two hours or longer), you will likely need to eat more carbohydrate and lower your insulin (if you take any). Longer rides will also use up more of your muscle glycogen stores, thus increasing your risk for low blood sugars later. If you cycle with lower insulin levels, either first thing in the morning or before meals, then your blood sugars may not drop as much. If they're high in the morning (more than 200 mg/dl, or 11.1 mmol/L), you may even need a small dose of rapid-acting insulin before exercise to prevent a rise in blood sugars if you cycle for an hour or less (or if you don't take insulin, make sure to eat something before exercise to stimulate insulin release). Higher blood sugars later in the day will usually respond better to exercise, and your blood sugars will decrease more then. See table 9.3 for further instructions on cycling.

Athlete Examples

Athletes decrease their insulin and increase their food intake to compensate for cycling. Prolonged cycling workouts invariably require greater regimen changes. For additional related examples, refer to the section on mountain biking in chapter 12.

Table 9.3   Cycling

Insulin: insulin pump	Insulin: basal-bolus regimen	Diet: insulin pump	Diet: basal-bolus regimen
• For shorter cycling distances, reduce your basal rates by 25–50% or suspend your pump. • Supplement with less carbohydrate for cycling in the morning before breakfast because of higher insulin resistance at that time of day. • For longer cycling (1–4 hours or more), reduce boluses by 30–50% before exercise, as well as for meals immediately afterward, depending on carbohydrate and basal insulin changes. • Consider reducing your basal rates starting 30–60 minutes before exercise and keep them lower for several hours (or even overnight) following longer rides to prevent lows.	• Exercise 2–3 hours after your last rapid-acting insulin to lower your circulating levels. • If cycling soon after a meal, reduce your rapid-acting insulin doses by 10–30% for shorter or more intense cycling. • For longer-duration cycling, reduce your preexercise meal doses by 30–50%, as well as your postexercise meals by 10–30% to prevent hypoglycemia later in the day. • After long cycling bouts, consider reducing your evening basal insulin doses by 10–20%.	• Consume up to 15–30 grams of additional carbohydrate every 30–60 minutes of cycling, depending on your exercise intensity. • Consume extra carbohydrate after prolonged cycling to prevent postexercise lows. • Consider eating an extra bedtime snack, especially if you don't lower your basal rates overnight, following prolonged bouts of cycling.	• You may need 15–30 grams of carbohydrate per 30–60 minutes of cycling, depending on your insulin reductions, especially if cycling after a meal. • For shorter cycling distances, you may not need much carbohydrate, especially if you exercise more than 2–3 hours after your last dose of rapid-acting insulin. • Consume extra carbohydrate following prolonged cycling to prevent postexercise hypoglycemia. • Consider eating an extra bedtime snack (especially if you don't lower your basal rates overnight) after long workouts.

Diet Changes Alone

Chris Mailing of Northbrook, Illinois, doesn't adjust his insulin during higher-intensity cycling. Instead, he eats an extra 30 grams of carbohydrate at the start of a ride and then takes in another 15 grams or so per hour.

A type 1.5 diabetic cyclist controlled on oral meds only, Robert King of Hanover, Pennsylvania, increases his carbohydrate intake during the hour before a ride and brings dilute sports drinks and glucose tablets with him as a precaution. He also eats low-sugar whey protein bars during extended rides of 45 to 60 miles (70 to 100 kilometers).

Similarly, Alan Miller, a resident of Woodinville, Washington, who has metformin-controlled type 2 diabetes, sometimes eats an oatmeal breakfast or a peanut butter and jelly sandwich right before a long ride of 50 to 100 miles (80 to 160 kilometers).

Thomas Gallagher of Wisconsin only uses metformin, so regular cycling is his main way to lower elevated blood sugars, and he bikes an average of 10,000 miles (16,000 kilometers) a year. In the summer, when he cycles over 300 miles (500 kilometers) a week, he can eat almost anything he wants without much effect on his blood sugars, but during the late fall and early spring when his cycling time is limited, he has to be more careful about his carbohydrate intake.

Another type 2 diabetic cyclist, Anne Moyers of Vancouver, Washington, usually eats about 15 grams of carbohydrate for every hour of intense cycling that she does. Although she takes only Starlix as a diabetes medication, she has experienced lows during strenuous cycling that includes speed or hills. She often has a 12-ounce (360-milliliter) or larger latte following a ride.

Combined Regimen Changes

A Boulder, Colorado, resident, Sara Kirkse usual keeps her basal rates the same during cycling but takes boluses that are only 50 to 75 percent of normal. If she starts trending low on a long ride, she drops her basal rate first to 75 percent of normal and then down to 50. Drinking whole milk before rides also helps her prevent lows during the activity, as does eating about 45 grams of carbohydrate per hour, more for long or strenuous rides.

San Diego, California, resident Peter Nerothin lowers his basal rate by 20 to 80 percent for rides lasting longer than 60 minutes. In addition, he consumes 60 to 90 grams of carbohydrate per hour without boluses. Typically, he reduces his basal dose incrementally as his heart and metabolic rates rise during cycling. He may not lower it until an hour after he starts; by two hours, he's usually down to 40 percent of normal; and by four hours, it's at only 20 to 30 percent of where it started. How quickly he lowers it depends on how active he has been during the hours and days leading up to his ride. Afterward, he boluses with 1 or 2 units, depending on what he consumed during his cool-down (taking the GI of the carbohydrate into account). More often than not, he takes another 2 or 3 units as a dual wave before eating some greasy, high-protein foods. His basal rate may stay reduced by 20 to 50 percent for up to 36 hours afterward, depending on how long and hard he works out, and he gradually increases it back to normal depending on how often he's having postexercise lows.

Charles Ferguson Sr. of Marshall, Missouri, uses the lowest of his three basal settings on his pump (a 20 to 25 percent reduction from normal) during long bike rides and eats some carbohydrate every 30 minutes. After 50-mile (80-kilometer) bike rides, he can remain more insulin sensitive for up to 5 days.

For easy rides, Tom Shearer of Carlsbad, California, sets his basal rates at least 50 percent lower starting 30 minutes beforehand. For hard rides, he has to lower it 75 percent or take off his pump, but he has to give a bolus about 15 minutes before stopping (for rides of 3 hours or longer) to replace most of his basal insulin. Otherwise, his sugars spike afterward. He usually eats at least once per hour during rides and drinks some Gatorade with his water.

David Panofsky of Madison, Wisconsin, focuses on mountaineering now but at one point was a competitive cyclist. For that activity, he made adjustments based on the length of his training rides. He lowered his basal rates by 60 percent during rides lasting up to three hours and supplemented with about 45 grams of carbohydrate. For longer rides, he used a 70 percent reduction and consumed 15 to 25 grams of carbohydrate per hour beyond the initial three.

A resident of Melbourne, Victoria (Australia), Jennifer Roche reduces her pre-meal NovoRapid by about 25 percent before long bike rides. She doesn't adjust her insulin that much, though, because she prefers to eat extra instead. She often eats toast and baked beans before rides, or she may drink orange juice or eat a handful of jelly beans, both of which shoot her blood sugars way up without exercise. She doesn't adjust her Levemir doses, though.

During road biking, Linda Olson of Eagan, Minnesota, sets her pump on a temporary basal that is 50 to 60 percent of normal, and she eats at least 30 grams of carbohydrate before she starts with a bolus that is 80 to 100 percent of her normal one. She again boluses at the end of exercise, this time about 50 percent of the basal insulin that she missed during the last two hours of her ride, to avoid a postexercise spike in her blood sugars. She doesn't eat much afterward, and five to six hours later she has to lower her basal rate the same amount again to prevent later-onset lows.

Gastroparesis adds another variable to the cycling that Keith LeMar of Memphis, Tennessee, does. Before biking 30 to 42 miles (48 to 68 kilometers), he has to reduce his basal rate by 70 percent starting an hour beforehand. He eats about 80 grams of carbohydrate (a PowerBar and Gatorade) without a bolus because he won't take any insulin before riding, and he consumes an additional 20 to 30 grams every 10 miles (16 kilometers), or about 40 minutes, of riding.

A type 2 exerciser from Berkeley, California, Janis Eggleston modifies her use of both Byetta and metformin for long-distance cycling. She can't cycle with any meds on board without developing hypoglycemia, so she takes no Byetta at all when biking longer distances of 65 miles (105 kilometers) or more in a day, and she takes metformin only at night. During cycling, she consumes up to 250 calories per hour of Hammer Perpetuem and gels.

Linda Frischmeyer, a resident of Vancouver, Washington, makes adjustments based on the duration of her ride. For rides of two hours or less, she consumes extra carbohydrate but usually doesn't change her insulin. For rides lasting longer than two hours, she reduces her basal insulin by about 50 percent and consumes an extra 60 grams of carbohydrate in the first hour; during each subsequent hour, she eats 30 grams of carbohydrate.

A Flagler Beach, Florida, resident, Jim Moore takes a reduced bolus (1.5 to 2 units less) for the meal before cycling and may decrease his basal rate during the ride by 40 to 50 percent, depending on its length and intensity. To start the ride with a blood glucose level of about 180 mg/dl (10 mmol/L), he increases his carbohydrate intake before and during cycling. He checks his blood sugars every hour or so and eats energy gels or bars as needed to prevent lows.

For Australia native Darcy Hughes, road cycling for five hours or longer requires him to lower his Lantus dose the night before (from 32 units down to 28) and to snack during the activity without taking any NovoRapid to cover the food. While cycling, he consumes PowerBars, gels, and sports drinks. When he is racing, though, he doesn't need as many snacks as usual because they drive his sugars too high during strenuous workouts that release adrenaline.

Michael Malone from Kilkenny, Ireland, eats carbohydrate without bolusing during strenuous cycling and lowers his basal rate by 0.3 unit per hour. If he exercises over a long period, he eats about 15 grams of extra carbohydrate (in the form of a snack bar) every 30 minutes. By checking his blood sugars frequently, he's able to start snacking before experiencing big drops, and he's also able to prevent highs that would limit his ability to cycle or do other types of exercise. If the weather is hot, he has to reduce his basal rate down to almost nothing for an hour to prevent lows.

Intensity, Duration, and Other Effects

Effect of exercise intensity and duration   For Spike Beecroft of Bellfield, Victoria (Australia), both how long and how hard he rides affect his insulin changes. For example, he generally reduces his basal rate to 60 to 80 percent of normal during cycling, but it varies with the type of riding he's doing, with lesser reductions for more intense rides. For longer rides, he needs to use a lower basal rate, and he then keeps it 10 to 15 percent lower for two days afterward.

A member of the 2007 Team Type 1 Race Across America (RAAM) Team, Robert Schrank of Gurnee, Illinois, bases his regimen changes on how long and hard he's riding. For rides under two and a half hours he doesn't adjust his insulin at all, but he eats every half to three-quarters of an hour. For moderate-pace riding, he keeps his basal rate at 60 percent of normal, whereas for short, intense rides, he ends up needing to take a bolus of insulin to bring down his hyperglycemia.

A RAAM 2007 teammate, Linda Demma of Atlanta, Georgia, finds that when she cycles for more than 2 hours, she needs to reduce her basal rate by only about 25 percent (as opposed to 50 percent during shorter rides) and eat 25 to 50 grams of carbohydrate per hour without bolusing for them. For 12-hour races, though, which require her to eat more carbohydrate, albeit less frequently, she sometimes has to give herself reduced boluses to cover them. In either case, she avoids taking Symlin before longer rides or races.

Elise Rayner of Colorado Springs, Colorado, finds that for prolonged rides and races lasting more than 10 hours, she has to reduce her basal Lantus dose by 20 percent (given the night before) and lower her breakfast NovoLog dose by 80 percent. Halfway into her ride, she also gives a bolus that is 50 to 80 percent reduced for food that she eats during the ride.

Effect of multiple days of exercise   Tom Seabourne, a type 1.5 diabetic cyclist from Mt. Pleasant, Texas, found that he had to decrease his basal insulin (Lantus, the only one he uses) during his solo attempt at doing the RAAM and take no Byetta at all. He also learned that consuming too much carbohydrate while biking long distances (night and day) could be as bad for his performance as taking in too few; when he cut back on his carbohydrate intake, his blood sugars stayed in a more normal range.

For Candace Dalton, a new-onset type 1 diabetic cyclist from Kirkland, Washington, doing multiple days of cycling really affects her insulin action. On the first day of long riding, she turns off her pump, but gives herself a 0.2-unit bolus every few hours. She also lowers her boluses by 10 to 25 percent for her meals that whole day and eats 20 grams of carbohydrate from Gu or Clif Shot Blocks every 25 to 35 minutes to prevent lows. On the second day, she again turns her pump off, although when she's done cycling, she sets her basal rates at 75 percent for the rest of the day and overnight, and keeps boluses at only 50 percent of normal.

After cycling for two or three days in a row, Chris Mailing reduces his basal rate by 25 percent for a day or two and increases his carbohydrate-to-insulin ratios (eating about 25 percent more carbohydrate for the same insulin). He goes back and recalculates this ratio each time that he has to eat an extra 20 grams of carbohydrate to compensate for low blood sugar after cycling.

MARATHONS

Participation in marathons involves high-mileage training and the ability to cover the distance of 26.2 miles (42.2 kilometers) at your maximal race pace. This activity is almost purely aerobic in nature, resulting in significant depletion of muscle glycogen in many different muscles because of how long it lasts. Your body will use a combination of carbohydrate and fat (more carbohydrate, though), and the harder you push yourself, the greater your carbohydrate use will be. Even non-diabetic athletes usually benefit from carbohydrate consumption during the event to prevent fatigue and hypoglycemia (yes, people without diabetes can experience exercise-induced lows during marathons).

For diabetic athletes, marathoning requires both additional carbohydrate and minimal circulating insulin because of its prolonged nature. The actual changes that you make will depend on factors like your race pace, how well trained you are (making you able to use slightly more fat), and how low your insulin levels are during the race. The key to maintaining your blood sugar levels during a marathon is having minimal insulin in your system, which you can accomplish by decreasing your basal insulin doses the evening before and the morning of the race, plus taking less insulin for anything you eat before you start. If you still make your own insulin, you can keep your insulin levels lower by avoiding eating higher GI foods before racing. See table 9.4 for further instructions on marathons.

Table 9.4   Marathons

Insulin: insulin pump	Insulin: basal-bolus regimen	Diet: insulin pump	Diet: basal-bolus regimen
• Generally, don't alter your basal rates until the morning of a marathon, when you may reduce them by 25–100% to minimize insulin levels. • Reduce your boluses for prerun meals by 25–75%, depending on your blood sugars. • Reduce boluses for meals later in the day by 25–50%. • To prevent late-onset lows, keep your basal rates at 10–25% lower for the rest of the day and overnight.	• Lower your insulin levels at the start of the marathon with a 10–25% reduction in your previous evening's dose of basal insulin (if taken in the p.m.), or lower your basal dose by 10–50% in the morning if you take one then. • Reduce your insulin doses for food eaten before the event by 25–50%, depending on your starting blood sugar levels. • Reduce your postmarathon evening dose of basal insulin to a lesser extent (10–25%), depending on your morning reduction. • Reduce your doses of rapid-acting insulin following the event by 25–50%, depending on blood sugar readings and carbohydrate intake during the race.	• Supplement with 15–30 grams of carbohydrate every 30–60 minutes, depending on your blood sugar levels and how much you reduce your basal insulin. • If your blood sugar starts out on the high side, you will usually need less carbohydrate, at least initially, during your run.	• Supplement with 15–30 grams of carbohydrate for every 30–60 minutes of exercise, depending on your blood sugar levels. • Starting with a higher blood sugar will usually require less supplementation, at least initially, during your run.

Athlete Examples

Diabetic marathoners have tried a variety of strategies to maximize their performance. All their regimen changes involve decreases in insulin and increases in carbohydrate intake. For additional examples, refer to the sections on running and jogging, triathlons, and ultraendurance events and training.

Combined Regimen Changes

Diabetic marathoner Bill King of Aston, Pennsylvania, supplements with 10 to 20 grams of carbohydrate (e.g., Clif Shot Bloks Chews, SportBeans, or Extend Bars) every 20 to 30 minutes while running a marathon. He also lowers his basal rates. For him, wearing an insulin pump is the key to staying more tightly controlled during long training runs and marathons. Before races, he finds that nervousness makes his sugars go up, which he counters with a temporary increase in his basal

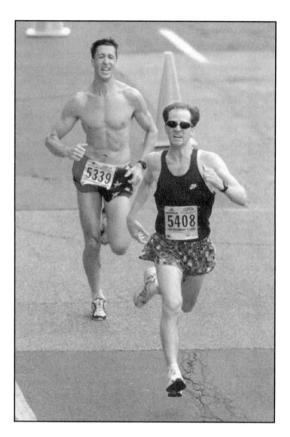

A marathon is almost purely aerobic in nature, resulting in significant depletion of muscle glycogen in many different muscles because of how long it lasts. Even nondiabetic athletes usually benefit from carbohydrate consumption during the event to prevent fatigue and hypoglycemia.

rate. He then lowers it to 40 to 60 percent of normal about an hour before a race or long run. As his conditioning improves with consistent training, his glucose levels climb 40 to 90 minutes into a longer, slower run, so he often either gives a small bolus or increases his basal rates before reaching the end of the 26.2-mile (42.2-kilometer) race to avoid postrace highs.

A Lantus and Humalog user, Tom Kingery of Delaware, Ohio, finds that for both marathon and triathlon training, he has to consume a lot of carbohydrate—both fast- and slow-acting ones—although he uses protein as his main recovery supplement. He normally takes only 1 unit of Lantus a day and 4 to 6 units of Humalog but doesn't take any insulin before or after a long training day or race.

When training for a marathon, Scott Wiebold of Cartersville, Georgia, makes adjustments based on how far or long he'll be running. He usually reduces his basal rate by 40 to 70 percent during training runs. If he's on the low side before starting, he may eat an energy bar to raise his blood sugars. When he eats energy gels while running, he doesn't bolus for them unless his sugars are too high, in which case he takes a half bolus. He also consumes about 16 ounces (480 milliliters) of a sports drink during long runs of two and a half to three and a half hours.

A type 1.5 diabetic runner from Italy, Cristian Agnoli finds that he runs best (doing marathons, half marathons, and more) when his starting blood sugar is in the range of 160 to 250 mg/dl (8.9 to 13.4 mmol/L), which he accomplishes by eating breakfast the morning of an endurance race without taking any NovoRapid unless his fasting sugars are over 100 mg/dl (5.6 mmol/L), in which case he takes only two-thirds of a unit. In addition, he lowers his basal dose of Lantus from 14 down to 10 units starting 2 days before the race. He drinks some carbohydrate (usually Coca-Cola or Maxim sports drinks) every 30 minutes during the race.

Jerry Nairn, a resident of Chandler, Arizona, reduces his basal rate by about 40 percent an hour before starting a long run or marathon. During this activity, he consumes an Accel gel (because it contains some protein) every 40 minutes or 5 miles (8 kilometers). If he wants to go longer without eating, he reduces his basal insulin rate more.

For David Walton of Newtown, Pennsylvania, many factors affect his blood sugar responses to marathon training. He always takes his pump off during runs of 3 to 13 miles (5 to 21 kilometers), although he keeps his basal rates normal until then. He reduces any bolus insulin that he takes before running by 75 percent as well. If it's hot or if he'll be running a longer distance (13 miles as opposed to 3, or 21 kilometers as opposed to 5), he usually needs to have a gel to treat or prevent low blood sugars. He also factors in whether he's running hills or just a flat, normal pace.

Intensity, Duration, and Other Effects

Effect of training   Peter Nerothin of San Diego, California, wears many athletic hats, from triathlete to wilderness adventure guide. For marathon training, he usually finds that as his training gradually intensifies (10 percent distance increase per week), his insulin doses decrease accordingly. But on one occasion when he ran a marathon without doing much training, his insulin strategy was different. Normally, he would have started the race with his basal rate at 50 percent or less, but that day he kept a normal basal rate without reducing it until about mile 10 (kilometer 16). As he says, many people are perplexed by race-day highs, but they happen, at least in part, because the runners have been tapering their training and their bodies don't respond to the shorter training distance as they do during their peak.

RUNNING AND JOGGING

Unless you're doing track events (covered in chapter 10) or all-out sprinting (chapter 11), these activities are generally aerobic in nature. The main fuels that your body uses for running are carbohydrate and fat, and your reliance on blood glucose and muscle glycogen increases with running intensity. Thus, how hard you run affects your blood sugars, as do how far you run, the time of day that you run, your insulin levels, and your starting blood sugar levels. Intense running releases more glucose-raising hormones, making it possible for your sugars to go up during intense 5K races or tough interval training. The longer you run, the more energy comes from your stores of muscle and liver glycogen, making it harder for you to maintain your blood sugars during long runs without eating some carbohydrate. Using more muscle glycogen also increases your insulin sensitivity afterward and increases your risk for lows later on.

If you run when your insulin levels are lower (generally before meals for most insulin users or first thing in the morning for everyone), your workout won't cause your blood sugars to drop as much because you'll be experiencing a more "normal" physiological response. Pump users can easily lower their insulin during exercise by suspending or reducing their basal rates. Your insulin levels are lower and your resistance greater early in the morning; therefore, if you run before breakfast (and before taking or releasing any insulin), you will have more stable blood sugars even without taking in extra carbohydrate. Conversely, if your blood sugars are high when you run, you may need a small dose of rapid-acting insulin to prevent a rise, particularly during morning workouts. See table 9.5 for further instructions on running and jogging.

Table 9.5 Running and Jogging

Insulin: insulin pump	Insulin: basal-bolus regimen	Diet: insulin pump	Diet: basal-bolus regimen
• Decrease or discontinue your basal insulin during runs. • For shorter runs of 3 miles (5 kilometers) or less, suspend your pump altogether to provide more normal insulin response to exercise and eliminate your need for extra carbohydrate. • Reduce your boluses by 10–30% for meals before and following runs to prevent low blood sugars, depending on changes in your basal rates and carbohydrate intake. • For longer runs, reducing your basal rates by 50–100% during the run, along with reducing your preexercise boluses, will help maintain your blood sugar levels. • You may need to keep your basal rates lower for several hours following your workout (or even overnight), especially after long or unusually strenuous runs. • For higher starting blood sugars, consider giving 0.5–2 units of rapid-acting insulin to prevent further increases in your blood sugars if you are going to run hard.	• Reduce your rapid-acting insulin by 10–30% for the meal before exercise for shorter runs or 20–50% for longer ones to prevent low blood sugars during a run. • After your workout, consider reducing your rapid-acting insulin by 10–30% as well. • For preplanned longer runs, reduce your morning dose of basal insulin by 10–20% to prevent later-onset lows or consume additional carbohydrate after running. • For higher starting blood sugars, you may need to inject 0.5–2 units of rapid-acting insulin to prevent further increases in blood sugars if you work out intensely.	• Consume 10–20 grams of carbohydrate every 30–45 minutes during long runs. • If you haven't reduced your basal rates during shorter runs, consume 15–30 grams of carbohydrate. • For runs of any length early in the morning before a meal bolus (especially intense running such as races or interval training), you may not need to eat or reduce your insulin much. • With a starting blood sugar of 200 mg/dl (11.1 mmol), you shouldn't need any extra carbohydrate during shorter runs or for the first 30–60 minutes of longer workouts.	• If your insulin levels are low, you won't need much carbohydrate for shorter runs of 3 miles (5 kilometers) or less. • Take in 10–20 grams of carbohydrate for every 30–45 minutes of running. • For runs of any length early in the morning before breakfast, you may not need any carbohydrate. • With a starting blood sugar of 200 mg/dl (11.1 mmol) or less, don't consume any extra carbohydrate initially. • For running longer than 45 minutes, you'll likely need some carbohydrate after the initial 30 minutes of running, depending on your blood sugars. • Running intense road races or doing interval training may require less carbohydrate to maintain your blood sugars, especially in the early morning.

Athlete Examples

Diabetic athletes use various regimen changes to compensate for running, depending on a number of factors. If weight loss is your goal, then try to compensate without having to eat a lot of extra carbohydrate that adds calories to your diet.

Insulin Changes Alone

Oak Park, Illinois, resident Stetson Siler has recorded his pre- and postrun blood glucose readings for years to figure out what works best for him. He runs every morning, first thing, usually 4 to 5 miles (6.4 to 8 kilometers) at a 9:00 (5:35) pace. If he wakes up with an elevated blood glucose level, he takes 1 unit of NovoLog for every 50 mg/dl (2.8 mmol/L) that he's above 120 (or 6.7). Ideally, he likes to wake up between 60 and 120 (3.3 to 6.7 mmol/L), for which he takes no insulin, but he usually experiences some increase in his blood sugars from running. Only if he is below 60 does he eat any carbohydrate before completing his run.

Diet Changes Alone

Roberta Voulon of Paris, France, usually tries to time her runs so that her insulin levels are lower; that is, she runs three hours after her last dose of NovoRapid for a meal. She doesn't adjust her insulin for the meal beforehand. Instead, she just takes her usual dose. Before 5K runs, she drinks orange juice with 22 grams of carbohydrate; for 7 kilometers, she additionally eats two Mentos (5 more grams); and for longer runs, she adds in a slice of bread and brings some sports gels along with her on the run. After the run, her blood glucose may go up a bit, which she corrects by adding a unit to her dinner meal injection.

Benny Privratsky of Carlsbad, California, prefers to consume gels and carry fluids with him to drink during long runs rather than adjust his basal rates or disconnect his pump. His routine is to run 3 to 8 miles (5 to 13 kilometers) three to four times per week, and as such, it's built into his normal insulin regimen. He prefers to start a run with a blood glucose level of 180 mg/dl (10 mmol/L) because running brings it down afterward; starting that high prevents him from experiencing lows during his runs.

For running 5 days a week, Nicolas Eisen of Poitiers, France, lowers his basal rate. He also takes in some carbohydrate every 20 minutes during intense running. He uses Ovomaltine chocolate bars to treat low blood sugars when he has them.

A type 2 runner from Des Moines, Iowa, Randall Maxey regularly runs five days a week and controls his diabetes by taking metformin ER (extended release) as well. Sometimes he eats a banana or another easily digested carbohydrate before doing heavy exercise.

Combined Regimen Changes

California resident Peter Nerothin reduces his basal by 20 to 100 percent when running for more than 45 minutes, but he leaves his pump connected even if he's not receiving any insulin. He finds that running has the greatest potential to drop his blood sugars fast and dangerously. To be prepared, he carries different types of foods with him—fast acting, medium acting, and long acting—but he avoids using the fast-acting carbohydrate to preserve them for emergencies. He has it pretty much down to an intuitive science at this point, and during runs, he rarely drops lower than 120 mg/dl (6.7 mmol/L) or goes higher than 200 (11.1). After long or intensive runs, he has to monitor his blood glucose closely during the hours and day following because he is much more likely to have nighttime lows or extreme insulin sensitivity through lunch the next day.

Murry Ahern of Dublin, Ireland, runs six days a week. When he plans on doing long runs of 15 miles (24 kilometers) or more, he reduces his evening Lantus dose the night before by about 25 percent, and he cuts back on his NovoRapid doses before and afterward. He primarily relies on Lucozade sports drinks before, during, and after his long runs, along with glucose tablets and gels to prevent and treat hypoglycemia.

For Meryl Ortiz of Dix Hills, New York, the adjustment she makes for running depends on her starting blood sugars and how long she's planning on running. Normally, she lowers her basal rate to 30 to 40 percent of her usual an hour before starting. During short runs, she doesn't eat anything unless her sugars are on the low side before she starts. For longer runs of 8 miles (13 kilometers) or more, she eats breakfast and gives half of her usual bolus an hour beforehand. She then consumes glucose tablets, gels, and Gatorade as needed during the activity.

A resident of Lincoln, Nebraska, Kimberly Burhoop finds that eating a high-fiber cereal (with 45 grams of carbohydrate) before her morning runs without taking any rapid-acting insulin works to keep her blood sugars stable during an hour-long run. She starts her runs 30 to 45 minutes after eating and checks her blood sugars a couple of times during the activity; only if she's too high near the end does she take any insulin. She keeps her basal insulin constant, though.

Gold River, California, resident Matthew Briel participates in distance running and triathlons. For a given workout or event, he decreases his basal rate starting 30 minutes beforehand and aims for his initial blood sugars to be around 150 mg/dl (8.3 mmol/L). If he exercises for less than an hour, he takes his pump off, whereas during longer runs and activities he drops his basal to 50 percent and frequently drinks some Cytomax or Accelerade during the activity. If he runs without his pump, he reconnects and boluses if his sugars are high and for a 20-gram carbohydrate snack he eats then (although his bolus is smaller if his sugars are on the low side). After longer runs, he eats twice as much carbohydrate. He avoids exercising if he has bolused more than 2 units in the past 2 hours.

Brent Bublitz of Centuria, Wisconsin, cuts back on his NovoLog doses by 40 percent before running 6 miles (10 kilometers) or longer. For this activity, he also eats a glucose tablet every 1 to 1.5 miles (1.6 to 2.4 kilometers) and a gel pack or Clif Shot Blok every 6 miles (10 kilometers). Afterward, he eats more protein.

A resident of Saint Louis Park, Minnesota, Karen Stark usually keeps her basal Lantus or Levemir insulin the same for running but lowers her postexercise meal insulin by at least 50 percent to compensate. She consumes fast-acting carbohydrate like sports drinks, raisins, crackers, or half a PowerBar before running to bring her preworkout blood glucose level to about 200 mg/dl (11.1 mmol/L). After runs that last 30 to 40 minutes, she ends with her blood sugars back to normal, and she monitors closely for later-onset lows. Sometimes after running, she lowers her evening dose of Lantus by a couple of units, or if she has been particularly active, she may completely skip her usual 5-unit dose.

Canada resident Martin Desbois makes adjustments for running based on exercise duration. For all lengths of running, he eats some carbohydrate beforehand so that his blood sugars are on the rise when he starts. As for insulin changes, he doesn't make any for running less than an hour; for 90 minutes of running, he lowers his basal rate to 50 percent for 2.5 hours; and for runs longer than 90 minutes, he turns off his pump from 60 minutes beforehand until the end of his run.

Type 2 diabetic exerciser Brenda Rossini from Winnetka, Illinois, jogs 6.5 (10.5 kilometers) miles three or four times a week. Following her runs, she always has a Powerade sports drink and plenty of water all day long. Her only medication is metformin, which she takes in the morning.

Intensity, Duration, and Other Effects

Effect of environment Scott McKinnon of Midlothian, Texas, finds that environmental conditions have a big effect on his blood sugar responses to his usual 3-mile (4.8-kilometer) run around his neighborhood. For example, the Texas heat and humidity can cause his blood sugars to drop by 100 mg/dl (5.6 mmol/L) during summertime runs, whereas a cold, dry winter day will have no effect at all (i.e., his blood sugars stay stable).

Effect of time of day Washington, D.C., resident Cynthia Kahn finds that her blood sugars are easiest to maintain if she runs in the morning. She usually lowers her basal rates by 60 to 75 percent during running and for 60 to 90 minutes afterward. She consumes glucose tablets as needed during her runs to keep her blood sugars normal.

Effect of exercise intensity Tom Gohl of Westminster, Colorado, finds that he has to reduce his basal rate for running or cycling longer than an hour but increase it for shorter, intense races like 10K distances (lasting 22 to 25 minutes) to as high as double his normal rate. He has also found, though, that overcorrecting for a postrace high blood glucose level can cause him to come crashing down within 1 or 2 hours afterward, so he gives himself a smaller bolus than he thinks he needs to correct it.

SWIMMING

This activity is mainly aerobic in nature, especially when swimming long distances rather than competing in short races. Longer endurance swims use a mixture of fat and carbohydrate, and as in running, your reliance on blood sugar and muscle glycogen increases with your intensity. Short sprints or racing competitions (covering distances of 200 meters or less) use mainly anaerobic energy provided by your phosphagen and lactic acid systems.

Your swimming intensity will affect the release of glucose-raising hormones; intense exercise, such as swim meets or other competitions involving short, intense efforts may raise your blood sugar levels rather than lower them as longer swims usually do. The more glycogen that you use, the greater your insulin action is afterward, so you'll have to work to prevent later-onset lows if your glycogen use is significant. If you swim when your insulin levels are minimal (more than two to three hours after your last insulin dose or with lower basal rates), your blood sugars will not decrease as much. For longer swims (lasting an hour or more), you will likely need to eat extra carbohydrate to offset the glucose-lowering effect of using much of your muscle and liver glycogen. If you swim before breakfast, you will have more stable blood sugar levels, but you may need to supplement with insulin, particularly if you start out with higher sugars. See table 9.6 for further instructions on swimming.

Table 9.6   Swimming

Insulin: insulin pump	Insulin: basal-bolus regimen	Diet: insulin pump	Diet: basal-bolus regimen
• If you remove your pump during swimming, you will need to eat little carbohydrate unless your swim lasts over an hour. • Short, intense swims (like at meets) may actually cause your blood sugars to rise, for which you may need a small bolus of insulin afterward. • If you wear a waterproof pump during swims, reduce your basal rates by 25–75% during the activity, depending on how hard your workout is and how long it lasts. • Reduce your premeal boluses by 10–30% to minimize insulin levels during your swim. • Reduce your bolus by 10–25% for meals afterward, especially following longer workouts. • Keep your basal rates lowered by 10–20% for several hours after the swim to prevent hypoglycemia after long swims.	• You won't need to change much for short swimming sprints, but you should give a small dose of rapid-acting insulin if your blood sugars go up from the activity. • Reduce your rapid-acting insulin doses by 10–30% before longer swims. • Reduce your insulin doses by 10–25% for meals after the swim, especially following more prolonged workouts. • Consider reducing your evening basal insulin doses by 10–20% following unusually long workouts or multiple days of swimming.	• Eat 15–30 grams of carbohydrate per hour for most swim workouts. • You will need only 0–15 grams of carbohydrate for early morning swims because of increased insulin resistance at that time of day. • Eat extra snacks (especially at bedtime) following prolonged swims to prevent lows.	• Increase your carbohydrate intake by 0–20 grams for shorter swims and 15–30 grams per hour for longer swims, depending on how much you reduce your premeal insulin. • Consume less carbohydrate (0–20 grams) for swims early in the morning (when insulin resistance is high), when your insulin levels are low, or for more intense swimming. • Eat extra snacks (especially at bedtime) after longer workouts to prevent later-onset hypoglycemia.

Athlete Examples

The following examples show that your duration and intensity of swimming, along with the time of day that you exercise, largely determine the regimen changes that you'll need to make to maintain control over your blood sugars.

Insulin Changes Alone

Greg Cutter of Norfolk, Virginia, normally swims a mile (1,600 meters) at least five days a week. Because he swims before lunch locally or before breakfast when traveling, he seldom becomes hypoglycemic during this activity because he has lower insulin levels at both of those times. His swimming is so consistent that he adjusts his insulin upward only for meals (to the higher end of his usual range of 4 to 12 units of Humalog) when he is traveling and doing less swimming, but he makes no changes to his evening Lantus or other doses.

For recreational swimming during the summer, preteen Kaylee Swanson of Long Beach, California, takes her pump off even though it is waterproof. She then reconnects once an hour and gives herself the basal amount that she missed as a bolus. If she eats anything while swimming, she reconnects and gives half of her usual bolus to cover it.

Before swimming, Julie Majuring of Indianapolis, Indiana, removes her pump. She also tries to make sure that she starts with a blood sugar in the range of 150 to 180 mg/dl (8.3 to 10 mmol/L).

Diet Changes Alone

A six-year-old resident of Etters, Pennsylvania, Andrew Steckel eats an extra seven grams of carbohydrate during every hour of swimming.

For lap swimming an hour at a moderate pace (about 2,250 meters), Sheri Ochs of Virginia Beach, Virginia, eats about 15 grams of carbohydrate (one-half of a cheese sandwich) to prevent lows if she starts out with normal blood sugars. Because she usually swims at least two or three hours after her breakfast and before giving any Humalog for lunch (with Lantus for basal coverage), her insulin levels are low during her swim. Accordingly, her blood sugars don't usually drop much during this activity; however, if her sugars are 150 to 180 mg/dl (8.3 to 10 mmol/L), she swims without eating anything first and ends up with normal blood sugar levels.

Combined Regimen Changes

A Hyde Park, New York, resident, Kyle Berg is a Division I competitive swimmer at his university. Three days a week he practices for two hours in the early morning and another two in the afternoon; on the other two weekdays he has only afternoon practices, and on Saturdays he has swim meets during the season. To compensate for practices, he usually eats 50 to 100 grams of carbohydrate beforehand uncovered by insulin, drinks Gatorade throughout practice, and eats a Gatorade energy bar one-quarter at a time. He also decreases the basal rate on his pump starting one and a half hours before practice and disconnects for the two hours that he's in the pool.

For Jennifer Broussard of LaPlace, Louisiana, swimming competitively year round is second nature because she has been doing it for a decade. To compensate for workouts, she sets a temporary basal rate on her pump (with lower levels) and eats either a snack before swimming or an extra piece of bread at lunch to compensate. If her sugars are low during practice, she eats three glucose tablets and waits 10 minutes before getting back in the pool.

Tyler Rockenfield of Janesville, Wisconsin, swims competitively on his high school team. Before swim practices, he eats one or two PowerBars, and he disconnects his pump while swimming. His basal rate also is lower during the entire swimming season on practice days, when he decreases it by about 30 percent to prevent lows. He also eats everything in sight during the season without having to change his insulin boluses much.

When he swims, Peter Nerothin of California disconnects his pump but never for more than two hours. Usually, he eats a granola bar or banana before entering the pool, along with possibly another 30 grams of carbohydrate after an hour during a longer swim. He always boluses with 1 or 2 units immediately afterward, which serves to cover the gap he had in his basal insulin.

A type 2 diabetic lap swimmer, Donna L. Johnson of Knoxville, Tennessee, takes a smaller dose of Starlix before breakfast or dinner, depending on which meal she swims after. She also finds that she needs to eat more carbohydrate before doing intense workouts to prevent lows.

Intensity, Duration, and Other Effects

Effect of exercise intensity Swim meets have a completely different effect from swim practices, as Kris Berg can attest. He tries to keep his blood sugars around 150 mg/dl (8.3 mmol/L) during meets, but the adrenaline release from the stress of competition and all-out sprinting during shorter events (50 or 100 meters) can easily make his sugars spike by 200 mg/dl (11.1 mmol/L) or more. He finds that events of 200 meters or longer still cause an increase in his blood glucose, but not as much as the sprint distances.

Effect of exercise duration and more Jen Alexander from Halifax, Nova Scotia (Canada), is the first swimmer ever to have done a double crossing of the Northumberland Strait, which lies between Prince Edward Island and the southern and western shores of the Gulf of Saint Lawrence in eastern Canada. To cross the strait twice, Jen had to do a continuous swim for 19 hours and 17 minutes. During the swim, she consumed about 30 grams of carbohydrate every 30 minutes, mostly in the form of Kool-Aid and Gatorade, while adjusting the basal rate on her insulin pump to compensate. She had to increase her basal rate after about 2 hours until about 10 hours (up to 25 to 75 percent above normal), after which she set it as much as 50 to 60 percent lower than normal. On several occasions when her sugars rose near the start and the end of her swim, she took 0.4-unit boluses to compensate. The latter increase was probably due to her suffering from hypothermia after swimming 18 hours in ocean water that averaged about 20 degrees Celsius (68 degrees Fahrenheit).

Effect of time of day Kris Berg decreases his basal rate starting 90 minutes before practices, but the amount is different based on the time of day. For early morning swimming, he lowers it from 0.9 unit per hour down to 0.7 before practice, whereas his changes are closer to a 50 percent reduction before afternoon swims. His morning practices are made up of an hour of weight training followed by an hour of swimming, whereas he just swims during his afternoon practices, which makes a difference as well.

Although Sheri Ochs usually swims before lunch, if she does her hour-long swim before breakfast instead, she has to give herself 0.5 unit of Humalog beforehand. Without that small dose, her sugars double from 75 mg/dl (4.2 mmol/L) to about 150 (8.3) during an hour of swimming, even without eating anything, because of her higher insulin resistance at that time of day.

For New York City resident David Weingard, the time of day when he swims has a big effect on the adjustments that he needs to make. For morning swims before breakfast, he gives 0.1 unit of NovoLog as a bolus if his blood sugars are between 100 and 130 mg/dl (5.6 to 7.2 mmol/L) to cover the 60 to 90 minutes that he swims. For sugars over 130, he takes 0.2 unit. Afterward, he takes another 0.2 or 0.3 unit to replace the missed basal, along with a larger-than-usual bolus (given 15 minutes before eating) for yogurt and his postworkout meal. When he swims in the evening, he eats a large lunch that doesn't require a square-wave bolus at least 5 hours beforehand to ensure that his insulin levels are minimal during this activity. Halfway through, he usually needs to consume one gel containing 20 grams of carbohydrate.

TRIATHLONS

Triathlons range in length from sprint and Olympic distance to half and full-length Ironman events. By nature, these prolonged activities use aerobic energy systems almost exclusively, regardless of their length. Your body relies on both fat and carbohydrate, although you'll use more carbohydrate the faster you go, and most events cause significant depletion of your glycogen stores. You can alter your insulin, diet, or both to compensate, but for the longer triathlons, if you take insulin you'll have to lower your doses to avoid hypoglycemia during and after the event.

The length of the triathlon will greatly affect your blood sugar responses. Sprint triathlons may be completed by doing an hour of intensive exercise. Sprint triathlons that result in a greater release of glucose-raising hormones may help keep your blood sugars higher throughout the event. Olympic, half, and full-length events, however, can last 3 to 12 or more hours, a duration that will have a more significant effect on your glycogen and blood glucose use. The more depleted your glycogen stores become, the more your body relies on your blood sugars. During longer events, you will have to take in extra carbohydrate throughout to prevent lows, along with lowering your insulin doses. Watch out for later-onset lows sneaking up on you after events of all lengths because of glycogen depletion. See table 9.7 for further instructions on triathlons.

Athlete Examples

Required regimen changes are largely determined by the length of the event. Longer triathlons require major insulin (if taken) and carbohydrate intake changes to prevent lows.

Diet Changes Alone

Type 2 diabetic exerciser Curtis Harter from Palm Beach Gardens, Florida, does triathlon training about 8 to 10 hours per week. Because he controls his diabetes with Amaryl only, he adjusts by eating 15 grams of rapidly absorbed carbohydrate per hour of exercise. He also eats more if his blood sugars are below 100 mg/dl (5.6 mmol/L).

Table 9.7   Triathlons

Insulin: insulin pump	Insulin: basal-bolus regimen	Diet: insulin pump	Diet: basal-bolus regimen
• Don't lower your basal rates or boluses until the morning of the competition. • Reduce your basal rate during the triathlon by 25–100%, depending on its length, possibly even starting 1–2 hours before exercise to lower your insulin levels. • For sprint triathlons, suspending or removing your pump altogether or dramatically lowering your basal rate is most effective. • Reduce your premeal insulin boluses before the event by 25–75% depending on your blood sugar levels, basal rate reductions, and triathlon length. • During the swimming portion, disconnect the pump or reduce the basal rate to a minimal amount (on waterproof pumps only). • Take smaller insulin boluses (20–50%) for carbohydrate that you eat after the event and up to 75% following prolonged events. • Consider reducing your basal rates by 10–25% during the rest of the day and overnight to lower the risk of postexercise, late-onset hypoglycemia.	• Reduce your morning rapid-acting insulin dose before the event by 25–75%, depending on your fasting blood sugar levels and the length of the triathlon. • Cut back your morning basal insulin dose by 10–50% (if you take one), depending on the duration of the triathlon, reducing it less for shorter events compared with longer ones. • Consider reducing your postexercise evening basal insulin by only 10–20%, especially if the reduction in the morning dose was large. • Reduce your doses of rapid-acting insulin afterward by at least 20–50%.	• Supplement with 15–30 grams of carbohydrate for every 30–45 minutes of exercise during the event, especially longer ones, depending on your blood sugars and insulin reductions. • You may not need to eat during sprint triathlons if you lowered your basal insulin enough. • You will likely need to eat a bedtime snack to prevent overnight lows.	• If your insulin levels are low, you may not need to take in any carbohydrate during sprint triathlons. • For longer events, consume 15–30 grams of carbohydrate every 30–45 minutes of exercise, depending on your blood sugar levels and insulin reductions. • Doing longer events will likely require you to eat a bedtime snack to prevent later-onset hypoglycemia.

For doing 8 to 10 hours a week of training for duathlons (10K run, 40K bike, 5K run events), Alan Dean of Horsham, West Sussex, United Kingdom, tries to start his workouts, which usually last 45 to 120 minutes, with his blood glucose levels at 12 mmol/L (216 mg/dl) or higher. If his levels are below that, he has a quick snack and a sports drink to raise them.

Thomas Pintar of Fort Wayne, Indiana, doesn't adjust his basal rates for doing triathlons or training for them. His typical adjustment is that when his workouts or events last longer than 40 to 60 minutes, he eats 25 to 40 grams of extra carbohydrate (PowerBars, Clif Bars, or PayDay candy). He always carries food and Gu with him. When he did the Ironman Wisconsin, he kept his basal the same mostly because he trained that way (taking about 1 unit per hour), but by hour 12 (mile 18, or kilometer 30, of the marathon portion), he was so tired of eating extra that he simply disconnected his pump during the final 8 miles (13 kilometers) of the race. Afterward, he reconnected and took a 50 percent lower bolus to cover a sub sandwich.

Combined Regimen Changes

San Diego resident Blair Ryan competes as a collegiate triathlete, for which she trains about 15 hours a week doing swimming, cycling, and running. For a long-distance training day, such as doing an 8-mile (13-kilometer) run at a moderate pace in the afternoon, she tries to get her blood sugars up to 200 mg/dl (11.1 mmol/L) preworkout by giving less insulin than normal for lunch. She finds that if she has eaten some longer-acting carbohydrate, her blood sugars are usually sustained. If she's too high at the start (over 240 mg/dl, or 13.3 mmol/L), she takes a small bolus of insulin (usually only 0.1 to 0.2 unit) because any insulin that she takes within an hour of starting her workout makes her sugars drop rapidly.

Boise, Idaho, resident Casey Boren uses an extended bolus on his pump to cover the 400 grams of carbohydrate (PowerBar gels and Hammer nutrition products) that he takes in during the 112-mile (180-kilometer) cycling portion of a triathlon, which takes him about five hours to finish. The bolus is 8 units, which is half of what he takes when not exercising. To complete the marathon-length run afterward, he cuts back his basal insulin by 30 percent during the first half of the run and by 80 percent for the second half.

To compete in Olympic-distance triathlons (1.5K swim, 40K bike, 10K run), Scott Sidener of Seattle, Washington, usually lowers his evening Lantus dose by 10 to 25 percent the day before and often in the evening afterward as well. He usually eats 25 grams of carbohydrate beforehand, along with taking 1 to 2 units of NovoLog, and he eats more afterward. During events or long training, he eats a carbohydrate gel at each transition (i.e., swim to bike and bike to run), along with drinking Gatorade during the biking and running portions.

For sprint triathlons that last less than 90 minutes, Boston, Massachusetts, resident Kathryn Cunningham eats protein and slow-acting carbohydrate an hour before the race starts and then removes her insulin pump during the event. Halfway through, when biking, she consumes a Gu gel and ends with her blood sugars between 100 mg/dl (5.6 mmol/L) and 160 (8.9).

During any type of high-intensity triathlon training, Julie Majurin of Indiana either suspends her insulin pump or lowers her basal rates to 10 to 30 percent of normal. She also consumes a gel every 45 minutes. Before long rides or runs, she also decreases her basal rates to 50 percent starting about 2 hours before exercising to lower her insulin levels. After finishing, she usually boluses with extra insulin to prevent highs, but she prefers adjusting afterward rather than having to treat a low while training.

Katie Johnson of Scottsdale, Arizona, adjusts her regimen based on which of the three training activities she's doing. Before run training, she boluses 50 percent of normal for food intake and then sets her basal rate at 50 percent for five hours if exercising in the morning, or for only one or two hours for any other time of day. Before cycling, she takes a 75 percent bolus for food and set her basal at the same percentage for one to two hours. Swimming requires her to take only a 25 percent bolus, and although she detaches her pump during this activity, she still has to drink some Gatorade to prevent lows. She lowers her boluses for any food that she eats after running, but not after cycling or swimming.

Sarah Faust of Middleton, Wisconsin, participates in triathlons of all lengths: sprint, Olympic distance, and half and full Ironmans. When exercising for 5 to 15 hours nonstop during triathlon events or training, she needs small amounts of insulin at the beginning but then usually none for the last 3 to 10 hours. If she has taken any insulin within 3 hours of exercising, she eats a snack before starting, depending on what her blood sugars are. Early in the morning or late in the afternoon (when her insulin levels are low), she usually doesn't eat before training unless her blood glucose is below 135 mg/dl (7.5 mmol/L). She consumes granola bars, Clif Shot Bloks, raisins, and caramels before and during exercise to maintain her blood sugars. Although she uses Levemir for basal insulin coverage and a pump for Humalog boluses, she usually doesn't adjust her basal insulin for exercise because it is so consistent from day to day.

Ed Liebowitz of New York City reduces his basal rate by 75 to 95 percent while doing a variety of triathlon training seven days a week. He also eats a Clif Bar without bolusing and an Accel gel before starting his workout. For him, swimming provides the biggest challenge to maintaining his blood sugars because he can't test while in the water.

Intensity, Duration, and Other Effects

Effect of time of day   David Weingard of New York City lowers his basal rates on his insulin pump for his triathlon training. He finds that exercising in the morning negates his normal need for extra insulin at that time of day. For long bike rides or runs, he eats and takes only 25 percent of his usual bolus to cover it, and he consumes extra carbohydrate on an hourly basis.

Effect of seasonal training   Springfield, Illinois, resident Jay Handy finds that when he increases his training for an Ironman event, both his body weight and his need for basal insulin decrease. He usually drops his Levemir dose from 14 units in his training off-season down to 11 when he's in full training. In addition, he tries to exercise with as little insulin in his system as possible, so he's always aware of when he last took any rapid-acting insulin because it can last up to three hours for him.

ULTRAENDURANCE EVENTS AND TRAINING

Ultraendurance activities include multiple days of strenuous exercise (such as cycling, running, walking, backpacking), as well as ultramarathons and other extremely long distance events. Prolonged events use aerobic energy systems almost exclusively, with a mix of muscle glycogen and blood glucose, circulating and intramuscular fats, and protein sources. Training for and competing in ultraendurance events can maximally stress the body's stores of energy, resulting in significant depletion. To participate effectively, you will need to lower your insulin (if you take it) and eat more during the event and for 24 to 48 hours afterward while your body is restoring what you used, particularly muscle and liver glycogen stores.

Your insulin sensitivity will generally be heightened during this time, and your risk for hypoglycemia will be greater. The only exception occurs when you have caused significant damage to your muscles, resulting in delayed-onset muscle soreness. While your muscles are repairing in the next couple of days, you may actually be somewhat more insulin resistant (an effect that happens even in nondiabetic people) because glycogen can't be restored until your muscles are repaired. See table 9.8 for further instructions on ultraendurance events and training.

Athlete Examples

These examples show the extreme regimen changes that are necessary for ultraendurance events and training. The type and length of the event or training determine your requisite changes, which usually include both insulin (if used) and food intake adjustments. For additional examples, refer to triathlons and marathons in this chapter, and to adventure and trail running, backpacking, and mountaineering in chapter 12.

Combined Regimen Changes

A world-class ultradistance runner and marathoner, Missy Foy of Cedar Grove, North Carolina, keeps her insulin regimen fairly constant despite training up to 120 miles (190 kilometers) per week during the peak of her training season. Although she uses Lantus for basal insulin and an insulin pump for her rapid-acting insulin delivery, she usually gives herself 2 units of Humulin R to cover her insulin needs when she does ultralong runs once a week. She finds that when she is at the peak of her training, her total daily dose of insulin is much lower even though she eats more than 4,000 calories a day then. During runs, she eats carbohydrate in the form of Gu, Clif Shot Bloks, Accel Gel, Crank, or others.

Jerry Nairn of Arizona reduces his basal rate on his insulin pump by 40 percent starting an hour before a 50K race. He also consumes an Accel gel every 5 miles (8 kilometers) or so, along with cheese crackers and a juice box.

During a 160-mile (260-kilometer) bike ride in Colorado that went over three mountain passes and took approximately 12 hours, John Moore of Boone, North Carolina, gave 50 percent of his usual boluses for breakfast and lunch but took no basal insulin (Lantus) at all before the ride. When using an insulin pump and participating in an ultramarathon race, he decreased his basal rate from 0.6 unit per hour to 0.3 and consumed up to 24 grams of carbohydrate every 30 minutes.

Table 9.8 Ultraendurance Events and Training

Insulin: insulin pump	Insulin: basal-bolus regimen	Diet: insulin pump	Diet: basal-bolus regimen
• You probably should not lower your basal insulin rates until the morning of the event or ultraendurance training. • Reduce your basal rate during the activity by 25–100%, depending on how long it lasts, possibly starting 1–2 hours before exercise to lower your insulin levels. • Cut back on your preexercise meal boluses by 25–75%, depending on where your blood sugar starts and how long you'll be exercising. • Lower your meal boluses by 25–50% later in the day, depending on your blood sugars and the duration of your exercise. • Reduce your basal rates by at least 10–25% during the rest of the day and overnight to lower the risk of developing later-onset lows.	• Reduce your morning rapid-acting insulin dose before the event by 25–75%, depending on your blood sugar levels and the length of your workout. • Cut back on your morning basal insulin dose by 0–50% depending on the expected duration of your activity. • For all carbohydrate that you eat afterward, reduce your insulin doses by 25–50%. • Consider reducing your evening dose of basal insulin by only 10–20%, especially if your morning dose was substantially lower than normal.	• During your activity, supplement with 15–45 grams of carbohydrate for every 30–45 minutes of exercise, depending on your blood sugar levels and insulin reductions. • Consume extra carbohydrate after the event (taking smaller boluses) and a bedtime snack.	• Eat 15–45 grams of carbohydrate for every 30–45 minutes of exercise, depending on your blood sugar levels and insulin reductions. • Take in extra carbohydrate afterward with smaller boluses to prevent later-onset lows and overnight hypoglycemia. Eat a bedtime snack.

For 400K or 24-hour cycling events, Roy Burnham of Columbus, Ohio, has to lower his basal rates to 70 percent of normal and increase his carbohydrate-to-insulin ratio. He eats a substantial amount of food every 2 hours during such events and drinks Powerade and consumes Gu packets at 45-minute intervals to prevent lows.

Bob Paxson of Sacramento, California, cycles as his primary activity. During rides he keeps a steady flow of 300 calories per hour coming in with a primarily liquid diet that includes 10 to 15 grams of protein. Usually, he finds that his exercise metabolism doesn't start kicking in until about 40 miles (65 kilometers) into a ride, which is usually when he lowers his basal to 50 percent. He boluses for carbohydrate only if his blood sugars rise over 150 mg/dl (8.3 mmol/L). But if he is doing a cycling tour during which he is riding day after day, he starts each subsequent morning with a slightly lowered basal rate. He normally leaves it reduced after ultradistance events (century rides or longer) for about two hours or as long as overnight for rides that are 200 miles (320 kilometers) or longer. A 50 percent reduction in his basal rates is the rule of thumb that he uses, but he may lower them further based on his blood sugar readings, particularly when cycling ultradistances.

Athlete Profile

Name: Missy Foy

Hometown: Cedar Grove, North Carolina, USA

Diabetes history: Type 1 diabetes diagnosed in 1997 (at age 33)

Sport or activity: Distance runner

Greatest athletic achievement: Olympic Marathon Trials (2000), top 10 world ranking for 50 miles (2005), U.S. 50 Mile National Championship second place finish (2007)

Current insulin and medication regimen: Humalog in insulin pump and Lantus for basal coverage

Training tips: Try everything in practice that might come up in a race; my coach always says, they call it practice for a reason. Also, don't always assume that diabetes is the problem. We still have to train our way to achievement and we end up with the same problems and injuries that athletes without diabetes encounter.

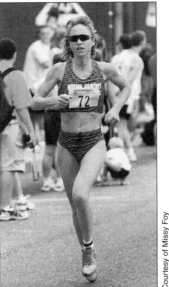

Courtesy of Missy Foy

Typical daily and weekly training and diabetes regimen:

▶ *Monday:* Morning: run 4 miles (6.5 kilometers) easy, do weights; afternoon: 8 miles (13 kilometers) easy, 30 minutes of stretching

▶ *Tuesday:* Morning: 4 miles (6.5 kilometers) easy, abs workout; afternoon: short workout, usually on the track, either (a) 3-mile (5-kilometer) warm-up, two or three sets of 4 × 400 meters at 75 to 80 seconds with 30 seconds of jogging and then 1 × 1 mile at 5:45, 3 miles (5 kilometers) easy cool-down; or (b) 3-mile (5-kilometer) warm-up, six sets of 1 × 1 kilometer at 3:36 to 3:40, 1 × 1 kilometer at 4:00 to 4:10 (run continuously, no stopping), 3 miles (5 kilometers) easy cool-down

▶ *Wednesday:* Morning: 4 miles (6.5 kilometers) easy; afternoon: 4 to 8 miles (6.5 to 13 kilometers) easy, weights, 30 minutes of stretching

▶ *Thursday:* Morning: semilong run, 12 to 20 miles (19 to 32 kilometers), no set pace; afternoon off except for 30 minutes of stretching

▶ *Friday:* Morning: 4 miles (6.5 kilometers) easy, weights and abs; afternoon: 8 miles (13 kilometers) easy, 30 minutes of stretching

▶ *Saturday:* Morning: either race or long run with embedded workout; for example, (a) 40-mile (64-kilometer) run with 15 to 20 × 1 mile at 6:10 to 6:30 with a 400-meter jog between miles (run on a 1-kilometer dirt trail loop), or (b) 35-mile (56-kilometer) run with the middle 15 miles (24 kilometers) run a little faster than marathon pace

▶ *Sunday:* Morning: off, sleep late; afternoon: run 4 to 10 miles (6.5 to 16 kilometers) depending on how I feel, followed by 30 minutes of stretching

It comes out to be about 100 to 120 miles (160 to 190 kilometers) per week of running, plus weights, abs, and stretching. During the off-season, I run about 35 to 70 miles (55 to 110 kilometers) per week, all easy and slow. My easy days are at a 7:30 to 8:30 per mile pace. My insulin schedule stays the same (except on Saturdays): a.m.: 8 to 9 units of Lantus; p.m.: 1 to 2 units of Lantus and 2.28 units of Humalog with an insulin pump (about 0.2 unit per hour with an increase to 1 unit per hour at 5:00 a.m. for 30 minutes and again at 6:00 a.m. for 30 minutes to combat dawn phenomenon). The Saturday schedule changes a little for my long run or race. I take 2 units of regular insulin when I disconnect from my insulin pump so that I have enough insulin while I'm training so hard for such a long time.

Other: Breakfast is usually four eggs and cheese with a 2-unit bolus of Humalog. Lunch is usually one or two sandwiches and chips with 4 units, and dinner is usually salad and chicken, fish, or beef with 2 units (so, about 20 units of insulin total per day). When I'm at full training and really fit, my total daily dose can drop as low as 15 to 16 daily units even though I eat 4,000 calories or more a day. I supplement carbohydrate while running by using a carbohydrate gel like GU, Clif Shot, Accel Gel, Crank, or others.

Other hobbies and interests: I'm a science geek. I like to go to the bookstore, sit down in the science aisle, and read anything odd that catches my eye. One of my training group partners, Elly Rono, is a math geek, so he and I will go to Barnes & Noble bookstore after practice sometimes for an hour; he'll be in the math aisle, and I'll be in the science one.

Good diabetes and exercise story: When I was first trying to qualify for Olympic trials, I was told over and over again that it couldn't be done, that if a diabetic athlete could qualify for Olympic marathon trials, it would have been done already. One evening after practice on the track, I was feeling discouraged. Walking back to my car, I saw what looked like a ticket on the front window. I thought to myself that maybe I really couldn't do this and that I should just quit. When I reached my car and took the paper off the front window, someone (probably one of the kids who had been watching practice that night) had left a note on my car that read, "Missy, you're my hero." Needless to say, it made my day, and I even competed in the Olympic trials.

CHAPTER 10

Endurance–Power Sports

We have all heard of Michael Jordan, John Elway, and Tiger Woods because of the popularity of endurance–power sports. But have you heard of Chris Dudley, Adam Morrison, Kendall Simmons, Jay Leeuwenberg, Jay Cutler, Michelle McGann, and Scott Verplank? Although they may not be as well known, they are just a few of the many professional athletes with diabetes who are playing football, basketball, golf, and other sports.

In general, endurance–power sports require short, powerful bouts of activity that are repeated at frequent intervals. In basketball, the action may involve a jump and a dunk of the ball and then a sprint down the court; in tennis, it may be a serve and a short volley. Power activities may have no effect on blood sugars or may actually raise them, but when the key movements are repeated many times over a prolonged period, they often have a cumulative effect on glycogen use and may require greater regimen changes to prevent your blood sugar levels from decreasing while you're doing them and later on.

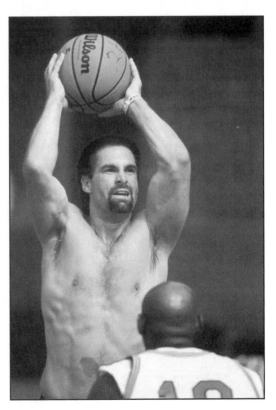

Power activities like basketball may not have much effect on blood sugars, but over an extended period, as during a full basketball game, they can have a cumulative effect on blood sugars, and you may need greater regimen changes to compensate both during and afterward.

Everyone can benefit from participating in team sports, either endurance or endurance–power sports. Kids can start to develop their coordination and skill by doing these various activities, and adults can stay youthful and active by participating. Check around your area for a local gym, recreation center, or sports league, and get the whole family involved in the sports covered in this chapter, including American football and rugby, basketball, field hockey and lacrosse, Frisbee (ultimate), golf, gymnastics, horseback riding (competitive), ice hockey, soccer, tennis, water polo, and wrestling, among others. Certain aspects of other sports, such as sprint swimming events, should technically be included in this chapter but are included with the endurance sports instead because of the long-duration training required to compete in them. The purely power sports like baseball and bodybuilding are included in the next chapter.

GENERAL RECOMMENDATIONS FOR ENDURANCE–POWER SPORTS

Most of these sports require power performances in the form of short, intense bouts of muscular activity. If the activity lasts less than 10 seconds, your first energy system alone provides the energy. Children are particularly suited for these types of short-burst activities because their other two energy systems are less well developed before they reach adolescence, particularly the lactic acid system (see chapter 2 for a review of these systems).

For any activity lasting up to two minutes (such as competitive cheerleading routines), your phosphagen system combines with the lactic acid system to provide muscular energy. ATP and creatine phosphate supply the immediate energy, and glycogen is broken down to supply the remainder. When you're working less hard (such as walking between holes in golf) or recovering from these activities, your body uses aerobic energy derived from the metabolism of fat and carbohydrate.

GENERAL ADJUSTMENTS BY DIABETES REGIMEN

The sport itself determines the diabetic regimen changes that you'll need to make. Intense activities can decrease, increase, or have no effect on your blood sugar levels. Generally, though, power moves performed intermittently over an extended period, as during a full basketball game, can have a cumulative effect, and you may need greater regimen changes to compensate both during and afterward.

Insulin Pump Users

For recreational endurance–power sports, your insulin adjustments have to be sport specific. You may require no insulin or diet changes for easy or brief play. For prolonged team practices or games, you may need to reduce your preactivity rapid-acting insulin boluses, as well as your basal insulin during the activity, by 10 to 50 percent, depending on how long and how hard you're playing. Your insulin reductions, however, will generally be less than you would need for straight endurance sports because of the intense, brief nature of the power portion of endurance–power activities. In some cases, your blood sugar levels may actually increase because of the glucose-raising effect of the hormones that your body releases, which may raise your need for insulin in the short run. For prolonged or intense participation, though, you may need 10 to 30 grams of carbohydrate per hour, depending on your insulin levels. You may also want to reduce your boluses by 10 to 25 percent after participating in certain sports, such as American football, basketball, soccer, and tennis; increase your carbohydrate intake; and reduce your basal insulin by 10 to 20 percent after the activity.

Basal-Bolus Regimens

For these types of sports, your insulin adjustments will depend on the sport. Short or easy play may require you to make no insulin or diet changes. Before longer practices or games, you may need to reduce premeal insulin doses by 10 to 50 percent. Keep in mind that you'll probably have to cut back less than you do for endurance sports, given the intense, brief nature of the power part of these activities. In some cases, your blood sugar levels may actually increase because of the high intensity of the activity, necessitating an increase in your insulin rather than a decrease. For prolonged or intense participation, you may need 10 to 30 grams of carbohydrate per hour, depending on your reductions in insulin and the time of your last dose. Following certain sports, you may want to reduce your bedtime basal doses by 10 to 15 percent, along with possibly eating a bedtime snack to prevent overnight lows when you've depleted a significant amount of muscle glycogen during the activity.

Noninsulin and Oral Medication Users

The power portion of these activities can actually raise your blood sugars (albeit temporarily), unless you do them for a long enough time. Doing an aerobic cooldown following these activities will help you counter any rise in your blood sugars. Later on, your blood sugars are likely to be better controlled, especially if you used up more muscle glycogen by doing the activity for longer. The heightened insulin action that follows these activities can persist for 24 to 48 hours, so be on the lookout for lows if you are taking certain medications like sulfonylureas (e.g., Diabinese, DiaBeta, Micronase, or Glynase).

Intensity, Duration, and Other Effects

How long, how hard, which sport, and how you play it (recreationally or competitively) can affect your blood sugar responses. Another factor to consider is what position you are playing. For instance, in soccer, midfielders may run significantly more during a game than defenders do. Being more active overall (and thus depleting more glycogen with repeated, powerful movements) can reduce your blood sugar levels more dramatically. Moreover, recreational play is usually less intense, but often more prolonged, than competitive matches or games. A short, intense competition like a wrestling match may cause your blood sugar levels to rise because of its intensity and brevity, whereas recreational softball may have no discernible effect on your blood sugars. Playing two hours of basketball, on the other hand, may cause a substantial decrease in your blood sugars during and afterward, and even overnight.

AMERICAN FOOTBALL AND RUGBY

Both of these sports are extremely anaerobic in nature. Most football plays last only 10 to 20 seconds and involve power moves, such as pushing with full force on the offensive or defensive line, throwing the ball, sprinting into position, running powerfully with the ball, or tackling an opponent.

Many factors affect your blood sugar responses to these activities. Whether you're involved in a practice or a game will determine some of the differences. During practices, you'll likely run more than you do during competitive games, when the plays are more intense and shorter and offensive and defensive units take turns on the field. Players in positions that require more running overall (e.g., wide receiver, running back, defensive back) may use muscle glycogen at different rates than those in "brute force" positions (offensive and defensive linemen) who just block or try to shed blocks and do anaerobic work during plays. All players will end up using a great deal of muscle glycogen by the end of a game (well, unless your usual position is benchwarmer), for which you'll need to eat extra carbohydrate (and take less insulin) following the activity.

In addition, preseason practices, especially twice-a-day sessions, will significantly increase your insulin action and require greater regimen changes compared with doing shorter, easier practices during the regular season, especially before upcoming games. For recreational play in these sports, you'll likely run more and work less hard, which means that your blood sugars are more likely to drop at some point during the activity. See table 10.1 for further instructions on American football and rugby.

Athlete Examples

These examples show that recreational football or rugby requires quite different regimen changes than more competitive games.

Insulin Changes Alone

Although he played college football with diabetes, Vic Kinnunen of Lawrenceville, Georgia, now engages in running, softball, weight training, and playing rugby only once a year. For his rugby games, he removes his pump, tests his blood sugars at halftime, and boluses to cover any lost basal insulin that has led his blood sugars to rise.

The main adjustment that preteen John Elwood of Indian Trail, North Carolina, makes for football practices and games is to remove his insulin pump. He monitors his blood sugars frequently and makes adjustments as needed during this activity. He treats lows with Gatorade or juice boxes.

Combined Regimen Changes

To play football on his high school team, Tyler Rockenfield of Janesville, Wisconsin, disconnects his pumps during games and practices, and lowers his basal rate for a couple of hours beforehand. Before football activities, he also drinks a Powerade, and he treats any lows with that drink, glucose tablets, or Hammer gels.

Table 10.1   **American Football and Rugby**

Insulin: insulin pump	Insulin: basal-bolus regimen	Diet: insulin pump	Diet: basal-bolus
• For afternoon practice sessions of 2–3 hours, lower your basal insulin rate during them by 25–50%. • If you remove your pump, check your blood sugars at least hourly and reconnect the pump and bolus as needed to correct for any significant rise in your blood sugars. • Reduce your premeal insulin boluses by 25–50% for practices or games within 2–3 hours. • Your basal rates should remain 10–20% lower for several hours following intense or prolonged practices or games (and possibly overnight). • Reduce your dinner insulin boluses by 10–30% after strenuous play to prevent lows.	• For afternoon practices lasting 2–3 hours, reduce your morning basal doses by 0–25%. • Reduce your premeal insulin dose by 25–50% depending on changes in your carbohydrate intake. • For practices when your insulin levels are low, don't lower your insulin at the meal before. • Reduce your dinner insulin by 10–30% following prolonged or intense practice sessions or games to prevent later-onset lows.	• Consume 15–45 grams of carbohydrate per hour depending on your insulin reductions and practice intensity. • Consume additional carbohydrate afterward and possibly at bedtime to prevent lows.	• Supplement with 15–45 grams of carbohydrate per hour depending on how much you lower your insulin and how hard you're working out. • Consume additional carbohydrate as necessary during and after the activity (and possibly at bedtime) to prevent later-onset lows.

Tommy Fluen of Christchurch, Canterbury (New Zealand), plays rugby. On game days he reduces his morning dose of Protophane (an intermediate-acting insulin) by about a third. He also eats a carbohydrate snack before playing if his blood glucose is below 6 mmol/L (108 mg/dl), just in case. His biggest challenge is that rugby games can differ from week to week. Sometimes he plays 80 minutes, and it may be very hot; other times he may be injured and play only 20 minutes, so he has to have a reactive plan to deal with unpredictable highs and lows.

To play flag football seasonally, Riley McCullen of Mechanicsville, Virginia, turns off his basal insulin when he starts to go low. He also always has quick carbohydrate snacks on hand, and he makes sure that his blood sugars are over 100 mg/dl (5.6 mmol/L) before he starts any exercise.

BASKETBALL

This court activity involves many stop-and-start movements and quick, powerful moves like shooting, passing, and dribbling. As a result, it is more anaerobic than aerobic. But when you play for an hour or more continuously, you'll use up a lot of muscle glycogen and blood glucose. Basketball also has an aerobic component when you run up and down the court at a moderate pace. You may need changes in both your insulin and carbohydrate intake to prevent a drop in your blood sugar levels during or after a game or practice.

How long you play and how much insulin you have on board are the factors that affect your blood sugars the most. If you can exercise with minimal insulin (i.e., two to three hours after rapid-acting insulin, early in the morning, or with lowered basal rates on your insulin pump), you will maintain your blood sugar levels more effectively while taking in less carbohydrate. If you play for a long time, your use of muscle glycogen will cause lower blood sugars later on that you can prevent with increased carbohydrate intake and possibly lower doses of insulin. See table 10.2 for further instructions on basketball.

Table 10.2 Basketball

Insulin: insulin pump	Insulin: basal-bolus regimen	Diet: insulin	Diet: basal-bolus regimen
• Remove your insulin pump or reduce your basal rates by 50–75% during the activity. • Reduce your preactivity meal boluses by 25–50% within 2 hours of playing. • Consider keeping your basal rates 10–15% lower for several hours (or even overnight) after strenuous or prolonged play.	• Reduce your rapid-acting insulin doses by 25–50% for play following meals. • For early morning exercise or when your insulin levels are lower, cut back on your insulin by only 10–25%. • Consider reducing your evening basal insulin (if you take it then) by 10–15% following extended playing to prevent overnight hypoglycemia.	• Consume 10–30 grams of carbohydrate per hour, depending on your insulin reductions. • Eat a bedtime snack following prolonged activity to reduce your risk of later lows.	• Consume an extra 10–30 grams of carbohydrate per hour, depending on your insulin levels. • Eat an additional snack at bedtime to prevent nocturnal hypoglycemia.

Athlete Examples

These real-life examples demonstrate that diet, insulin, or both can be modified to maintain your blood sugar control during and following basketball play.

Insulin Changes Alone

A preteen basketball player from Sterling, Virginia, Joey Sweeney sets a temporary basal rate that is 60 percent of his normal level during playing. If he gets low, he treats it with glucose tablets, Gatorade, or orange juice.

A resident of Los Lunas, New Mexico, Baylee Glass uses basal Lantus once a day, which she reduces by 1 unit on days that she plays basketball. Although her sugars tend to run high during practices and games, they come down two to five hours afterward, at which point she needs to eat extra snacks.

Jenny Vandevelde, a resident of San Diego, California, simply removes her pump when she plays basketball and uses gummy bears to treat lows, if she has any.

Diet Changes Alone

When Rory McFarland of East Wenatchee, Washington, plays basketball, he doesn't have to make many adjustments because of its intensity. But he has to increase his carbohydrate intake two to four hours afterward to prevent later-onset hypoglycemia.

John Elwood of North Carolina keeps his pump on while playing this sport and doesn't usually adjust his basal or bolus doses. He does, however, eat more carbohydrate as needed to prevent lows while playing. He has never missed a game because of diabetes.

Combined Regimen Changes

Akachi and Cheokie Okereke, brothers from Charlotte, North Carolina, both of whom are type 1 diabetic basketball players, remove their insulin pumps to play. They then check their blood sugars every hour and treat highs or lows with extra insulin or food, respectively. They treat lows with milk, Snickers bars, and other carbohydrate-rich foods, but they also try to eat protein with carbohydrate after playing to prevent later-onset lows.

A resident of Falls Church, Virginia, Rick Philbin regularly plays basketball for exercise and fitness. To compensate, he reduces his basal rate by 50 percent while playing, and he adjusts the duration of his temporary setting based on how long and hard he plays. In addition, he eats 15 to 30 grams of carbohydrate every 30 to 60 minutes that he exercises, treating any lows with juice or glucose tablets.

When playing basketball in a men's league, Gary Scheiner of Wynnewood, Pennsylvania, finds that he has to make unusual adjustments compared with what he does for kickboxing or running. He has to give himself a small insulin bolus before starting to prevent an adrenaline-induced rise in his blood sugars, and then he has to snack frequently while playing to prevent lows. He also doesn't take Symlin if he's going to play shortly after eating a meal.

COMPETITIVE CHEERLEADING AND DRILL TEAM

Most cheerleading or drill team routines last for only a couple of minutes, but they can involve powerful moves like jumping and explosive arm movements. Moreover, competitive cheerleading also includes aspects of gymnastics that require powerful moves (e.g., back flips and cartwheels). Because practices can last for one to two hours, this sport is considered an endurance–power one. Although practices are more likely to cause your blood sugars to drop than doing short routines during competitions or athletic games, the amount of glycogen that you use will determine which adjustments you'll need to make afterward to prevent later-onset lows.

Athlete Examples

These examples show that competitive cheerleading and drill team practices and competitions usually require food and insulin adjustments to compensate.

Combined Regimen Changes

Maggie Hudson of Glen Allen, Virginia, has seven hours of competitive cheerleading practices a week, which also involve working out on the trampoline and practicing her gymnastics. To compensate, she frequently checks her blood sugars and sets lower basal rates on her pump or eats snacks, as needed. In addition, she sometimes has to take her pump off, and then she corrects using NovoLog if her sugars start to rise after a while.

For cheerleading, Kelsey McGill of Bear, Delaware, takes her pump off but checks her blood sugars every 30 minutes to make adjustments in food or reconnecting to bolus, or she may keep it on but lower her basal rates during it. Before this activity, she tries to eat a healthy, light snack to keep her blood sugars stable.

A Memphis, Tennessee resident, Lindsey O'Hare was the captain of her high school drill team. Their activities varied greatly from day to day, sometimes involving only stretching but on other days including two hours of high kicks. She kept her blood glucose monitor nearby and paid close attention to how she was feeling. During intense workouts, she often reduced her basal rate by 20 to 50 percent, occasionally keeping it lower for 60 to 90 minutes afterward. Before morning practices, she often ate a small breakfast (toast and an orange) without bolusing.

FIELD HOCKEY AND LACROSSE

Depending on the position that you play, field hockey and lacrosse involve a combination of stop-and-start movements and longer sustained runs that involve both anaerobic and aerobic components, although lacrosse players may use their arms a bit more (holding their sticks up and handling and throwing the ball) than field hockey players do. Both are most similar to soccer play when compared with other endurance–power team sports, and playing them can cause you to use a great deal of your muscle glycogen and blood sugar.

The position that you play will greatly affect your overall activity level (e.g., goalies will run a lot less than the field players do), so you will need to make adjustments based on what position you play and how much time you play during the games. Playing longer will require you to eat more carbohydrate and reduce your insulin more before, during, and after playing. During practices, the activity levels among positions may be more similar if all team members do continuous running, throwing, or shooting drills. During the playing season, you will generally need to decrease your basal insulin doses compared with what you do in the off-season. See table 10.3 for further instructions on field hockey and lacrosse.

Athlete Examples

These examples show that insulin and food adjustments may be necessary, both for playing field hockey and lacrosse and for maintaining correct blood sugar levels during the season.

Table 10.3 Field Hockey and Lacrosse

Insulin: insulin pump	Insulin: basal-bolus regimen	Diet: insulin	Diet: basal-bolus regimen
• During any field hockey or lacrosse practice or game, reduce your basal rates by 25–100%. • A midfielder who runs more continuously for an hour-long game may need a larger reduction (50–100%) than a goalie does (25%). • Lower your preactivity insulin by 20–40% as well. • Following prolonged or intense play, consider reducing your insulin for the next meal by 20–30% and lowering overnight basal insulin rates by 10–15%.	• For practices and games, decrease your doses of insulin by 20–30%. • After prolonged or intense games or practices, reduce your next meal insulin by 20–30% and consider reducing your evening basal insulin doses by 10–25%.	• Consume up to 15–30 grams of additional carbohydrate per hour. • Eat an additional bedtime snack to prevent overnight hypoglycemia following prolonged or strenuous play, especially if you don't lower your basal rates.	• Depending on your insulin reductions, consume 15–30 grams of carbohydrate per hour. • Consider eating a bedtime snack, especially following prolonged or strenuous play.

Insulin Changes Alone

Victoria Thorn of Melbourne, Victoria (in Australia), recognizes that field hockey has a large effect on her blood sugars. After a game of full-field (outdoor) field hockey, she finds that she is much more insulin sensitive the next day, so she has to lower her basal rates on her pump to compensate. Although her blood sugars often go up during strenuous play, they always come down later, so she has to eat right after games, no matter what her blood glucose is, to prevent lows. If her sugars are below 8 to 10 mmol/L (144 to 180 mg/dl) before a game, she eats some sweets then and always drinks Gatorade during games.

Michael Blackwell of Midlothian, Virginia, finds that he doesn't need to lower his basal rates for lacrosse games because of the number of kids on his team (which limits his individual playing time). If he is running low on a given practice day, though, he may reduce his basal rate by 80 percent for an hour starting 30 minutes beforehand.

Combined Regimen Changes

Joe Fiorucci from New York lowers his overall basal (Lantus) insulin doses during the lacrosse season and eats just enough food during practices and meets to prevent lows. He prefers not to run high at all before competing because doing so negatively affects his performance.

Riley McCullen of Mechanicsville, Virginia, turns off his basal insulin when he starts to go low during lacrosse practices and games. He eats to make sure that his blood sugars are over 100 mg/dl (5.6 mmol/L) before starting any play, and he treats his lows with juice or various candies.

FRISBEE (ULTIMATE)

This activity involves periods of sprinting, running, and standing and is considered an endurance–power sport, much like other team sports played on a field (e.g., soccer, field hockey, and lacrosse). Recreational games of Frisbee may not require many changes in your diabetes regimen but competitive games will. The more you run and the longer you run, the less insulin and the more carbohydrate your body will need to prevent hypoglycemia. Following particularly long or intense play, you may want to consider eating an extra snack at bedtime and lowering your basal insulins (if you use them) overnight.

Athlete Examples

How intensely you play Frisbee will affect your required regimen changes. Just throwing a Frisbee around may not require many adjustments, compared with playing a game of ultimate Frisbee.

Insulin Changes Alone

An Indiana resident, Sarah Soper sets a temporary, lower basal rate during Frisbee play that is 45 percent of normal for two hours. If she needs to bring her sugars down before playing, she gives a correction that is only 33 to 50 percent of the amount that her pump recommends.

Diet Changes Alone

A resident of Scottsdale, Arizona, Katie Johnson doesn't make too many adjustments before ultimate Frisbee games. Sometimes, she drinks Gatorade without taking any insulin if she is running a lot while playing. She finds that games are extremely unpredictable. She may do constant short sprints for 5 to 10 minutes and then sit on the sidelines for the same amount of time. Because adjusting insulin in advance is problematic, she usually doesn't do it.

Flip Bethavas of Scotch Plains, New Jersey, plays Frisbee at least once a week. As a type 2 exerciser, he controls his blood sugars with metformin only, but he usually has a low-carbohydrate breakfast before working out in the gym or playing Frisbee. He usually works out at the gym for two to three hours before going to play, so he makes sure to drink plenty of water during the activity.

GOLF

This activity requires short bursts of energy for hitting, driving, and putting, which are anaerobic in nature and mainly use the first energy (phosphagen) system. Walking the golf course is aerobic in nature, and carrying your own golf clubs increases the work that you're doing. Of course, driving a golf cart doesn't require much work at all. The amount of walking that you do has the greatest effect on your blood sugars, and walking the entire course requires you to make greater regimen changes, especially if you play 18 holes instead of just 9. Playing in hot and humid conditions lowers your blood sugars more because you body must use more glucose to cool itself. See table 10.4 for further instructions on golf.

Table 10.4　Golf

Insulin: insulin pump	Insulin: basal-bolus regimen	Diet: insulin	Diet: basal-bolus regimen
• If walking, reduce your insulin boluses by 10–50% for any meals before or during golfing. • Reduce your basal insulin rates by 25–50% as well during the activity. • Hotter conditions or longer play may require greater insulin reductions or carbohydrate intake.	• Reduce your insulin doses by 10–50% for any meals before or during golfing, if you walk. • You probably won't need to reduce your basal insulin doses. • If it's hot or you play for longer, consider reducing your insulin more or consuming carbohydrate.	• Consume 0–15 grams of carbohydrate per hour, depending on the reductions in basal insulin.	• Increase your carbohydrate intake by 5–15 grams per hour when walking the course.

Athlete Examples

The amount of walking you do, the air temperature and humidity, and the duration of your play affect what adjustments you'll need to make.

Insulin Changes Alone

When Spencer Band of Stittsville, Ontario (Canada), plays golf, he either suspends his pump or lowers his basal rate during 9 or 18 holes, depending on what his starting blood sugars are, when he last boloused, and how much insulin he gave.

Combined Regimen Changes

For golfing, Rose Pisano of Chicago, Illinois, lowers her basal rate on her insulin pump by 50 to 75 percent for two hours before starting and during the activity. In addition, she eats 15 grams of carbohydrate when she starts playing if her blood glucose level is 120 mg/dl (6.7 mmol/L) or lower.

A Howell, Michigan teenager, Christopher Pentescu plays golf four or five times a week, during which he tests his blood sugars every three holes when walking the course. He eats small, frequent snacks with carbohydrate and protein during the activity and decreases his overnight basal rate following play.

When golfing for four hours, Adelaide Lindahl of Bloomington, Minnesota, usually reduces her basal rate to 0.5 unit for the first three hours of play but then returns it to normal during the last hour or so. During long rounds of golf, she often has a 20-gram carbohydrate snack (like a granola bar) and takes little or no bolus for it.

Julie Haverly of Richmond, Virginia, reduces her basal rate by 50 percent before golfing. She also eats before playing without making any insulin adjustments.

Intensity, Duration, and Other Effects

Effect of environment   Rose Pisano walks when golfing, usually carrying her clubs but sometimes pulling a cart. If the course is hilly, her sugars go lower than when it's flat, and if it's hot and humid, they usually come down faster than normal as well.

GYMNASTICS

Doing gymnastics requires mainly short, powerful movements both during practices and competitions to complete routines of two minutes or shorter on various pieces of equipment. The first two energy systems supply most of the energy because of the intensity and duration of the activity. Prolonged practices can result in drops in your blood glucose levels, but gymnastics routines themselves may require minimal changes in your diabetes regimen because of their nature. Doing several short routines during a meet may have little effect on your blood sugars or even raise them, but two or three hours of practice will likely have more of a glucose-lowering effect because of your greater use of muscle glycogen over time. See table 10.5 for further instructions on gymnastics.

Table 10.5   Gymnastics

Insulin: insulin pump	Insulin: basal-bolus regimen	Diet: insulin	Diet: basal-bolus regimen
• Decrease your basal insulin rates by 10–50% during gymnastics practice. • Remove your insulin pump completely during short routines. • If you keep your pump off for longer than an hour, monitor your blood sugars closely and reattach your pump to administer boluses if your blood sugars begin to rise. • Consider reducing your insulin boluses by 10–20% for this activity following a meal. • Reduce your overnight basal rates by 10–15% after prolonged or strenuous practices.	• If your activity follows a meal, reduce your rapid-acting insulin doses by 10–30%. • Keep your basal insulin doses the same unless your practices are unusually long and strenuous, after which you may lower your evening doses by 10–20% to prevent lows.	• Increase your carbohydrate intake by 0–15 grams per hour for extended gymnastics activity. • Eat an extra bedtime snack (if you don't lower your basal insulin) following exceptionally strenuous or prolonged practices.	• Increase your carbohydrate intake by 5–15 grams per hour during extended gymnastics activity. • Eat an extra bedtime snack following exceptionally strenuous or prolonged practices.

Athlete Examples

Required changes vary with the length and intensity of the gymnastics or other related activity, as well as whether you're involved in a practice or a competition.

Diet Changes Alone

For 90-minute ballet, jazz, and gymnastics classes, youngster Juliana Kotsifakis of Ocean City, Maryland, usually eats enough beforehand to get her blood sugars into the 150 to 200 mg/dl (8.3 to 11.1 mmol/L) range. Usually her blood glucose level is around 70 (3.9) when she finishes.

Combined Regimen Changes

During gymnastics classes that last 90 minutes, Kelsey McGill of Delaware takes her pump off but checks her blood sugars every 30 minutes to make adjustments in food or to reconnect to bolus. She eats a healthy, light snack beforehand to help keep her blood sugars stable.

Maggie Hudson of Virginia also frequently takes off her pump during gymnastics practices and meets. If she keeps it off for several hours, her blood sugars start to rise, so she takes an injection using a Novopen to bring them down. She also snacks before starting practices.

A Yukon, Oklahoma, resident, Meredith Bussett does three hours of gymnastics most days of the week, during which she disconnects from her pump. She tests frequently during the activity and reconnects to give boluses as necessary, and she eats a 15-gram carbohydrate snack before starting her practices.

Shannon Triller of Madison, Wisconsin, participates in nine hours of gymnastics a week throughout the year. Before practices, she makes sure that she has eaten well, but she decreases her prepractice boluses so that she only takes 1 unit of insulin for every 30 grams of carbohydrate instead of her usual 20 grams. In addition, after practices she doesn't use a correction factor for elevated sugars.

Delaine Wright of Hopkinton, Rhode Island, participates in training for trapeze and aerial fabric work through the New England Center for Circus Arts (www.necenterforcirucusarts.org). She takes her pump off during workouts because keeping it on it would hinder her performance, but she tests every 30 minutes and reconnects to bolus as needed. During this activity, she usually needs more insulin than for others that she routinely does (like treadmill running) because of the greater anaerobic and strength components that the activity requires and the adrenaline release that it causes. She also does quite a bit of trampolining, which she finds drops her sugars quite rapidly and requires a lowered basal rate if she jumps with her pump on.

Intensity, Duration, and Other Effects

Effect of competition   Even without eating anything, Shannon Triller often experiences large increases in her blood sugars during gymnastics competitions because of the mental stress of competing, along with the intense, short routines that she does. She tends to run low the morning after meets, though.

HORSEBACK RIDING, COMPETITIVE

This activity is usually of high intensity and short duration, especially during competitions. You use contractions of your postural muscles to keep yourself on top of the horse while it's moving through the competitive course. The faster the horse is moving, the more energy you'll have to use to stay on. The physical stress of this event, combined with the psychological stress of competition, may actually cause your blood sugars to rise. While practicing for such events, though, you'll repeat these movements many times, resulting in a glucose-lowering effect for which you may need to increase your carbohydrate intake slightly or lower your insulin doses.

Athlete Examples

For competitive riding, you will usually need to make adjustments to compensate, depending on the length and intensity of the activity.

Diet Changes Alone

While riding dressage, Delaine Wright of Rhode Island usually experiences a slight rise (50 mg/dl, or 2.8 mmol/L) in her blood glucose levels, which she tries to prevent with a basal rate that is higher by 0.2 unit per hour. She always feels better without having food in her stomach during short-duration exercise, so she avoids eating beforehand.

Combined Regimen Changes

To ride her pony Pal competitively during shows, Juliana Kotsifakis of Maryland eats snacks to increase her blood sugars to 130 to 150 mg/dl (7.2 to 8.3 mmol/L), and she then takes less insulin during the day because she's usually active and outdoors all day. For 90-minute lessons or riding on her own, she tries to start out a bit higher, between 150 and 200 mg/dl (8.3 and 11.1 mmol/L).

For competitive horseback riding (jumping), Maggie Drysch of Coto de Caza, California, usually has to give more insulin in the morning when she's competing and mentally stressed, but after she has been riding for a while, her blood glucose starts to come down. If she drops below 100 mg/dl (5.6 mmol/L), she eats a snack with 10 grams of carbohydrate in it. If she decides to take her pump off for a while, she gives a 0.3-unit bolus before disconnecting to cover the basal insulin that she'll be missing. Otherwise, her blood sugars will start to rise after a couple of hours. Overall, she needs less insulin for practices than for competitions.

ICE HOCKEY

Ice hockey involves short, power moves like shooting the puck and skating quickly to another position. The activity can be intense, however, resulting in significant use of muscle glycogen and blood sugar when you play for an extended time. Depending on how long and how hard you play, you may need to make some regimen changes. Practices may require more changes because of their prolonged, less intense nature compared with games. A confounding variable is that ice hockey competitions and practices often occur at unusual times (e.g., early morning practices, late-evening games). Early morning practices when your insulin levels are low may require you to make fewer adjustments. At other times of day (especially during evening games) or when you play for longer periods, you may need to increase your carbohydrate intake more and take less insulin for preexercise meals. See table 10.6 for further instructions on ice hockey.

Athlete Examples

These real-life scenarios show that ice hockey participation usually requires a combination of diabetes-related adjustments to compensate.

Combined Regimen Changes

Teenager Spencer Band of Canada takes off his insulin pump when he plays hockey because of the physical contact that playing entails. He usually removes it 30 to 45 minutes before his hour-long games start. On the bench, he has Gatorade during the games. He tends to have a delayed effect from the activity, and his sugars often drop by 6 mmol/L (108 mg/dl) overnight.

To play ice hockey on a travel team, Michael Blackwell of Virginia has to adjust for the games by setting a temporary basal rate on his pump that is 20 percent of his normal, starting 30 minutes before his games or practices and continuing for an hour. He tries to avoid eating really high-carbohydrate snacks afterward (like french fries) because his sugars tend to be higher right afterward. Because of his tendency to drop about 4 hours later, though, he doesn't give any insulin for his postexercise elevations. He also plays roller hockey, an activity that makes regulating his sugars a bit harder because there is no ice to cool him off.

To play hockey once a week on an adult league, Brian Witschen of St. Albert, Alberta (Canada), has to lower his preactivity insulin dose by 2 units (20 percent of his dinner dose) and drink a juice box halfway through to prevent lows.

Table 10.6 Ice Hockey

Insulin: insulin pump	Insulin: basal-bolus regimen	Diet: insulin	Diet: basal-bolus regimen
• Remove your insulin pump or reduce your basal rates by 50–75% during the activity. • Reduce your meal boluses by 25–50% if taken within 2–3 hours of playing. • Reduce your basal rates by 10–20% overnight following extended play later in the day.	• Decrease your rapid-acting insulin by 25–50% for activity after meals, less for activity first thing in the morning. • Following extended playing, reduce your evening dose of basal insulin by 10–15%.	• Consume 15–30 grams of carbohydrate an hour, depending on your playing time and intensity. • Eat a bedtime snack after prolonged activity, particularly in the evening.	• Consume an extra 15–30 grams of carbohydrate per hour depending on how hard you're working. • Consider having a snack at bedtime to help prevent nighttime hypoglycemia, especially when your games or practices take place in the evening.

INDOOR RACKET SPORTS (BADMINTON, HANDBALL, RACQUETBALL, AND SQUASH)

Racket sports involve quick, powerful moves, such as hitting or throwing the ball and moving into position, that are mostly anaerobic in nature. How hard and how long you play, along with your skill level, largely determine what changes you need to make for these activities. Playing longer will have more of a glucose-reducing effect, even if you're playing intensely, simply because you're doing more total activity. In addition, better players are more skilled at ball placement and may end up running less than their less-skilled opponents do. Well-placed, point-winning serves may also result in more waiting time and less active playing time. See table 10.7 for further instructions on indoor racket sports.

Table 10.7   Indoor Racket Sports: Badminton, Handball, Racquetball, Squash

Insulin: insulin pump	Insulin: basal-bolus regimen	Diet: insulin	Diet: basal-bolus regimen
• For shorter durations (30–60 minutes), reduce your rapid-acting insulin doses by 10–25% before playing. • Reduce your basal insulin rates by 25–50% or remove your pump altogether during the activity. • For longer games lasting 1–2 hours, reduce your boluses by 15–40% before exercise, and reduce basal rates by 50–75% during play.	• For shorter durations (30–60 minutes), reduce your rapid-acting insulin doses by 10–25% before playing, depending on how hard you're playing. • If playing when your insulin levels are lower (before a meal), make minimal insulin reductions and increases in carbohydrate intake. • For longer games lasting 1–2 hours, reduce rapid-acting doses by 15–40% before playing.	• Consume an additional 15–30 grams of carbohydrate per hour depending on your reductions in basal insulin rates and bolus doses. • Consume additional carbohydrate for longer games as needed, depending on your insulin reductions.	• For shorter durations, take in an additional 15–30 grams of carbohydrate per hour, especially if your insulin levels are higher (within 2–3 hours following a meal). • For longer games, increase your carbohydrate intake.

Athlete Examples

These examples show that court sports are intense enough to require some regimen changes to prevent hypoglycemia. Prolonged play has more of an aerobic effect as well.

Diet Changes Alone

To play badminton, type 2 exerciser Carys Jones of Chilliwack, British Columbia (Canada), does not need to change her doses of metformin. If she needs a snack while playing, she usually eats about 30 grams of carbohydrate.

Combined Regimen Changes

When Susan Greenback of Australia plays squash for an hour, she takes her insulin pump off 30 minutes before she begins and keeps it off until she is done playing. If she eats within 2 hours of playing, she doesn't bolus for less than 20 grams of carbohydrate; otherwise, she reduces her premeal bolus as well.

To compensate for playing squash for an hour, Toronto, Ontario (Canada), resident Michael Riddell usually reduces his preactivity bolus for a meal by 50 percent. He may also eat some carbohydrate during playing and more afterward, covering the postexercise carbohydrate with half of a usual bolus amount. If his starting blood sugar is above 10 mmol/L (180 mg/dl), though, he waits until it drops down to half that before eating any extra carbohydrate.

ROLLER DERBY

An American-invented contact sport, roller derby takes place on a circuit track onto which two teams send five players at a time: three blockers, one pivot, and one jammer (the only scorer). The contest involves three 20-minute periods that include 2 minutes of intense activity at a time (called jams), during which the teams attempt to score points. Players at certain positions (i.e., jammers) will generally work harder (and use up more glycogen) because they alone have to attempt to pass the pack during the jams and lap around as many times as possible. The other players on each team bunch together in a pack and skate at a slower speed. Because of the mix of anaerobic and aerobic work involved, this sport requires changes in carbohydrate intake and insulin doses to prevent lows.

Athlete Examples

The intensity of this sport can vary greatly during games and competitions, making regimen changes harder to predict.

Combined Regimen Changes

To participate in roller derby practices and competitions, Abigail Tinker of Somerville, Massachusetts, eat about 30 grams of carbohydrate without bolusing. She may also reduce her basal rate by 50 percent staring an hour before exercise and throughout the activity. She finds that in this sport the intensity of activity is not constant, so the effect on her blood sugars is hard to predict. Her biggest challenge is dealing with adrenaline-enhanced spikes in her blood sugars on competition days. To compensate for all these variables, she checks her blood glucose levels often and consumes glucose if her sugars fall below 120 mg/dl (6.7 mmol/L).

ROWING

Also called crew, outdoor rowing involves rhythmic, intense, full-body workouts over the length of a course or race on the water. Teams generally have one, two, four, or eight rowers per boat, and races usually consist of 5 to 8 minutes of all-out rowing for a standard-length event, which is 2,000 meters for the Olympics and 1,500 meters for U.S. high school races. But race distances can vary from 500-meter sprints to marathon or ultramarathon lengths.

Your regimen changes (insulin and diet) will depend on the intensity and duration of your practices and events. Longer, less intense crew practices may require greater regimen changes to maintain blood sugar levels. Wind conditions can increase the intensity of rowing because stronger winds will increase resistance. In addition, crew regattas (races on open water) may be more intense and have a larger anaerobic component, making your blood sugars more stable or even elevated during them. See table 10.8 for further instructions on rowing.

Table 10.8 Rowing

Insulin: insulin pump	Insulin: basal-bolus regimen	Diet: insulin	Diet: basal-bolus regimen
• For shorter, more intense rowing, reduce your basal insulin during the activity by 25–50%. • If you remove your pump, your blood sugars may rise during intense rowing; if this happens, give a small bolus of insulin when you reconnect. • You may need small reductions in meal boluses (10–20%) before rowing. • For longer rowing lasting 30 minutes or more, reduce your basal rates by 25–100% and premeal boluses by 20–30%.	• Reduce your insulin doses by 10–20% before shorter, more intense bouts of rowing. • For longer, less intense rowing (30 minutes or more), reduce your rapid-acting insulin by 20–50%.	• Supplement with 15–30 grams of carbohydrate per hour, depending on your insulin reductions. • If you reduce your insulin enough, you won't need much carbohydrate during intense rowing.	• Depending on how long you row and your preactivity insulin reductions, consume up to 15–30 grams of carbohydrate per hour. • For intense exercise with low insulin levels, you may need only 0–15 grams of carbohydrate.

Athlete Examples

These examples show that the intensity and duration of rowing activities have the biggest effect in determining what regimen changes you'll need to make.

Combined Regimen Changes

Olympic rower Chris Jarvis from Victoria, British Columbia (Canada), watches his glucose trends and pays attention to what his insulin levels are, how much carbohydrate he's eating, how strenuous his workouts are, and how mentally stressful competitions are, all of which affect his blood glucose levels. He may practice more than once a day, but for morning practices, he reduces his bolus for what he eats prepractice down to 0.5 unit per 125 grams of carbohydrate, with 0.6 unit of basal insulin per hour. During warm-ups, he may lower his basal further and take Power Gels to prevent lows. Thirty minutes before finishing his practice, he brings his basal back up to 1.25 units per hour. He boluses after practice with 1 to 3 units, waits 30 to 45 minutes, and then eats breakfast.

A varsity team rower for Georgetown University, Samantha Stevens (of Washington, D.C.) gives only 25 percent of her boluses before practices that last 3 hours (starting in the early morning), and she uses a square-wave bolus on her pump for any meals or snacks that she eats beforehand. If necessary, she takes in 15 grams of carbohydrate every 30 minutes during practice.

When Susan from Gander, Newfoundland (Canada), was part of a rowing team for three years, she found it to be a strenuous activity. She had to lower her insulin and eat an additional snack at bedtime to prevent overnight lows.

SOCCER (OR NON-AMERICAN FOOTBALL)

Depending on the position that you play, soccer is a combination of stop-and-start movements, power moves such as kicking or throwing the ball, and long runs. Midfielders and strikers may do sustained running, whereas fullbacks and goalkeepers may do only short bursts of intermittent activity. During practices, almost all team members may do continuous running or shooting drills.

You will likely need changes in both insulin and carbohydrate intake for most soccer play, but the adjustments will vary with your position and the duration of your play. You may need 30 to 45 grams of carbohydrate per hour, depending on your insulin levels, your intensity, and the duration of play. Longer practices or more playing time during games will cause greater use of your muscle glycogen stores and blood sugar, thus requiring some carbohydrate intake and reductions in insulin before and possibly after playing. During the soccer season, you will probably need to reduce your basal insulin doses as well. See table 10.9 for further instructions on soccer.

Athlete Examples

These examples show that combined insulin and diet changes are often, but not always, necessary to compensate for soccer play.

Diet Changes Alone

Spencer Lee Jones of Raleigh, North Carolina, plays soccer at least two hours a day, participating in both the club team at his university and in various adult leagues. He does not usually adjust his insulin intake before training, but he usually eats raisins or granola bars then.

Table 10.9 Soccer

Insulin: insulin pump	Insulin: basal-bolus regimen	Diet: insulin	Diet: basal-bolus regimen
• During any soccer play, reduce basal rates on your insulin pump by 25–100%. • A midfielder who runs more continuously during a game may need greater reductions (50–100%) than a goalkeeper does (25%). • For morning play, reduce your breakfast boluses by 10–30%, depending on how much you plan to lower your basal rates. • For soccer practices and games in the afternoon, reduce your lunchtime insulin boluses by 20–30% if playing within 2–3 hours. • Following prolonged or intense play, reduce your boluses for the next meal by 20–30 and reduce overnight basal insulin rates by 10–25% as well.	• For morning practices and games, lower your breakfast doses of rapid-acting insulin by 10–40%. • For soccer practices and games in the afternoon, decrease your prelunch doses of rapid-acting insulin by 20–50% if you'll be playing within 2 hours. • After long practices or intense playing, lower your insulin doses for your next meal by 20–30% and reduce evening basal insulin doses (if you take them) by 10–20% as well.	• Consume 15–30 grams of carbohydrate per hour for soccer play, depending on reductions in insulin basal rates and boluses and the intensity and duration of playing. • Consume more carbohydrate after intense or long workouts, and consider having a bedtime snack to help prevent lows overnight.	• Take in 15–30 grams of carbohydrate per hour for practices or afternoon games, depending how much you lower your premeal doses and how long and hard you play. • Consume extra carbohydrate afterward and an additional bedtime snack to prevent later-onset hypoglycemia.

A resident of Huntington Beach, California, Madison Muirhead eats extra carbohydrate to participate in soccer practices and games. She uses a sliding scale for her carbohydrate that changes with her starting blood sugars, but when starting in a normal range, she usually consumes about 20 grams. She usually doesn't adjust her Humulin N (intermediate-acting insulin) or Humalog doses.

Insulin Changes Alone

J.P. Delisio of Virginia takes his pump off during soccer games to compensate. If he has a low while playing, he drinks a juice box.

To play in an adult soccer league in Chesapeake, Virginia, Kirsteen Mitchell tries to start games with a blood glucose reading of 150 mg/dl (8.3 mmol/L). She then takes her pump off during the game.

Combined Regimen Changes

Before soccer games, John Moore of North Carolina takes 50 percent or less of his usual meal insulin, although he keeps his basal dose of Lantus the same. He may have to eat up to 25 grams of carbohydrate per half hour as well, depending on how hard he's playing.

If Michigan resident Christopher Pentescu has elevated glucose levels before playing soccer, he corrects with only half his usual dose of rapid-acting insulin. He additionally lowers his basal rate on his pump to 80 percent overnight, and he eats a small snack with carbohydrate and protein before playing.

To play high school soccer, Ethan Wehrly of Dayton, Ohio, usually needs to drink Gatorade during practices and games, and he eats a high-protein snack beforehand. Although he is often on the high side afterward, his sugars drop later, requiring him to cut back on his Lantus dose at bedtime and give a smaller amount of NovoLog for his bedtime snack on days when he plays games or has long practices.

Jake Sheldon of Maryland plays competitive soccer year round on a travel team. When he has practices right after dinner, he reduces his meal bolus by 20 to 25 percent and then takes off his pump during the activity. If he has a game scheduled midmorning or midafternoon, he eats a snack with protein and carbohydrate in it 30 minutes before starting and removes his pump during the game. After this activity, he only uses half corrections for high blood sugars because he's likely to drop later, for which he compensates by cutting back his basal rates by 50 percent for up to 8 hours after a practice or game.

For United Kingdom resident Joel Quinn, playing "football" (soccer in the United States) requires him to set a temporary basal rate that is 80 percent lower than normal starting 40 to 60 minutes before the activity. In addition, he eats a cereal bar with 15 grams of carbohydrate or a banana beforehand, and he may consume up to a bottle of Lucozade while playing.

A resident of Norwood, New Jersey, Michael Luzzi tries to have his blood sugars around 150 mg/dl (8.3 mmol/L) before soccer games. After games, he takes only half of his usual NovoLog doses but doesn't adjust his bedtime Lantus. He eats his usual meal before practices, and before games he consumes about 15 grams of carbohydrate.

Jenny Vandevelde of San Diego, California, plays indoor, beach, and regular soccer in several adult leagues. She takes her insulin pump off during all soccer play. Because beach soccer is extremely strenuous, she eats 30 to 40 grams of carbohydrate before she plays it.

For playing soccer, six-year-old Andrew Steckel from Pennsylvania cuts back on his premeal NovoLog by 0.5 unit and eats a snack after the game if he plays right after a meal. For practices or games at other times, he drinks a juice box halfway through. He doesn't adjust his bedtime Lantus, though.

Intensity, Duration, and Other Effects

Effect of position   Kirsteen Mitchell of Virginia finds that not wearing her pump works well when she plays forward, a position that requires a lot of running. When she ends up playing a defensive position, though, she has a much harder time keeping her blood sugars under control without any basal insulin.

TENNIS

Playing tennis involves short, powerful moves like serving, returning serves, moving into position, and hitting the ball, but extended periods of waiting occur between actions. Because of its stop-and-start nature, tennis is a mix of anaerobic and aerobic activity. The intensity depends on whether you're playing singles or doubles, because playing alone on your side of the court will usually force you to run farther and more overall. Both how long and how hard you play will affect your blood sugar responses and the adjustments that you'll need to make, and substantial differences are likely to be present between playing competitive and recreational tennis. Longer tennis games or practices will generally have more of a glucose-reducing effect than shorter ones. The skill level of the players can affect exercise intensity because being more skilled may mean that you end up running less as well. High-level serving can additionally result in more waiting and less active playing time. See table 10.10 for further instructions on tennis.

Table 10.10 Tennis

Insulin: insulin pump	Insulin: basal-bolus regimen	Diet: insulin	Diet: basal-bolus regimen
• Reduce basal insulin rates by 25–50% or remove the pump altogether while playing. • Reduce your premeal boluses by 10–25% before playing. • For tennis games or practices lasting 1–2 hours, reduce your boluses by 15–40% with similar basal rate changes.	• For playing less than an hour, lower your premeal insulin doses by 10–25%. • For longer tennis games or practices lasting more than an hour, reduce your doses by 15–40% before playing.	• Consume 15–30 grams of carbohydrate per hour, depending on your insulin reductions. • Increase your carbohydrate intake more for longer durations, if needed.	• Increase your carbohydrate intake to 15–30 grams per hour, especially if insulin levels are higher. • Playing tennis for longer may require greater carbohydrate intake to prevent lows.

Athlete Examples

The following examples show that you can make many regimen changes for tennis, depending on the length and type of tennis.

Combined Regimen Changes

Teenager Hortense Thomas of France plays competitive tennis. Before tennis training, which she does five times a week for an hour and a half, she lowers her basal rate by 30 percent, and if she eats within two hours of playing, she reduces her premeal bolus by 2 units. After doing her training, she cuts back her boluses by another 1 to 2 units for meals. To boost her blood sugars during practices or matches, she eats cereal bars.

Susan Greenback of Australia usually plays tennis for an hour for singles and 2 hours for doubles. For playing an hour, she takes her insulin pump off 30 minutes before her exercise, but for doubles lasting twice as long, she simply reduces her basal rate to 25 percent of normal 30 minutes beforehand and keeps it there during play. If she eats within 2 hours of playing, she doesn't bolus for less than 20 grams of carbohydrate, or she reduces it for more.

A USTA-ranked tennis player since the age of 14, Dan Anzel of Los Angeles, California, still plays tennis daily even though he is in his 70s. To compensate, he always has sweet drinks with him courtside, which he consumes as needed. He also takes a small amount of insulin before playing if his sugars are too high, but he does not adjust his Levemir doses.

Ten-year-old Joel Quinn of the United Kingdom plays competi-

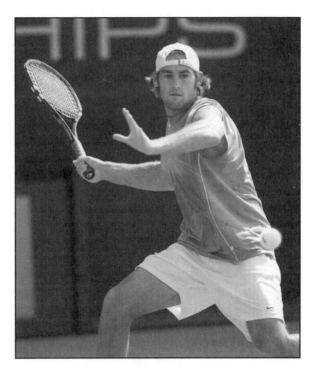

Longer tennis games or practices will generally have more of a glucose-reducing effect than shorter ones.

tive tennis and compensates for practices and tournaments by using a basal rate that is 70 percent lower than his normal rate, starting 40 to 60 minutes before he plays. He also eats a cereal bar with 15 grams of carbohydrate or a banana, along with three-fourths to a full bottle of Lucozade while practicing or competing.

A teenage resident of Phoenix, Arizona, Carter Gillespie participates in tennis practices and tournaments. His practices are after dinner for two hours, so at that meal, he reduces his NovoLog doses for the amount of carbohydrate that he eats from 1 unit for every six grams (1:6) to 1 unit for every eight (1:8). About an hour into practices, he drinks a 12-ounce (360-milliliter) bottle of Gatorade. Tournaments are generally more intense for him, so he uses a 1:10 ratio before them and sips Gatorade at each changeover, taking in about 18 ounces (540 milliliters) total during a match. He adjusts only his NovoLog doses for exercise, not his basal Lantus.

A type 2 diabetic tennis player and a USTA state champion in 2006, Connie Hilliard of Greensboro, North Carolina, plays on a couple of tennis teams that have competitive matches a couple of times per week. She sometimes adjusts the time of day that she takes her Amaryl if she has a match (she normally takes it at breakfast, along with metformin twice a day); otherwise, the only adjustment she makes is using glucose tablets to bring up a low blood sugar.

Another type 2, Richard Bell of Watkinsville, Georgia, plays tennis in a mixed doubles league a couple of times a week. By doing this activity and walking on a treadmill three days a week, he has been able to eliminate his Actos medication and now takes only metformin. He usually works out in the morning before he takes any medications to prevent lows, and he eats five small meals a day and 100 to 150 grams of protein daily.

Alan Kent Teffeteller from Athens, Tennessee, is a wheelchair athlete who adjusts for playing tennis by lowering his basal rate and giving smaller insulin boluses for carbohydrate before he plays. He also eats Extend bars if he needs to during games.

A Maine resident, Steffi Rothweiler uses a lower basal rate while playing tennis and drinks some juice before playing. Similarly, Katie from Harrison, New York, drinks some orange juice before playing if her sugars are on the low side, but then she removes her pump while playing.

TRACK EVENTS (400 TO 1,600 METERS)

Most track events are short, lasting from 45 seconds to 5 minutes or so and requiring a near-maximal effort. (Sprinting for less than 45 seconds is covered in the next chapter.) These types of events rely primarily on anaerobic energy sources. Longer track events such as 800-meter runs require more energy production from the lactic acid system but are still primarily anaerobic. Runs lasting longer than 2 minutes start to use a greater proportion of aerobic sources of energy, and track practices that involve running longer distances or repeated intervals are more aerobic in nature than track meets during which athletes run only shorter distances.

The diabetic regimen changes that you will need to make are determined more by the duration of aerobic activities and are less affected by anaerobic events. Your blood sugars will tend to decrease more following track practices or meets when muscle glycogen is restored than during the activity itself, when you're releasing glucose-raising hormones that keep your blood sugars higher. You may need more regimen changes to maintain your blood sugars both during and after practices when running for longer (compared with meets).

Athlete Examples

These examples demonstrate the usual types of regimen changes required for track practices and competitive meets.

Combined Regimen Changes

A San Diego resident, Blair Ryan has participated in collegiate track, running 800-meter and 4 × 400-meter relay events. For interval workouts on the track, she believes that she does her best running with blood glucose levels between 180 and 200 mg/dl (10 to 11.1 mmol/L). Longer-distance warm-ups (e.g., 3 miles, or 4.8 kilometers) bring her sugars down because of their lower intensity and duration compared with her track events. For interval workouts, she ends up taking in carbohydrate drinks during the warm-up and between intervals. The 6 × 800-meter portion of her training (with two-minute rest periods between intervals) can make her blood sugars drop as well, for which she consumes more carbohydrate drinks, but they also sometimes cause them to rise, for which she may take a 0.1-unit bolus of insulin.

Svati Narula of Maryland takes her pump off during all track running events. She finds that her blood sugars skyrocket during meets, so she doesn't need to eat much to compensate, particularly if she hasn't taken any insulin boluses within a few hours of racing.

Katie from New York usually does either 400- or 800-meter runs in the middle of track meets and then another 800 in a relay near the end of the meet. To compensate, she takes her pump off during each event, from the time that they call her event until afterward, or about a half hour at a time. She usually runs high after the events, but she boluses with enough NovoLog to bring her back down. Because track meets last all day, she eats and boluses normally. If she's low before one of her events, she simply drinks some orange juice to bring her sugars up.

WATER POLO

Water polo involves a combination of aerobic activity and anaerobic sprints, especially during competitions. Overall, this sport is primarily aerobic because it involves constant motion in the water to stay afloat using an eggbeater motion with your legs. You will encounter the anaerobic component when you have to do a sprint when play shifts from one end of the pool to the other or when you throw the ball. Training for water polo involves doing some distance swimming as well as shorter sprints.

Athlete Examples

The duration and intensity of water polo play usually requires adjustments to both food intake and insulin doses to compensate. For a comparable sport, refer to the section on swimming in chapter 9 and focus on the more intensive swimming recommendations and athlete examples.

Combined Regimen Changes

Because water polo practices involve two hours of nonstop treading water and some swimming, preteen Jake Adams of Carlsbad, California, disconnects from his pump during the sessions. He checks his blood sugars before practice, and if they're over 150 mg/dl (8.3 mmol/L), he boluses with 0.1 unit before disconnecting. After practices, he gives himself another 0.3 unit after reconnecting. If his prepractice blood sugars are under 100 mg/dl (5.6 mmol/L), he eats a snack with 15 grams of carbohydrate.

WRESTLING

This activity involves short, powerful muscle contractions and is almost purely anaerobic in nature. A wrestling meet may require few regimen changes to maintain your blood sugars because matches are brief and intense. On the other hand, wrestling practices may lower your blood sugar levels because of the cumulative effects of repeated bouts of activity. See table 10.11 for further instructions on wrestling.

Athlete Examples

Wrestling is a short-duration, intense sport that can be effectively compensated for in different ways.

Table 10.11   Wrestling

Insulin: insulin pump	Insulin: basal-bolus regimen	Diet: insulin	Diet: basal-bolus regimen
• You can maintain your blood sugars during wrestling meets by removing your insulin pump during each of your matches. • Remove your pump during longer practices or reduce your basal rates by 25–50% during practices and for up to 1–2 hours afterward. • If your blood sugars increase with your pump off for more than an hour, reconnect and bolus a small amount periodically. • For longer practices, consider lowering your insulin boluses after workouts by 10–20%. • Consider lowering your overnight basal rates by a small amount (10–15%).	• Your blood sugars may drop very little during intense wrestling matches and may even rise somewhat. • Reduce your rapid-acting insulin doses by 10–20% before and after longer practices. • Following especially strenuous or prolonged workouts, consider reducing your evening basal insulin doses by 10–15%.	• Consume up to 15 grams of carbohydrate per hour for this activity. • Consider eating an extra bedtime snack following extended workouts.	• Depending on your insulin levels and exercise intensity, consume up to 15 grams of carbohydrate per hour for wrestling. • Consume more carbohydrate in the following meal and at bedtime to prevent nighttime lows.

Diet Changes Alone

Columbia, Missouri, resident Andy Bell participates in submission wrestling practice and tournaments. His main strategy is to have very little insulin in his body when he wrestles, which is challenging when he enters a tournament in which he can be called at any time to start. If he can, he finishes a full meal at least three hours beforehand, but when called to compete sooner, he supplements with honey. He also prefers to eat peanut butter crackers or skim milk–based protein shakes before exercise because of their longer-duration effect in keeping his blood sugars stable.

Combined Regimen Changes

Joe Fiorucci from Shirley, New York, often goes days with eating little to no food to make a weight class in wrestling. Although likely still in his honeymoon period then, he has gone up to three months without taking any insulin to prevent lows associated with a low carbohydrate and food intake. He relies on Gatorade, other drinks, or meal bars to prevent lows during practices and meets.

*A*thlete *P*rofile

Name: Jake Sheldon

Hometown: Millersville, Maryland, USA

Diabetes history: Type 1 diabetes diagnosed in 2005 (at age eight)

Sport or activity: Competitive soccer (year-round regional travel team), as well as basketball, baseball, tennis, and golf during the summers

Greatest athletic achievement: Participating on a competitive travel soccer team despite having diabetes

Current insulin and medication regimen: I currently use an Animas insulin pump with Humalog.

Training tips: Test your blood sugars often. I need to know my blood sugar numbers before, during, and after practices and games. If you don't want your diabetes to get in the way of playing sports, you need

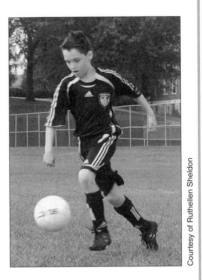

Courtesy of Ruthellen Sheldon

to eat properly and test a lot so that there aren't any surprises and your sugars are always in a good range. One thing that helps is eating my usual foods before games. During our last tournament, my mom got the entire team to visit Chik-Fil-A because their food is very predictable for me, but usually she packs my lunch and brings it in the car. I never want to have to miss even a minute of a game or practice because of diabetes.

Typical daily and weekly training and diabetes regimen (soccer season):

▶ **Monday:** I eat dinner 45 minutes before my 90-minute practices and bolus 20 percent less than my normal carbohydrate bolus and correction. During practices, I take my pump off the whole time. I used to test halfway through, but now I only do when I feel low. After practice, I reconnect my pump and test again. When I eat a snack afterward (usually a bowl of cereal), I decrease my bolus a little (maybe 10 percent). At bedtime, if I'm less than 150 mg/dl (8.3 mmol/L), I eat a snack (15 to 30 grams of carbohydrate and some protein). If I'm lower than 150 (8.3) at bedtime or during the night (my parents usually test me at their bedtime and 2:00 a.m.), my pump may be off for a couple of hours or my basal rates may be lowered 10 to 20 percent all night. If I'm ever high during or after practice (above 275, or 15.3), I correct with 50 percent of my usual dose because my sugars may only be temporarily high from a tough practice.

▶ **Tuesday:** Before I used a pump, I got lows the morning after practice at school, but not anymore.

▶ **Wednesday:** Same routine as Monday with a 90-minute soccer practice.

▶ **Thursday:** Just regular activities at school and afterward.

▶ **Friday:** Same routine as Monday with a 90-minute soccer practice (or sometimes no practice).

▶ **Saturday:** Usually a day off, except for an occasional soccer game or two.

► *Sunday:* For games, we have 45 minutes to warm up and hour-long soccer games, but the time when my team plays always changes. My parents like it best when my games are right after a meal because then it's like doing a practice. I bolus 20 percent less than recommended and eat 45 minutes before I start playing. For midmorning games, I eat an extra snack (30 grams of carbohydrate and some protein) and bolus less. Thirty minutes into our warm-up, I test and eat if I'm less than 150 (8.3)—something like 15 grams of carbohydrates in grapes or in drinkable yogurt, or maybe just a roll of Smarties. My parents like me to start a game with my blood sugar between 150 (8.3) and 250 (13.4). If I'm over 250 (13.4), it's probably just from excitement and I don't treat it, but my parents worry more! At halftime, one of my parents tests me again while the coach is talking to the team. The other kids know I have diabetes and don't care, but if I have to eat some Smarties or Skittles with our halftime fruit (like if I'm under 100, or 5.6), a few of the boys will put out their hands for extras. If I'm over 275 (15.3) at halftime, I eat the fruit but take a 50 percent correction bolus. During the games, I just drink ice water only because my pump is off. I can run low for up to 8 hours after a game, so I keep testing often and eating when I need to.

Other hobbies and interests: I love watching professional and college sports. My favorite teams are the Boston Red Sox and the Michigan Wolverines. I'm a straight A student and have an older brother (Tom) and a Pug named Shorty. I love to eat, especially pizza, hot dogs, soda, and Slurpees. I also like kneeboarding during the summer.

Good diabetes and exercise story: Three days after I got diabetes on July 4, 2005, I had to play in a baseball tournament. I was really new to the daily routine of testing my blood sugars and taking insulin injections, but I got out there and played. I even pitched two innings for the first time in a game situation and didn't give up any runs during that first inning. My parents wanted me to test every 20 minutes, but it didn't phase me—I stayed focused on the game.

I also attend a weeklong soccer camp that runs from 9:00 a.m. to 3:00 p.m. during the hottest part of the summer. My parents were cool enough to let me go the summer after I was diagnosed, and I managed OK. The first day of camp, though, it was so hot that my glucose meter stopped working. I didn't panic, just bolused for my food and assumed that because I was feeling fine I wasn't low. My parents sent me to camp the next day with a cooler for my meter!

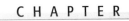

Power Sports

Power sports require you to perform short, powerful bouts of activity. In baseball, the activity may involve hitting the ball and sprinting to first base. In field events, it may be the high jump or discus throw. Recently, athletes with diabetes have excelled at playing baseball professionally. They have even been doing well in bodybuilding and power-lifting events, including winning Mr. Universe and other titles without using steroids or other performance-enhancing drugs. This chapter discusses some of these power sports and activities, including baseball and softball, bodybuilding, fencing, field events, power lifting and Olympic weightlifting, sprinting, and volleyball (indoor and beach).

GENERAL RECOMMENDATIONS FOR POWER SPORTS

For most power sports, the requisite bursts of activity last less than 10 seconds, which means that your phosphagen system (composed of ATP and CP) alone provides the energy that your muscles need to contract. If the activities last longer (up to 2 minutes), you'll also be getting some of the ATP through your lactic acid system, which is the one that you know is working hard when you start to feel the burn in your muscles. The burn results mainly from the breakdown of glycogen and the buildup of acids as a by-product. The resulting drop in pH in your muscles causes the discomfort.

GENERAL ADJUSTMENTS BY DIABETES REGIMEN

The power sport or activity that you're involved in will determine what changes you need to make in your regimen. Intense activities can decrease, increase, or have no immediate effect on your blood sugar levels. Their potential use of glycogen, though, can cause a lowering of your blood sugars later on, particularly when you do a power activity intermittently over an extended period. For example, the occasional hits, sprints, and throws required to play baseball can have a cumulative effect on glycogen use, and you may need to watch out for later-onset hypoglycemia when that glycogen is being restored.

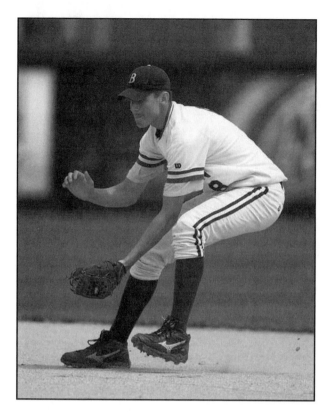

The occasional hits, sprints, and throws required to play baseball can have a cumulative effect on glycogen use, making it necessary to watch out for later-onset hypoglycemia when that glycogen is being restored.

Insulin Pump Users

For doing power sports recreationally, your insulin adjustments must be sport specific. You may require no changes for easy or brief play. But for prolonged play like team practices, you may need to reduce your rapid-acting insulin boluses and your basal rates during the activity by 10 to 50 percent, depending on the intensity and duration of your workout. You'll need to reduce your insulin less than you would for endurance sports, however, because of the intense, brief nature of power activities. If they cause a great enough release of glucose-raising hormones, your blood sugars may increase, and you may need more insulin to compensate. If you participate in these sports and activities for an hour or more, you may have to consume 10 to 30 grams of carbohydrate, depending on your insulin changes. You may also have to reduce your insulin boluses or basal rates by 10 to 25 percent following activity in certain sports, as well as eat more.

Basal-Bolus Regimens

For power sports, your insulin adjustments will depend on the sport. If you're doing short or easy activities, you may not need to adjust anything in your regimen. Working out for longer, though, such as when you're involved in team practices for an hour or more, may require that you reduce your preactivity, rapid-acting insulins by 10 to 50 percent. If you do cut back on your insulin, you'll need a smaller reduction than you use for more aerobic sports because the brevity and intensity of power activities often cause your blood sugars to go up temporarily instead of down (meaning that you may need some insulin to bring your sugars back down). For prolonged participation, you may need 10 to 30 grams of carbohydrate per hour, depending on how much you reduce your rapid-acting insulin and how much insulin is in your system. Following certain activities, you may choose to reduce your bedtime doses of basal insulin by 10 to 15 percent and have a bedtime snack to prevent lows when you've depleted a substantial amount of muscle glycogen.

Noninsulin and Oral Medication Users

The powerful nature of these activities is likely to raise your blood sugars (albeit temporarily), which happens even in athletes without diabetes. If you do these activities intermittently over an extended period, however, your blood sugar should come back down. As with the power–endurance sports, doing an aerobic cool-down of any length afterward will bring down elevations more quickly. In the day or so following these activities, your blood sugar may tend to stay lower while your body is using glucose to restore the muscle glycogen that you used up. You may be more insulin sensitive for 24 to 48 hours afterward. If you take certain longer-lasting oral medications (i.e., Diabinese, DiaBeta, Micronase, or Glynase), check your blood sugars if you ever start to feel any symptoms that you associate with getting low.

Intensity, Duration, and Other Effects

The level of effort, the duration, and the type of power sport (recreational or competitive) together have the biggest effects on your blood sugar levels. Recreational play is usually less intense but more prolonged than competitive play. Being more active overall, and thus depleting more muscle glycogen from repeated, powerful movements, can reduce your blood sugars, whereas an intense competition like throwing a shot put (field event) may cause them to rise from the release of glucose-raising hormones. On the other hand, recreational softball may have no effect on your blood sugar levels. But if you play for two or more hours, your softball activity can eventually cause a decrease in blood sugar levels, and doing any power activities enough times can cause them to be lower following the activity and overnight.

BASEBALL AND SOFTBALL

These activities usually require only short bursts of movement like sprinting, hitting, and throwing, so they are extremely anaerobic in nature. As a result, you may not use much energy doing them or need to make many adjustments for diabetes. But these activities help younger participants improve hand–eye coordination and fine motor skills and are useful for stimulating overall motor development.

How hard you're playing and at what level (i.e., recreational or competitive) will affect your blood sugar responses. For example, in baseball or softball, the catcher and pitcher are more active than the other fielders are because the former two are involved in almost every play. A recreational softball game can be quite sedentary because only one player at a time is up to bat for half the inning, and during the other half, most players are not directly involved with every play. Doing conditioning drills during practices will increase the potential glucose-lowering effects of these activities, as will doing any drills more continuously. See table 11.1 for further instructions on baseball and softball.

Table 11.1   Baseball and Softball

Insulin: insulin pump	Insulin: basal-bolus regimen	Diet: insulin pump	Diet: basal-bolus regimen
• Reduce your insulin boluses by 10–20% before more prolonged play like team practices. • If you're playing long or hard, alternatively or additionally reduce your basal rates by 10–15%.	• Reduce your preactivity insulin doses by 10–15% for practices and longer play.	• Increase your carbohydrate intake by 0–15 grams depending on your insulin reductions during longer games. • Consume 10–25 grams of carbohydrate for team practices involving running and other activities.	• Supplement with 5–15 grams of carbohydrate for intense or prolonged games. • Consume 10–30 grams of carbohydrate for practices involving aerobic training activities.

Athlete Examples

The following examples show that recreational play may require minimal changes but that longer, more intense practices can reduce your blood sugars to a greater degree.

Insulin Changes Alone

To compensate for playing baseball, Jake Sheldon of Millersville, Maryland, reduces his before-practice insulin boluses by 10 to 15 percent. If he needs to, he may set a lower basal rate for a while after a game or practice.

When playing baseball, J.P. Delisio of Midlothian, Virginia, keeps his pump on without adjusting anything except when he's up at bat. If he gets low, he treats it by drinking 4-ounce (120-milliliter) juice boxes.

Baylee Glass of Los Lunas, New Mexico, plays softball, and on the days that she plays she decreases her Lantus dose by 1 unit (down from 12 units). Usually her blood sugars are stable until two to five hours after games or practices, when they drop.

A resident of Long Beach, California, Kaylee Swanson pitches fast-pitch softball, during which she leaves her insulin pump on. Sometimes, she will give her hourly basal amount as a bolus before disconnecting.

Diet Changes Alone

North Carolina resident John Elwood plays baseball at the middle school level. For this activity, he leaves his pump on and doesn't adjust his insulin doses unless a pattern of lows is evident. Normally, he simply eats more carbohydrate to compensate for the activity.

An exerciser with type 2 diabetes, Chris Simmonds of Abingdon, Maryland, is a baseball umpire on weekends. He tries to eat some carbohydrate before every game because although he controls his diabetes with metformin as his only medication, his blood sugars often drop when he is refereeing, especially when he refs multiple games.

Combined Regimen Changes

Kate Zender of Enumclaw, Washington, plays fast-pitch softball, for which she usually lowers her basal rate by 50 percent. Occasionally, she takes her pump off during games when she is extremely active. She also makes sure to have some carbohydrate and protein before starting to play, and she may drink some Gatorade to prevent lows during games.

Phoenix, Arizona, resident Debbie Shisler plays softball on scholarship at her university in California. She finds that she doesn't have to take much NovoLog to cover her food during the softball season because she's a pitcher and practices a lot. To prevent lows when pitching, she consumes Oreos and orange juice. She usually takes Lantus in the morning and the evening, but she may take less of an evening dose on days that she has been very active.

Brandon Hunter of West Plains, Missouri, usually disconnects from his pump during baseball practices and games. He generally eats a snack with about 15 grams of carbohydrate before playing and often eats some more during games. When he can, he monitors his blood sugars, and if they start to rise during two-hour games, he reconnects and gives a small bolus of insulin to counter it.

To play cricket (similar to baseball) in the United Kingdom, Joel Quinn of Bath, Somerset, usually sets a temporary basal rate on his pump that is 50 percent lower starting 40 to 60 minutes before the activity. He also usually eats a cereal bar with 15 grams of carbohydrate or a banana beforehand, along with drinking Lucozade (about one bottle) while playing for 2 hours.

New York City resident Gayle Brosnan always turns off her insulin pump an hour before she starts playing softball during the spring and summer months. She likes her blood glucose levels to be at least 160 mg/dl (8.9 mmol/L) when she starts playing, and she will take in carbohydrate if it drops down to 130 (7.2) or below.

BODYBUILDING

This activity depends on anaerobic energy sources for the muscle-building portion but also includes a more aerobic component than activities like power lifting or weight training. Bodybuilding competitions themselves, depending on which division you've entered, may have little effect on your blood sugars other than from mental stress. The more prolonged training for these events is similar to high-resistance weight training, and the resulting increases in muscle mass can greatly increase your overall insulin sensitivity, causing you to need less insulin. Aerobic workouts undertaken to lower your body fat levels, though, are entirely different and more likely to cause reductions in blood sugar levels.

Heavy weight training causes a large release of glucose-raising hormones, and your blood sugars may actually rise rather than fall during this activity. Doing a prolonged weight-training session, though, can use up a lot of muscle glycogen, thus increasing your risk of later-onset hypoglycemia. For specific regimen changes for higher-intensity workouts, refer to the section on weight training in chapter 8. Combining weight workouts with some cardio training can effectively lower your blood sugars. For the cardio portion, your regimen changes will depend primarily on the intensity and duration of your workout. Refer to chapter 8 for recommendations for specific aerobic conditioning machines as well. See table 11.2 for further instructions on bodybuilding.

Table 11.2 Bodybuilding

Insulin: insulin pump	Insulin: basal-bolus regimen	Diet: insulin pump	Diet: basal-bolus regimen
• When weightlifting, keep your basal rates the same or reduce them only slightly. • During bodybuilding competitions, disconnect your pump but give a bolus when reconnecting if your sugars have gone up. • If you combine weight training with aerobic workouts, you may choose to disconnect your pump during both activities if they last less than an hour, or reduce your basal rates by 25–50%. • When resistance training after a meal, reduce your meal bolus by 10–20%.	• You will need minimal changes to your rapid-acting insulin doses to maintain your blood sugar levels during this activity. • For weight training soon after eating, doing prolonged training of 2 hours or more, or combining it with aerobic workouts, reduce your premeal insulin by 10–30%. • Doing this activity alone (with no aerobic workout) when your insulin levels are low may cause your blood sugars to rise, for which you may need to take some insulin afterward. • You will not generally need to change your basal insulin doses for this activity.	• For workouts of less than an hour, you may not need extra carbohydrate, depending on how much you lower your insulin. • For prolonged training sessions of 2 hours or more, consume 5–20 grams of carbohydrate per hour.	• For shorter workouts, consume 5–10 grams of carbohydrate per hour, depending on your insulin reductions. • For prolonged training, consider consuming 10–20 grams of carbohydrate per hour.

Athlete Examples

The following examples show that training for bodybuilding can have different effects than those that occur in competition.

Insulin Changes Alone

Because she follows a strict bodybuilding diet (high in protein), Lisa Harlan of Kettering, Ohio, mainly adjusts for bodybuilding with her insulin regimen. She exercises consistently by lifting weights regularly and intensely and by doing one hour of cardio work a day. Because her routine is set, she only has to lower her insulin by 0.5 to 1 unit when doing a particularly draining workout. She believes that the posing part of competitive bodybuilding is extremely difficult and draining, although the cardio training is most likely what causes her blood sugars to drop.

Combined Regimen Changes

Kansas City, Missouri, resident Kim Seeley is a professional fitness competitor in the IFBB, the International Federation of Body Builders. She finds that high-intensity lifting makes her blood glucose levels rise, whereas the cardio training portions lowers them. She also finds that when she's dieting down (eating "clean") over 9 to 12 weeks for a show, her body fat gets extremely low and her overall insulin requirements drop by at least 30 percent. But she also has to watch how many calories she's eating to continue losing fat. When she is getting ready for a competition, she switches to using Lantus and Humalog instead of a pump because when her body fat gets low, she doesn't have any suitable places to insert her pump infusion sets. The only time that she has to increase her Humalog instead of lowering it is on leg workout days and during competitions when her stress levels cause her blood sugars to rise.

Mr. Universe title holder Doug Burns from Menlo Park, California, agrees with Kim's experiences with body fat levels and insulin requirements. He finds that his training schedule differs drastically when he's just training to stay healthy compared with when he is preparing for a show. He adjusts his insulin doses slightly based on his body weight and body fat levels. His also finds that the leaner he becomes for a show, the less insulin he needs to take. He alters his diet when he's trying to get lean for a show, which also affects his insulin needs.

A resident of Auckland, New Zealand, Nev Raynes finds that when he does hard weight training and bodybuilding workouts, he has to lower his NovoRapid doses by 2 to 3 units (about 25 percent of his normal) to prevent lows. Unless he has some insulin in his body when he trains, his blood sugars rise rather than fall. To prevent lows, he usually sips fruit juice throughout his workouts or training sessions. To prevent overnight lows, he sometimes lowers his bedtime Protophane (intermediate-acting) insulin on days when he has been more active.

FENCING

One of only four sports that have been featured at every modern Olympic games, fencing involves short, powerful thrusts and jabs and quick movements, as well as constant leg movement during a given round of competition. Training for this activity usually involves a combination of power and endurance movements. Doing well in fencing requires a good level of general fitness that can be achieved through a combination of yoga, weight training, and other cardio and endurance workouts—even jump rope training and plyometrics. The glycemic effect will vary most with the duration and intensity of your training. Working harder for longer produces the greatest chance of lowering your blood sugars. If you're competing, your blood sugars may go up instead of down because of the intensity of the match and the mental stress of competition.

Athlete Examples

Because of its brief but extremely intense periods of activity followed by lengthy down times, this activity can be compensated for in a variety of ways.

Combined Regimen Changes

Adrian Connard of Victoria, Australia, takes half his usual meal bolus if he eats within two hours of the start of a fencing bout but otherwise makes no adjustments to his NovoRapid or Protophane (intermediate-acting insulin) doses. He substitutes sports drinks for water during a competition because he finds that he can't eat anything while competing.

FIELD EVENTS

Most field events (at track and field competitions) are short, requiring either a near-maximal muscular contraction (like throwing a shot put or throwing a discus) or near-maximal full-body effort (e.g., long jump). These types of events use anaerobic energy sources almost exclusively. The intensity and brevity of events during competitions should make your blood sugar levels easy to maintain, although they may decrease more when your muscle glycogen is being restored afterward. You may need more regimen changes to maintain your blood sugar levels both during and after practices (compared with meets) because of doing more prolonged activity then. See table 11.3 for further instructions on field events.

Table 11.3   Field Events

Insulin: insulin pump	Insulin: basal-bolus regimen	Diet: insulin pump	Diet: basal-bolus regimen
• Decrease your basal rates by 10–50% during practices, depending on how long they are and how hard you are working. • Reduce your boluses by 10–20% for practices following a meal as well. • During most field competitions, you can remove your pump during your events, reattaching it to give boluses if you keep it off longer than an hour at a time. • You will likely need to make limited changes for competitive events because of their intensity.	• If your training follows a meal, reduce your premeal doses by 10–20%. • Make minimal insulin changes for competitive meets, because the events are short and intense.	• Consume no extra carbohydrate for short, intense field events. • Increase your carbohydrate intake by up to 5–15 grams per hour for extended practices.	• Consume no extra carbohydrate for field events and competitions. • Consume 10–15 grams of carbohydrate per hour during extended practices, if needed.

POWER LIFTING AND OLYMPIC WEIGHTLIFTING

These activities rely on short-term energy sources like ATP and CP to fuel maximal lifts lasting no more than 10 seconds. But power lifting and Olympic weightlifting competitions are different sports; power lifting involves doing maximal lifts in the squat, bench press, and dead lift, whereas Olympic weightlifting consists of only two lifts, the snatch and the clean and jerk. Both activities may initially cause a rise in your blood sugars because of their intensity, but your blood sugars may drop later. Doing prolonged training for these events is similar in many ways to high-resistance weight training. Increases in your muscle mass resulting from this training, however, can greatly increase your overall insulin sensitivity, which means that you will need less insulin. For specific regimen changes for higher-intensity weight workouts, refer to the section on weight training in chapter 8.

Athlete Examples

Depending on how intense your training is and how long you train, you may have to make various adjustments to manage your blood sugars effectively with these activities.

Insulin Changes Alone

A type 1.5 diabetic Olympic weightlifter from Aloha, Oregon, Keith Knight turns his pump off completely before starting high-intensity weightlifting workouts that last 45 to 60 minutes. Usually, he doesn't turn the pump back on until 2 to 3 hours after exercise. He does not start weightlifting unless his blood sugar is 140 mg/dl (7.8 mmol/L) or higher.

Diet Changes Alone

Type 2 diabetic exerciser Bob Duncan of Richmond, Virginia, finds that doing power-lifting routines maintains his blood sugars more effectively than doing aerobic workouts does. He consumes a protein powder, a banana, and dried fruit before his lunchtime workouts.

SPRINTING

Although a true power sprint would be running at your maximal speed until you can't keep up the pace any longer (usually for 5 to 10 seconds), sprinting can be done for different lengths and intervals. For example, 800-meter runs require more energy production from the lactic acid system and are still primarily anaerobic, whereas runs lasting longer than 2 minutes will begin to use a greater proportion of aerobic sources of energy. When you practice running longer or do repeated intervals, your recovery is mainly aerobic, although the actual sprint or faster intervals may not be. If you do a single sprint, your blood sugar may go up (as a means to keep blood sugars higher at the end of an aerobic workout, as discussed in chapter 2). If you do repeated sprints, the immediate effect will be a rise in your blood sugars, followed by a drop later when your body is restoring glycogen and other fuels that your body used. When sprinting, worry more about preventing later-onset lows than having them in the short-term. See table 11.4 for further instructions on sprinting.

Athlete Examples

These examples show that the primary effect of sprinting is an increase in your blood sugars rather than a decrease, at least while you're working out.

Table 11.4 Sprinting

Insulin: insulin pump	Insulin: basal-bolus regimen	Diet: insulin pump	Diet: basal-bolus regimen
• During short sprinting efforts, make no changes in your insulin. • Give a small bolus if sprinting causes a rise in your blood sugar levels.	• You will not need to make any adjustments for sprinting. • If the activity causes your blood sugars to rise, give a small dose of rapid-acting insulin, if desired.	• Make no adjustments for sprinting, unless you do repeated sprints that use up more muscle glycogen, for which you may need to eat a carbohydrate snack later to compensate.	• You should not need any extra carbohydrate for sprinting, but if you do multiple sprints eat a snack later to prevent later-onset lows.

Insulin Changes Alone

When Felix Kasza of Redmond, Washington, does maximal-intensity sprinting, he finds that he needs to give himself about 1 to 1.5 extra units of insulin per hour.

A Newtown, Pennsylvania resident, David Walton finds that sprinting at the end of a long run raises his blood sugars. For example, during a 3-mile (4.8-kilometer) run that he did at a fast pace, when he practically sprinted the entire last .5 mile (.8 kilometer), his blood sugars rose by 30 mg/dl (1.7 mmol/L), although they would have dropped had he not done the all-out pace.

Doretta Reily of Atlanta, Georgia, does sprinting intervals at least once a week, but for those, she doesn't adjust her food intake. Instead, depending on her blood glucose levels before exercise, she usually reduces her insulin doses for snacks and meals before working out. On the days that she does sprint intervals, she may need more orange juice to treat lows compared with what she takes in during her weight-training workouts.

VOLLEYBALL AND BEACH VOLLEYBALL

This activity involves short, powerful moves (serving or hitting the ball) and is generally anaerobic in nature. Your overall energy expenditure may be relatively low, depending on how long and hard you play, but beach volleyball may cause you to expend more because you'll be walking and running on loose sand. Generally, practices require more energy than games, simply because practices usually last longer. Moving to and hitting the ball require only short bursts of activity, and you will need to make fewer changes for volleyball than you do for more active court sports like basketball. If you play volleyball or the beach variety recreationally, you may not need to make many adjustments to your diabetes regimen because the intensity is usually low and you may not be actively involved in every play. Higher-level play may initially raise your blood sugars, but if you play hard or long, be on the lookout for later-onset lows. See table 11.5 for further instructions on volleyball and beach volleyball.

Table 11.5 Volleyball and Beach Volleyball

Insulin: insulin pump	Insulin: basal-bolus regimen	Diet: insulin pump	Diet: basal-bolus regimen
• Consider removing your insulin pump during more active play. • If you keep it on, reduce the basal rates of your pump by 25–33% during competitive play. • Reduce your premeal boluses by 10–20% if taken within 2–3 hours of playing.	• Decrease your insulin doses by 10–25% before more strenuous play. • For easy or recreational play, make minimal (if any) rapid-acting insulin reductions.	• Consume 0–20 grams of carbohydrate per hour, depending on how hard you're playing. • You may need no extra carbohydrate intake for recreational play, although the beach variety may lower your blood sugars faster than playing indoors on a court does.	• Consume an extra 10–20 grams of carbohydrate per hour depending on your insulin levels and the intensity of your activity. • Make minimal increases in your carbohydrate intake for recreational play, unless you're playing on loose sand on the beach.

Athlete Examples

The following examples demonstrate that the intensity of play has the greatest effects on your blood sugar response to volleyball.

Insulin Changes Alone

Jenny Vandevelde from California lowers her basal rate on her insulin pump to 20 percent of normal when she plays volleyball and treats lows with gummy bears.

Similarly, Julie Majurin of Indianapolis, Indiana, decreases her basal rate to 25 percent of her normal rate when playing volleyball.

Richard Feifer of California reduces his basal to 10 percent of normal starting 30 minutes before playing until 30 minutes before he stops.

A Canada resident, Tania Knappich of Brampton, Ontario, disconnects her pump when she plays, as does Leannne Lauzonis of Albuquerque, New Mexico. Leanne usually plays for one or two hours and then has problems with her blood sugars dropping afterward.

Combined Regimen Changes

To play on her high school's varsity volleyball team in Ashland, Virginia, Taylor Thornton usually has to decrease the amount of NovoLog that she takes on days when she does extreme amounts of exercise, but she doesn't adjust her Lantus doses. She also drinks Gatorade while playing to prevent lows.

Christa, a preteen from Palm Springs, California, plays volleyball year round. When she eats a meal before playing, she cuts back on her Humalog dose by 1 to 2 units, and she may take a unit less later after playing. If she starts to feel low while playing, she eats a Zone bar (the strawberry kind) because they have carbohydrate and protein in them.

*A**thlete** P**rofile***

Name: Doug Burns

Hometown: Redwood City, California, USA

Diabetes history: Type 1 diabetes diagnosed in 1972 (at age seven)

Sport or activity: Power lifting and bodybuilding

Greatest athletic achievement: Setting an American record in the bench press, winning the overall Natural Mr. USA (2004) and Natural Mr. Universe Tall Class (2006) titles

Current insulin and medication regimen: NovoLog in an Animas insulin pump

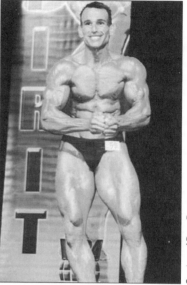

Courtesy of Doug Burns

Training tips: First, set your own goals, ones that are specific and ones that you believe in, ones that you own. Your training then has purpose. Second, train your hardest to bring them about. If I can do it, I know that you can! Give yourself the freedom to make mistakes and laugh them off, even the bad ones. All of us with diabetes make mistakes, either with our training, our performance, or by having rough blood sugar days.

Typical daily and weekly training and diabetes regimen: My training schedule differs drastically between "healthy training" and "contest training." I adjust my insulin dosages, slightly but consistently, based on my body weight and body fat levels (the leaner you are, the less insulin you need). Here is my standard healthy training schedule:

▸ **Monday:** Cardio early in the morning, usually for 30 to 45 minutes, and lifting in the evening using chest, shoulders, triceps, and abdomen (three to five sets of two to four exercises per body part)

▸ **Tuesday:** Hills in the late afternoon (outdoor cardio for 50 minutes) and leg workout (four to six sets of three to four exercises per body part, including squats and leg curls)

▸ **Wednesday:** Cardio early in the morning, usually for 30 to 45 minutes, and lifting in the evening using back and biceps (three to five sets of two to four exercises per body part)

▸ **Thursday:** Cardio workout for 40 minutes and leg workout (five sets of three exercises per body part)

▸ **Friday:** Cardio 30 for minutes and upper body (combined exercises)

▸ **Saturday:** Normal activities only

▸ **Sunday:** Rest day

Other hobbies and interests: I love to read and hike to places I've never been. I have an entrepreneurial spirit and keep looking for ways to excel.

Good diabetes and exercise story: Born in Washington, D.C., and raised in Long Beach, Mississippi, I was diagnosed with type 1 diabetes at the age of 7. Before the advent of blood glucose monitors and effective ways to monitor the disease, I spent my first few years in and out of various hospitals because of having extremely poor diabetes control. At the age of 10, I was admitted to the emergency room of Johns Hopkins Medical Center at a body weight of only 53 pounds (24 kilograms) and with a blood glucose reading of 1,153 mg/dl (64.1 mmol/L). Because of my emaciated appearance and consistent hospitalizations, I was picked on regularly by other children and was told that I couldn't participate in team sports.

Finding a picture of a muscular Sampson with a lion in a headlock, I was inspired to begin lifting weights anyway on my own (often using chunks of concrete and other homemade weights) and dedicated myself to getting stronger. At first nothing changed, but through persistence and within a few years, I went from being the kid in school known as "the bag of bones" to a champion who set state, regional, and American records in drug-free power lifting. Realizing the benefits of aerobic activity, I then shifted my focus to physique development and, to date, have the won the Southern States Championships, Mr. California, Mr. USA, and Natural Mr. Universe Tall titles.

CHAPTER 12

Outdoor Recreational Activities and Sports

Have you ever dreamed of walking or cycling across mountains and deserts, backpacking for weeks in the mountains, scuba diving in crystal blue waters, or whitewater rafting down a dangerous river? Maybe you have watched the Winter Olympics and seen athletes skiing down mountains at incredible speeds and wished that you could try that. Or maybe the slower pace and scenery of hiking is more to your liking. In any case, people with diabetes have done all those activities and many more, all while controlling their blood sugar levels.

This chapter gives recommendations for regimen changes and real-life examples for many outdoor physical activities and sports, including hiking and backpacking, rock climbing, mountain biking, boogie boarding, scuba diving and snorkeling, snowboarding, sailing, skateboarding, and many others—even yard work, adventure racing, and dog mushing. These recreational sports and activities vary widely in intensity. Some activities are brief, primarily fueled by ATP and CP, whereas others involve the lactic acid system and some muscular endurance, such as rock climbing. Most of these activities rely on aerobic energy sources, however, especially prolonged activities such as backpacking and mountaineering.

GENERAL RECOMMENDATIONS FOR OUTDOOR ADVENTURES

Giving overall general recommendations for regimen changes for all these activities is problematic because they run the gamut from extremely low-level activities to intense ones, from short activities to prolonged ones, and some activities themselves vary greatly (e.g., downhill skiing). For each sport or activity, however, you'll find general recommendations and real-life examples of diabetic athletes' specific regimen changes.

General Adjustments for Type 1 and Type 2 Diabetics

For lower-intensity activities like horseback riding with a trail guide, you will usually not need to reduce your insulin doses or increase your carbohydrate intake. For more intense activities like mountain biking, you probably will need to eat more and reduce your insulin (if you take it), depending on how long you do it. If you're mountaineering or backpacking, you will definitely need to make greater changes to keep your blood sugars stable during and following the activity.

Intensity, Duration, and Other Effects

As mentioned, this wide array of outdoor and recreational activities will elicit many different blood sugar responses depending on how long and how hard you're working and even how hot, cold, or high you are. Low-intensity activities like snorkeling may have minimal effect on your blood sugars unless you do it for several hours, whereas dog mushing will definitely require diligence on your part to prevent lows throughout the activity (especially if you're participating in the Iditarod Race). In fact, the effects of heat, cold, or high altitude can be sizable, causing greater than normal use of your muscle glycogen and blood glucose and occasionally a higher level of insulin resistance, managed only with regimen changes.

Dealing with Environmental Extremes: Heat, Humidity, Cold, and Altitude

Many people have noticed significant effects on blood sugar while exercising in extreme environments, which increase your metabolic rate, along with your reliance on carbohydrate. Warm or hot environments may also speed up your insulin

---

Tips for Dealing With Glucose Meters and Insulin Use in Extreme Environments

Colorado resident Lisa Seaman shares her experiences while mountaineering and more: "In my experience, all glucose monitors function poorly at low temperatures. Our (mountaineering group's) solution to this problem was to design a small fleece bag that straps onto your base layer with a chest harness system. This keeps your meter and insulin warm and accessible. I usually have a strip of Velcro on the back of my meter and on the bag so that I don't have to worry about dropping it; also, the lancet is tied to it with a little piece of cord. I try not to keep my strips all in one container in case I drop it (I keep some extras in my first aid kit or pack). Using this system, the meters tend to be within operational temperature range even in the worst of conditions."

For hot climates, I have a different system altogether. I spent a year in Costa Rica as a guide for Outward Bound. I used a little pelican box designed for cameras to carry my meter. They are completely waterproof, so I could even wear it in my personal flotation device when kayaking or rafting. I again use Velcro on the inside of the box and on the back of my meter, and I keep my strips and lancet in there as well. For insulin, I use the FRIO bags, which are really great! They just need to be wet and they will keep your insulin cool in hot temperatures."

absorption by increasing blood flow to your skin (for sweating and cooling purposes). The more prolonged your activity is, the greater the effect may be on your blood glucose and muscle glycogen use. Exactly how extreme an environment is affects your responses as well; hot and humid conditions increase your glucose use more than hot ones alone, windchill exacerbates the effects of a cold environment, and high altitudes cause effects that you won't experience at lower elevations. Refer to specific activities for athlete examples of regimen changes under environmental extremes.

ADVENTURE RACING AND EXTREME TRAIL RUNNING

These activities are highly aerobic in nature. For regular trail runs lasting an hour or two, you can follow the recommendations given for running in chapter 9. For extreme events that may involve grueling and unusual environmental conditions, and sleep deprivation during the longer events, the most analogous activity is ultradistance running (also covered in chapter 9), but even that doesn't come close to comparing directly with adventure racing. If you take insulin, you may get by using mostly basal doses without a need for rapid-acting insulin to cover most of the carbohydrate that you eat. In any case, you'll need to consume more carbohydrate to cover for the glycogen and blood glucose that you're using to fuel your activity, along with protein and fat to replace all the calories that your body is expending. Expect that the effects on your insulin action may last for two to three days beyond when you finish your event, especially if it is prolonged or physically grueling.

Athlete Examples

Because of the intensity and duration of these activities, you'll likely have to eat more and modify your medications to participate effectively. For some other ideas about how to compensate, refer to the section on ultradistance training and events in chapter 9 and mountaineering and backpacking in this chapter.

Combined Regimen Changes

Tim Godfrey of Seattle, Washington, participates in adventure racing, which can last from 5 to 24 hours per event, although some take 3 or more days. Typically, these events include a water portion (e.g., kayaking), mountain biking, and trekking or trail running. All you know when you start is the approximate amount of time it should take to finish but not the actual length of each leg, the order in which they'll occur, or where you'll be going (hence the "adventure" part of these races). To compensate, he almost never takes any Humalog during them, and he cuts his basal Lantus dose by a third to a half of his usual the night before racing. He finds it easiest to take in Hammer gels and Perpetuem, taking in about 50 grams of carbohydrate per hour, and he checks his blood glucose levels frequently. Because of the erratic nature of such racing, he tends to let his sugars climb to as high as 200 mg/dl (11.1 mmol/L) without correcting them to prevent lows, and he stays hydrated with electrolyte drinks that don't contain any carbohydrate.

Edwin Sherstone of Southport, Lancashire (United Kingdom), participates in fell racing, a sport that originated in England and involves mountain running run over high, remote ground. Participants have to use mountain navigational skills to choose the best route to follow. The terrain covered can vary widely but usually include significant ascents and rocky ground, making these races much harder than straight trail running. For fell races lasting three to seven hours, he reduces his fast-acting insulin by 1 to 2 units for food that he eats in the hour or two before starting, and he reduces his morning dose of Levemir (basal insulin) by 1 to 2.5 units as well. In addition, he increases his morning carbohydrate intake by 30 to 50 grams.

Canada resident Michael Riddell participated in a five-and-a-half-hour urban adventure race around Toronto (involving mountain biking, trail running, and canoeing) for which he consumed about one gram of carbohydrate per kilogram of body weight per hour, half of it before and during the event and the other half afterward. For this event, he had a hydration pack containing a sports drink on his back during the race. Before starting, he lowered his prebreakfast injection of Humalog by 50 percent, and he used correction boluses as needed during the race. For the carbohydrate that he consumed postrace, he again gave half his usual insulin. Following races like this one or on other active days, he consumes a Glucerna bar or shake at bedtime.

A Cambridge, England resident, Jean Sinclair marshals at adventure races about six weekends per year, which involves walking several miles (about 5 kilometers) over rough terrain (which is not nearly as grueling as participating in the race itself). Following this activity, she often reduces her intermediate-acting insulin at bedtime by as much as 25 percent and reduces the amount of Humalog that she takes for meals by 33 to 80 percent, depending on how much carbohydrate she eats and how active she has been. She carries sweets, dried fruits, and muesli bars along with her to eat as needed. When she has done adventure races herself, she finds it difficult to predict how her blood sugars will react or how much time the race will take.

For trail running, Bend, Oregon, resident Jamie Flanagan cuts back his basal rate by 25 to 50 percent. He also takes his blood sugars many times during exercising and always has enough food with him to prevent lows. He tries to keep his sugars around 130 to 150 mg/dl (7.2 to 8.3 mmol/L).

AIRSOFT AND PAINTBALL

A new craze, particularly among teenagers and preteens, airsoft and paintball are variable in nature, sometimes requiring burst of running and other times being more sedentary. Airsoft tournaments involve eliminating your opponents (i.e., other participants) by shooting them with plastic ball bearings (BBs) launched from airsoft guns. Organized tournaments may involve using replicas of real guns, tactical gear, and other accessories used by military and police. Paintball is similar, but it involves marking your opponents by shooting them with paintballs shot from a compressed gas-powered gun. The duration of play varies widely, as does how much running you'll do, which will affect your blood sugars the most. Almost all airsoft games are held outdoors, whereas paintball can take place indoors or outside.

Athlete Examples

Because these activities can be sporadic but also prolonged, regimen changes will depend on how much you run and how long you play.

Combined Regimen Changes

Carter Gillespie of Phoenix, Arizona, occasionally participates in organized airsoft and paintball games that are miniwar scenarios lasting up to 8 hours. The games are set up in facilities with buildings, military vehicles, and more. Playing time averages 3 to 4 hours, involving 15 minutes spurts of running and then short breaks. To compensate for these physically active games, he usually lowers his carbohydrate ratio beforehand and eats snacks containing 15 grams of carbohydrate two to three times without taking any NovoLog to cover them. He also has to check his blood sugars more often the day after games because he tends to run low then.

CANOEING AND KAYAKING

Canoeing and kayaking on relatively calm water (not whitewater) are prolonged and aerobic in nature, especially when done at lower intensities. Whitewater activities, which can be more intense and cause greater use of anaerobic energy sources, are addressed later in this chapter. For low-level paddling, you will need minimal changes, but the longer you do it (especially if you're working hard), the more regimen changes you may need to make to maintain your blood sugar levels. For example, for longer or more intense paddling, you may eat more carbohydrate and lower your insulin doses to prevent lows. For multiday trips or outings, you may benefit by lowering your basal insulin by 10 to 20 percent because you'll have glycogen to replace in your upper-body muscles, making you more insulin sensitive. See table 12.1 for further instructions on canoeing and kayaking.

Athlete Examples

These examples show regimen changes depending on the duration of canoeing or kayaking. For more intense whitewater sports, refer to the section found later in this chapter.

Diet Changes Alone

A type 2 diabetic triathlete, Charlie Dunn of Conway, Arkansas, also kayaks, an activity for which he has to make few changes compared with doing Ironmans. Because he controls his diabetes with oral medications only (Avandia and metformin), he carries a Gu pack with him when he exercises but doesn't have any problems with lows during kayaking. Generally, he finds that doing this (and other activities) after meals helps lower his blood glucose levels.

Nancy Vranich is a type 1.5 diabetic exerciser who controls her diabetes with Janumet. For kayaking, she usually consumes a larger carbohydrate load to get her through 6-hour or longer kayaking trips. When she does, her blood glucose levels

Table 12.1   Canoeing and Kayaking

Insulin: insulin pump	Insulin: basal-bolus regimen	Diet: insulin pump	Diet: basal-bolus regimen
• Reduce your basal rates by 25–50% during these activities, if done intensely. • Reduce boluses by 10–20% before less intense paddling and by 20–40% for prolonged or harder workouts. • If you remove your pump, reconnect every hour and bolus to prevent hyperglycemia. • Possibly reduce your basal rates overnight by 10–20% after prolonged activity or if you're on multiday canoeing or kayaking trips.	• Reduce your preactivity insulin doses by 10–20% for shorter, less intense activity or by 20–50% before prolonged or intense activities. • Lower your basal insulin doses overnight only if you're doing prolonged or multiday trips.	• For low-level paddling, increase your carbohydrate intake by 0–10 grams per hour. • For more intense paddling, consume about 10–20 grams of carbohydrate per hour, depending on your insulin reductions.	• Consume 0–15 grams of carbohydrate per hour for low-level canoeing or kayaking. • Increase your carbohydrate intake by 10–25 grams per hour during more intense paddling.

stay stable despite her higher carbohydrate intake. On other days when her sugars are running high, she adds a 30-minute walk to bring them down.

For kayaking for longer than an hour, AnneLisa Butcher of Stockton, California reduces her basal rate to 65 percent. In addition, if her blood sugars are normal to start, she eats an extra snack.

Combined Regimen Changes

For kayaking, Marin Desbois of Montreal, Quebec (Canada), who is also a marathoner, reduces his basal to 50 percent. Normally, he kayaks four hours a week during the summer months, but he has also participated in six-day kayak expeditions. During those trips, he often eats additional carbohydrate without bolusing. He treats low blood sugars with glucose gels and fruit juices.

DOG MUSHING

Dog mushing is a sport unto itself. The most famous of the dog sled races, the Iditarod, is run across the state of Alaska. The goal is to be the first to get from Anchorage to Nome with your team of 12 to 16 dogs pulling you and your gear on a sled. As the official Iditarod Web site states, this is "a race over 1,150 miles of the most extreme and beautiful terrain known to man: across mountain ranges, frozen rivers, dense forests, desolate tundra, and windswept coastline. Add to that, temperatures far below zero, winds that can cause a complete loss of visibility, the hazards of overflow, long hours of darkness, and treacherous climbs and side hills, and you have the Iditarod."

As you can imagine, this activity includes many elements that potentially affect your blood sugars: extreme environmental conditions, lack of sleep, higher-intensity exercise, multiple days of prolonged activity in a row (the average time to compete the race is 10 to 17 days), and more. For this activity, you will need little insulin in your system, and you will need to eat almost continually to maintain your blood sugars and body temperature.

Athlete Example

Because of the extreme nature of this sport, diabetic dog mushers have to adjust both food and insulin intake during training for and competing in events like the Iditarod.

Combined Regimen Changes

A resident of Kasilof, Alaska, Bruce Linton takes in more carbohydrate during periods of exercise, which includes doing Ironman triathlons and the Iditarod dog sled race. He takes much less insulin when doing the Iditarod because he runs the race on little sleep, sometimes needing no insulin at all during the day when sled racing (or when doing an Ironman race). In addition, racing outdoors across Alaska in March exposes him to extremely cold temperatures, for which he has to eat more just to maintain his body temperature. His first Iditarod took him more than 15 days to complete; doing repeated days of activity during the race also heightened his insulin action.

DOWNHILL SKIING AND SNOWBOARDING

These activities use a mix of anaerobic and aerobic fuels, depending on skill level. A skilled skier or snowboarder going down difficult slopes may ski more intensely, and if you're constantly shifting and moving, you'll rely more on your muscle glycogen and blood glucose; conversely, skiing straight downhill and letting gravity do most of the work will have minimal effect on your blood sugars. Spending time in chairlift lines, on the chairlift, or in the lodge warming up will also reduce your blood glucose use. Snow conditions (powdery versus icy), outside temperature, and wind chill on the slopes can also affect how your body responds, with more extreme conditions causing you to use more blood glucose to stay warm and dictating greater regimen changes. See table 12.2 for further instructions on downhill skiing and snowboarding.

Table 12.2 Downhill Skiing and Snowboarding

Insulin: insulin pump	Insulin: basal-bolus regimen	Diet: insulin pump	Diet: basal-bolus regimen
• Reduce your boluses by 10–30% for all-day or intense skiing or snowboarding. • Reduce your basal rates by 25–50% as well during the activity.	• For longer or intense participation, reduce your insulin doses by 20–50% for meals eaten right before or while you're doing these activities.	• If needed to prevent lows, consume 10–15 grams of carbohydrate per hour, depending on your insulin reductions.	• You may need up to 15–25 grams of extra carbohydrate per hour during the activity if your insulin levels are high.

Athlete Examples

The reported regimen changes vary widely with the intensity and duration of skiing or snowboarding as well as the environmental conditions. For regimen changes for cross-country skiing, refer to chapter 9.

Insulin Changes Alone

For downhill skiing, Jeff Mazer of Bozeman, Montana, reduces his basal rates on his pump by 20 percent during the activity. Likewise, Annie Auerback of Madison, Connecticut, reduces hers by 50 percent and tests her blood sugars often.

Combined Regimen Changes

A professional snowboarder, Sean Busby of Draper, Utah, reduces his basal insulin for this activity. The amount that he adjusts usually depends on the altitude and temperature, but he generally uses a 30 to 40 percent reduction. He also carries extra prefilled syringes in his coat during competitions and training in case he can't access his pump quickly under his clothing. To treat lows, he uses honey (especially if on a chairlift), and he generally eats a granola or energy bar every 45 to 60 minutes depending on how hard he's working. During competitions, though, he usually lowers it by only 10 to 20 percent because the release of adrenaline keeps his sugars higher.

Jamie Flanagan works as a professional ski patroller, for which he cuts his basal rate by 25 to 50 percent because it's a demanding, high-energy job. He also keeps a lot of food with him and snacks frequently. Although he patrols mostly on his snowboard, once or twice a week while working he does telemark skiing, also known as free-heel skiing, a more efficient mode of backcountry travel than snowboarding.

Karen Stark of Minnesota finds that downhill skiing has a profound effect on her blood sugars. To compensate, she often takes her basal insulin but no NovoLog while skiing. She grazes on food throughout the day, and her blood glucose levels stay fairly constant.

When Matt Green of East Longmeadow, Massachusetts, goes skiing or snowboarding, his blood sugars tend to rise even though he keeps his pump on. If he starts out with a blood glucose level of 150 mg/dl (8.3 mmol/L), he does not make any adjustments initially. He tests frequently, however, to pick up trends (up or down) and react to them.

Teenager Alex Oppen from Wisconsin finds that snowboarding drops his blood sugars faster than many other activities that he does. Sometimes he reduces his basal rate by 10 percent but more likely he just eats some extra carbohydrate to compensate. He treats lows with Jones soda.

Preteen Rory McFarland of East Wenatchee, Washington, has to consume additional carbohydrate and often more fat in the meal (e.g., toasted cheese sandwiches) before he skis to prevent lows. In addition, he often has to lower his basal rate on his pump.

Intensity, Duration, and Other Effects

Effect of environmental conditions and multiple days of activity To compete in snowboarding professionally, Sean Busby often trains extremely hard over several days. When he does so, he reduces his basal rate further (70 to 80 percent total). He usually makes large reductions during cold spells (–20 to 10 degrees Fahrenheit, or –29 to –12 Celsius), because he finds that his blood sugars drop faster in colder temperatures.

Massachusetts resident Matt Green's biggest problem during downhill skiing or snowboarding is using his blood glucose meter in the cold. If he takes his meter out of his jacket pocket into the cold, condensation often forms inside its plastic housing. As for his insulin pump, he keeps it close to his body underneath at least one base layer of clothing to protect it from the weather.

GAMING (FISHING, HUNTING, AND SHOOTING)

These activities are largely endurance related, but they are usually low level and may involve periods of inactivity interspersed with movement. Because you do them outdoors, environmental extremes (e.g., heat, humidity, coldness, and altitude) can affect your blood sugar responses. Fly fishing may be done standing in a cold stream or river and is more active, so it may cause your blood sugar levels to decrease more than hunting or other types of fishing if you're stationary.

Athlete Examples

A resident of Honokaa, Hawaii, Scott Dunton enjoys hunting and fishing when he's not surfing. To compensate for these gaming activities, he usually just snacks more, particularly if he's walking a lot while hunting.

For duck hunting, Thomas Pintar of Fort Wayne, Indiana, always carries glucose tablets with him to take if he gets low. Otherwise, he doesn't make any changes because the activity is low intensity compared with his training for triathlons.

Brandon Hunter of West Plains, Missouri, does both hunting and fishing. Because he may be outside for extended periods by himself when doing these activities, he usually takes extra food and drinks along with him. He doesn't adjust his insulin dosing, though.

Mike McMahon of Petersburg, Alaska, works on commercial fishing boats during the summers, an activity that involves a lot of manual labor. A morning Lantus user, he has to decrease his dose by about half (from 24 units down to 12) to avoid lows while working, and he eats extra snacks throughout the day to compensate as well.

HIKING AND BACKPACKING

Both hiking and backpacking are extremely aerobic in nature, requiring the endurance to cover long distances at a relatively slow pace. They are often done carrying

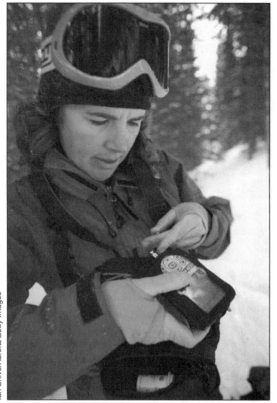

Ian Shive/Aurora/Getty Images

Many outdoor activities, like hiking and backpacking, pose extra concerns for diabetics. Along with the intensity and duration of the exercise, higher altitudes and colder temperatures will increase your blood glucose use, making it a good idea to test often.

extra weight, especially in the case of backpacking. At slower speeds, your body may be able to use quite a bit of fat as fuel, but increasing your speed, going uphill, or climbing increases your use of blood glucose and muscle glycogen. For hiking, you can simply eat more carbohydrate or lower your insulin, but if you take insulin, you will usually need to make changes in your intake of both insulin and carbohydrate for backpacking. Of course, the duration of these activities (hours or days), the amount of extra weight that you carry, the temperature, and the altitude can all affect your blood sugar responses and the adjustments that you'll need to make to prevent lows.

Higher altitudes and colder temperatures will increase your blood glucose use. Hot and humid conditions can predispose you to dehydration (mainly through increased sweating), as can high altitude (due to faster breathing rates), so you should be especially careful to drink plenty of fluids because being dehydrated can make your blood sugar readings come out higher. The terrain can also affect your blood glucose; uphill climbing requires more energy (in the form of carbohydrate) than downhill portions. Your risk for later-onset lows, especially at night, following such strenuous activities means that you may need to lower your insulin levels overnight and possibly eat a bedtime snack, particularly when doing several days of hiking or on longer backpacking trips. See table 12.3 for further instructions on hiking and table 12.4 for further instructions on backpacking.

Athlete Examples

These examples show the changes that you may need to make for hiking and backpacking, especially under harsher environmental conditions. Backpackers who use insulin can't get by with making diet changes alone (without insulin adjustments), although hikers often can. For additional backpacking examples in more extreme environments, refer to the section on mountaineering found later in this chapter.

Table 12.3 Hiking

Insulin: insulin pump	Insulin: basal-bolus regimen	Diet: insulin pump	Diet: basal-bolus regimen
• For short hikes of up to 2 hours, reduce your basal insulin by 25–50%; lower it 50–75% for longer hikes. • Reduce your preexercise boluses by 10–30%. • Lower your overnight basal rates by 10–25% after doing strenuous hikes or during multiday hiking trips.	• For short hikes of 1–2 hours, reduce your insulin doses by 10–30%. • For longer hikes of 3 or more hours, reduce your premeal insulin doses by 25–50%. • Reduce your overnight basal insulin dose by 10–25%, especially following unusually strenuous exercise or multiday hiking trips.	• Consume 5–20 grams of carbohydrate per hour during a short hike. • Consume more carbohydrate without insulin boluses for long hikes, depending on your insulin reductions and the difficulty of the terrain.	• For short hikes, consider consuming 10–25 grams of carbohydrate per hour. • During long hikes, consume more carbohydrate without taking any additional rapid-acting insulin if your insulin levels are not low enough.

Table 12.4 Backpacking

Insulin: insulin pump	Insulin: basal-bolus regimen	Diet: insulin pump	Diet: basal-bolus regimen
• Set your basal rate up to 50% lower while backpacking, depending on altitude and temperature. • Decrease your boluses by 25–50% for anything you eat during and following the activity. • Reduce your basal rates at night by 10–30%, especially during multiday trips.	• Reduce your basal insulin doses by 25–50% before starting the activity, depending on the altitude the temperature. • Lower your insulin doses by 25–50% for meals or snacks during and following the activity. • Cut back on your overnight basal insulin doses by 10–30% following the activity.	• Consume 10–30 grams of carbohydrate per hour, with extra protein and fat before bedtime.	• Consume 15–30 grams of carbohydrate per hour during the activity, with extra carbohydrate, protein, and fat as a snack at bedtime.

Insulin Changes Alone

Jeff Mazer of Bozeman, Montana, usually reduces his basal rates on his pump by 40 to 50 percent for hiking and may lower his boluses as well. If everything goes as planned with his pump settings, he makes minimal adjustments to his carbohydrate intake. During climbing, however, he reduces them by only 20 to 40 percent because of its higher intensity.

The main change that Andrea Limbourg of France makes for hiking is to reduce her basal rate by about 15 percent during the activity, testing occasionally and making adjustments as needed. Janet Switzer of Millstadt, Illinois, likewise lowers her basal rate to 30 percent of normal and starts her hike with a blood glucose reading of at least 150 mg/dl (8.3 mmol/L). Susan Shaw of Canoga Park, California, lowers her basal to 60 percent if she is going to hike for longer than an hour.

For hiking, Adelaide Lindahl of Minnesota reduces her basal rate by 0.5 unit per hour. But she also has to take a bolus for small meals or snacks (e.g., granola bars) at least every four hours to prevent her blood sugars from rising over time.

Diet Changes Alone

When hiking in the Colorado mountains, David Mendosa of Boulder, Colorado, usually takes trail-type foods with him to eat along the way. Although he takes Byetta twice a day, he doesn't adjust it for this activity. Another type 2 diabetic hiker, Cindy of Griffin, Georgia, carries carbohydrate or Snickers bars with her while hiking or backpacking sections of the Appalachian Trail.

For hiking or walking, Linda Frischmeyer of Vancouver, Washington, eats extra carbohydrate without adjusting her insulin doses. Similarly, Pat Shermer of Rapid City, South Dakota, exercises regularly and already has her insulin adjusted for it, so only when she is hiking does she take in extra carbohydrate to compensate.

Japan resident Renée McNulty finds that high-altitude hiking (above 2,000 meters) makes her nauseous. She simply drinks a watered-down sports drink to keep her blood sugars up during this activity.

Combined Regimen Changes

A National Outdoor Leadership School (NOLS) backpacking instructor, Jared Sibbitt of Flagstaff, Arizona, often takes 30-day trips during the summer. When he's doing them, he reduces his bedtime Lantus dose by 10 percent and takes smaller Humalog doses (10 to 40 percent lower) with every meal (mainly breakfast and dinner). When actively backpacking, he eats small snacks all day long without bolusing for them, mostly trail mix, gorp, sesame sticks, nuts, and some low-glycemic-index carbohydrate foods.

For hiking, Jedidiah Reeser of Trenton, Florida, usually sets the basal rate on his pump at 70 percent for 2 hours, at which point he checks his blood sugars and adjusts it up or down as required. He also eats a snack whenever he exercises for long than 20 minutes.

When doing an eight-day hiking trip, Australia native Susan Greenback kept her basal rates on her insulin pump set to 50 percent for the whole trip, except for when she was actually walking, when she often kept it as low as 10 percent of normal. She also vastly decreased her boluses for meals and snacks during the activity.

For backpacking about a week of every year, Garrick Neal of Canada finds that the adjustments he needs to make depend on the number of hours he's hiking each day and the elevation gain. Usually he makes about a 40 percent reduction in his morning Lantus, bedtime Humulin N, and Humalog for meals and snacks. He also finds that the lead time he needs for his Humalog injections is cut by the same percentage, so he waits only 12 minutes to start eating instead of his usual 20 when not backpacking.

For hiking or backpacking, Jude Restis of Kent, Washington, lowers his basal rates by 40 to 60 percent. In addition, he increases his carbohydrate intake to 20 to 40 grams per hour. To treat lows, he uses glucose tablets, Clif Shot Bloks, and Hammer gel.

Doug Bursnall of Colorado Springs, Colorado, enjoys a variety of sports, including backpacking, mountaineering, and climbing. For full-day or weekend events, he decreases his basal Lantus doses, taking from 0 to 10 units in the evening (along with less than his usual 30 units in the morning) and giving less Humalog for his meals. He also snacks throughout the activity.

Intensity, Duration, and Other Effects

Effect of training   Jamie Flanagan of Oregon recently backpacked across the entire state of Oregon on the Pacific Crest Trail (about 550 miles, or 900 kilometers) in 30 days. He struggled with some lows during the first week, but after that his body adjusted to the daily hiking even though he covered 15 to 18 miles (24 to 30 kilometers) a day wearing a 30- to 40-pound (14- to 18-kilogram) pack.

HORSEBACK RIDING, RECREATIONAL

This activity is usually low intensity, mainly requiring you to use your postural muscles to stay on top of your horse. The faster the horse goes, the more energy you'll have to expend to remain in the saddle. Recreational riding will generally not affect your blood sugar much, but going on all-day trail rides or riding while your horse is cantering or galloping may have a significant effect. Increase your carbohydrate intake to keep your blood sugars stable or slightly lower your basal insulin (if you take it).

JET SKIING

This activity mainly involves holding on to the handlebars of your jet ski on the larger ones. On certain smaller models, you may stand as well. The intensity of jet skiing has the greatest potential effect on your blood sugars. Short, intense bouts on your jet ski will maintain your blood sugars, but if you ride for long periods, you'll likely experience a decrease. For comparable activities, refer to athlete examples for snowmobiling and water skiing.

MOTORCYCLE RIDING AND RACING (OFF ROAD)

This activity mainly involves holding on to the handlebars of your motorcycle and navigating across frequently rough terrain, which can involve prolonged contractions in your arms and legs. The biggest effect on your blood sugars during this activity likely comes from the release of adrenaline because of the thrill and danger involved. In the short run, the release of this hormone and others will keep your blood sugars stable or higher, but if you ride for long enough, your blood sugars may drop over time.

Athlete Examples

Because of the nature of this activity, adjusting your insulin doses to compensate may be easiest. If you don't use insulin, you may or may not need to eat additional carbohydrate.

Insulin Changes Alone

Greg Cutter of Norfolk, Virginia, enjoys the adrenaline rush associated with doing off-road motorcycle racing. He always checks his blood sugars before doing this activity, but because getting low during the activity could be fatal, he errs on the high side with his blood sugars (staying greater than 150 mg/dl, or 8.3 mmol/L) when he's riding. To accomplish this, he takes a minimal amount of Humalog at breakfast before riding but doesn't adjust his bedtime Lantus dose. Also, he finds that the adrenaline release tends to keep his blood sugars higher while racing.

United Kingdom resident Kathryn Latham also enjoys off-road motorcycle riding. She has noticed that she has higher blood sugars during riding when she becomes excited, and she finds it difficult to control her stress hormone release during the activity.

Alex Oppen of Wisconsin does a related sport—junior drag racing. He finds that he needs to test his blood sugars often during this activity because adrenaline release raises them, but he also avoids going too low, which would affect his ability to focus and race well. For this latter reason, he is cautious about making too many adjustments that may lower his blood sugars while racing.

MOUNTAIN BIKING

This activity is mostly a prolonged endurance sport, but it requires occasional bursts of anaerobic energy to climb hills and inclines. The adjustments that you'll need to make depend mainly on how long and hard you bike and the terrain that you cover. More intense biking, such as what you do during climbs or over difficult terrain, may maintain your blood sugars better from greater release of glucose-raising hormones, but you'll have to watch out for lows after you stop. Mountain biking for long periods will use more of your glycogen stores and blood glucose, increasing your risk for hypoglycemia both during and following the activity. You will need to consume more carbohydrate and reduce your insulin doses to compensate. See table 12.5 for further instructions on mountain biking.

Athlete Examples

These examples show that mountain biking usually requires changes in both insulin and diet to compensate. For additional cycling examples, refer to the cycling section in chapter 9.

Diet Changes Alone

A resident of Denville, New Jersey, Joe LoCurcio finds that he can usually prevent hypoglycemia with basal rate changes alone. The changes that he makes depend

Table 12.5 Mountain Biking

Insulin: insulin pump	Insulin: basal-bolus regimen	Diet: insulin pump	Diet: basal-bolus regimen
• Reduce your basal rates by 15–40% during the activity and premeal boluses by 10–30%. • For rides longer than an hour, lower your basal rates by 25–50% during the activity and possibly for 1–2 hours before biking. • Reduce your premeal boluses by 25–50% before and after the activity. • Lower your basal rates overnight by 10–20% following strenuous biking.	• Lower your rapid-acting insulin by 10–30% for meals before biking and lower by 25–50% for prolonged excursions. • Consider reducing your morning basal insulin by 10–20% in anticipation of prolonged biking of 2 hours or longer. • Reduce your doses of insulin by 10–30% for the meal following your activity and possibly reduce your evening basal insulin by 10–20% after prolonged or strenuous biking.	• For biking 1 hour or less, increase your carbohydrate intake by 10–30 grams per hour, depending on your insulin reductions. • Consume 15–40 grams of carbohydrate per hour for longer rides. • Consider eating a bedtime snack to prevent overnight lows after prolonged biking.	• For short biking excursions, increase your carbohydrate intake by 15–30 grams. • For longer rides, consume 15–45 grams per hour, depending on your insulin reductions. • Eat a bedtime snack to prevent overnight lows, especially if your biking was strenuous or prolonged.

on how much insulin he has on board. If he boluses for a meal within an hour of riding, he may suspend his pump during a 45- to 120-minute ride. The longer and more intense his workouts are, the more likely he is to get low blood sugars. Following an intense 2-hour workout, he keeps his basal rate reduced for more than 4 hours, and his carbohydrate ratio may at 50 percent of normal for up to 8 hours.

Combined Regimen Changes

Kerry White of Vail, Colorado, finds that her strength is doing 24-hour mountain bike races and other long events (such as the cycling Race Across America in 2007 as part of Team Type 1). For long rides or races, she reduces her basal Lantus doses the night before and the morning of the event by 1 to 3 units each. She often doesn't need to take any Humalog all day during it, although she snacks on PowerBars and drinks Gatorade. Although she normally uses Symlin with her meals, she doesn't take it on race days because it can slow the treatment of any lows that she has during mountain biking or road cycling.

North Carolina resident Jimmy Dodson participates in long-distance mountain biking. To maintain his blood sugars, he generally eats 30 to 45 grams of carbohydrate beforehand and supplements at least every 30 to 60 minutes with another 30 to 60 grams of carbohydrate. He starts a lower, temporary basal rate (50 to 70 percent of normal) on his pump 20 to 45 minutes before starting, depending on the activity that he'll be doing, his expected intensity, the weather, and more.

A resident of Augusta, Georgia, Troy Willard challenges himself with mountain biking endurance races, including 12- and 24-hour, 100-mile (160-kilometer), and off-road events. He typically eats a breakfast higher in fat and protein at least 3 hours before starting to balance out his blood sugars early in a race. During it, he sets his basal rate at 50 percent and consumes Hammer gels and Clif Bars throughout, about 30 to 45 grams per hour, but he avoids simple sugar-based gels and bars. For training rides, he mixes up a recovery drink containing four times more carbohydrate than protein (usually 100 grams of carbohydrate and 25 of whey protein), for which he boluses with 8 to 10 units of NovoLog, depending on his postexercise blood sugars, to speed his recovery. He finds that these shakes help his legs feel fresher during his ride the next day.

Elise Rayner of Colorado Springs, Colorado, rides daily, doing either road cycling or mountain biking. For her daily workouts lasting 45 to 90 minutes, she reduces her NovoLog by 50 percent for any meal that she eats within 2 hours of riding, but if she rides more than 2 hours later, she makes no changes in premeal insulin. For rides longer than 2 hours and 30 minutes, she reduces her premeal doses by 80 percent but does not adjust her basal Lantus doses. Every 45 minutes, she takes in 15 to 20 grams of carbohydrate (typically gels); if her rides last more than 2 hours, she consumes that much carbohydrate every 30 minutes instead and alternates sips of water and Heed (an electrolyte drink) every 15 minutes. Often, she has to give a postmeal bolus of 1 to 3 units to cover postride spikes after strenuous rides.

For Renée McNulty of Misawa, Japan, mountain biking for long periods requires adjustments in insulin and food intake. She decreases the basal rates on her pump by almost 60 percent 60 to 90 minutes before starting exercise that will last more than 2 hours, and if she bikes for 3 or more hours, she keeps it reduced for another 12 hours or so. She eats a banana or the equivalent right before she begins riding, along with a 25-gram carbohydrate gel every hour, switching to a 40-gram bar every 3rd hour. Because her postexercise highs frequently resolve themselves, she doesn't always treat them immediately after stopping.

A collegiate mountain biker, Justin Taylor of Boulder, Colorado, reduces his basal rates by 60 to 90 percent, depending on the intensity of his biking. He eats before riding, takes in 15 to 30 grams of carbohydrate every hour during the activity, and eats enough carbohydrate afterward to replenish his glycogen stores. To prevent lows while riding, he prefers to consume Hammer gel products or Heed sports drinks.

Kent Loganbill of Tucson, Arizona, sets his basal rate at 0.5 unit per hour while riding a mountain bike. In addition, he consumes a Hammer gel or energy bar every half hour or so, and he eats raisins if his blood sugars are too low.

For mountain or road biking, Carrie Czerwonka of Blanchardville, Wisconsin, reduces her basal rate by 50 percent a half hour before starting and then takes her pump off during two-hour rides. Afterward, she keeps her basal at 50 percent. She mainly eats when disconnecting from and reconnecting to her pump. For longer rides, she leaves her pump on at a basal rate that is 30 to 50 percent below normal, and she eats during the ride. Following these workouts, she may have heightened insulin sensitivity for two or three days afterward.

For this activity, B.A. Smith reduces his bolus rates by 15 to 20 percent, and if the riding is vigorous, he reduces his boluses by 10 percent for several hours afterward. He also drinks 15 to 20 grams of carbohydrate in the form of orange juice before riding.

Intensity, Duration, and Other Effects

Effect of time of day and stress Jimmy Dodson finds that mountain bike races cause him to have an adrenaline kick at the start that raises his blood sugars. The problem is bigger during races that start early in the morning when his strong dawn phenomenon is still in effect and he has already reduced his basal rates for the event. Occasionally, he has to give a small bolus (about 1 unit of Humalog) to counter this effect; otherwise, his sugars rise into the high 200s (15 to 16 mmol/L) and stay there for too long. After his insulin resistance decreases during such races and his blood sugars start trending downward again, he begins his normal carbohydrate intake of 30 to 60 grams per hour depending on the intensity and duration of his ride.

A resident of Atlanta, Georgia, Linda Demma enjoys both mountain biking and road cycling. Her adjustments depend mostly on what time of day it is and what she ate for her last meal. For early morning cycling, she usually has a lower-carbohydrate snack (e.g., a granola bar) and turns her pump off. For afternoon workouts, she eats a higher-carbohydrate snack and drops her basal rate by 50 percent. She normally takes Symlin but foregoes it when she exercises after a meal because its effect on gastric emptying results in unpredictably high sugars two to three hours after eating when she exercises.

Effect of exercise intensity Chad Lawrence, a resident of Kingston, New York, enjoys all sorts of bicycling, including road cycling and racing, racing mountain bikes downhill, racing dual slalom, and doing cross-country mountain biking. Dual slalom is a head-to-head competition down a man-made course usually with gated turns (much like ski racing), and with obstacles such as berms, jumps, bumps, and occasional drops or rock piles. Many of these activities are short and intense (about 30 seconds per dual slalom run), and he finds that the adrenaline rush from doing them competitively often raises his blood sugars, which he offsets with an increase in his basal rates. He loads with carbohydrate before endurance events, however, and usually has to lower his basal rates depending on how intense and long the ride will be.

MOUNTAINEERING

Mountaineering is similar to backpacking but generally includes more intense elements. Also known as alpinism in Europe, this activity involves walking, hiking, trekking, and climbing mountains. At first, people just tried to reach the highest points of unclimbed, unconquered mountains, but the sport has now become specialized into rock craft, snow craft, and skiing, depending on whether you go over rock, snow, or ice. On ice you can wear crampons, spiked footwear that you attach to your boots to give better traction. On snow you can wear snowshoes or skis. Trips can last for days, and you have to carry all your gear to traverse these hazards; you may also have to contend with freezing temperatures, sudden snowstorms or thunderstorms, and more. In the United States, many people try to climb all the 14ers, mountains that are at least 14,000 feet (4,267 meters) above mean sea level, of which there are 54 in Colorado alone.

Mountaineering requires you to deal with high altitude and cold temperatures, both of which can affect your blood sugar responses. In general, physical stressors like these can increase your insulin resistance, keeping your sugars higher overall. If being at altitude gives you mountain sickness, you may not feel like eating, may become dehydrated more easily, and may experience high blood glucose levels. But being really cold may increase your risk of hypoglycemia, particularly if you are shivering (which counts as muscular activity). Any type of mountaineering requires significant carbohydrate intake during the activity, along with altered insulin levels to prevent hypoglycemia or hyperglycemia, depending on the conditions.

Athlete Examples

These examples show the extreme changes in food and medications that you will likely need to make for mountaineering. They also point out how some other factors, like altitude and cold, may affect your glycemic balance.

Combined Regimen Changes

A participant in various aspects of mountaineering, including hiking, rock and ice climbing, and high-altitude climbing, David Panofsky of Madison, Wisconsin, enjoys reaching the summit of mountains and helping other diabetic athletes do the same (starting with IDEA 2000, the International Diabetic Expedition to Aconcagua). From personal experience, he knows that this activity involves juggling many factors along with diabetes, including high altitude, cold weather, lack of sleep, emotional stress, and malfunctioning diabetes equipment in a harsh environment, just to name a few. In general, he finds that the trekking approach to a mountain (backpacking to the base camp) requires a 75 percent decrease in basal insulin rates, followed with some boluses or a slight increase over eight hours. For the high-altitude mountaineering portion, he may need either to decrease or to increase his basal rates by 25 percent. During certain aspects of mountaineering (e.g., leading, soloing, scrambling), he believes that letting his blood sugars stay slightly higher may be safer than risking a hypoglycemic reaction at those times. Although eating extra is important throughout the activity, he treats lows with licorice, Clif Bars and gels, Shot Bloks, soda, and sports drinks.

David Craycraft of San Diego, California, has reached at least 43 of the 50 United States highpoints (the highest point in each of the 50 states) and has ascended over a dozen 14ers since retiring. To compensate for climbing, he usually lowers his Humalog before meals while active and reduces the Humulin N (intermediate-acting insulin) that he takes in the evening. While hiking he grazes on granola bars, raisins, and gummy bears (if low) and rewards himself afterward with an occasional hamburger and french fries.

Intensity, Duration, and Other Effects

Effect of environment A resident of Raleigh, North Carolina, Jimmy Dodson finds that his biggest challenge with mountaineering is adjusting to the altitude. Until he acclimatizes to a new altitude, his blood sugars run higher as if he were sick (he does experience acute mountain sickness). For elevations above about 8,000 feet (2,400 meters), he has to increase his basal rates by 20 to 40 percent of normal for one to three days. He monitors his body's acclimatization by checking his resting heart rate (when he wakes up) and his basal insulin needs, both of which go back down to normal when his body adapts to a certain altitude.

For Jared Sibbitt of Arizona, mountaineering or climbing at altitudes above 14,000 feet (4,300 meters) makes him more insulin resistant. Despite doing heavy aerobic work while backpacking, he usually keeps his insulin doses close to normal under those conditions.

Lisa Seaman of Silverthorne, Colorado, finds that high-altitude mountaineering challenges her with the many variables that she has to consider to maintain her blood sugar levels, including eating unusual foods while on trips, dealing with the effects of high altitudes and low temperatures, and keeping her insulin from becoming too hot or cold.

ROCK AND ICE CLIMBING

Outdoor rock or ice climbing has some aerobic aspects, but much of the movements that it requires is quick and intense (e.g., grabbing and pulling). Rest periods between moves make it more of a strength-related, endurance activity. Normally, you'll need to use gear and safety equipment while you ascend difficult rock faces, particularly when they're covered in ice, and carrying gear can weigh you down and increase the intensity of your workout. More difficult climbing may initially maintain your blood sugars better (because of greater hormonal release), but you'll use more muscle glycogen and have greater risk for later-onset lows. Prolonged climbing will also increase your muscle glycogen use and require you to make greater regimen changes. The more intense your climbing activity is and the longer it lasts, the greater the risk is for hypoglycemia during the later stages and afterward. See table 12.6 for further instructions on rock and ice climbing.

Athlete Examples

You can use changes in insulin, diet, or usually both to compensate for this activity. The regimen adjustments differ when you climb for longer periods or more intensely.

Table 12.6 Rock and Ice Climbing

Insulin: insulin pump	Insulin: basal-bolus regimen	Diet: insulin pump	Diet: basal-bolus regimen
• Cut back on your insulin boluses by 25–50% before climbing. • Reduce your basal rates by 0–30% during short, active climbing and lower them slightly more (by 10–20% more) during all-day climbs.	• Reduce your premeal insulin by 25–50% before starting to climb. • For all-day climbing, reduce your morning doses of basal insulin by 10–20% (if possible).	• Consume 0–15 grams of carbohydrate right before climbing, depending on your insulin reductions. • Consume up to 30 grams of carbohydrate per hour during longer climbs.	• Take in 0–15 grams of carbohydrate before climbing to maintain blood sugar levels. • Consume an additional 10–30 grams of carbohydrate per hour for prolonged climbing.

Diet Changes Alone

While rock climbing a few times a month, Jared Sibbitt of Arizona doesn't make many adjustments because it is more of an anaerobic activity for him compared with backpacking, marathon training, or cycling to work. When climbing at high altitude, he actually experiences some insulin resistance, which keeps his blood sugars from dropping as much, so he keeps his insulin about the same as usual.

For free climbing, Mauro Sormani of Italy leaves his basal rates the same as normal because the physical and emotional stress associated with this activity keeps his blood sugars from dropping while he's doing it.

Combined Regimen Changes

A Wisconsin resident, David Panofsky finds it important to eat more during both ice and rock climbing to prevent lows and even to keep his blood sugars slightly higher during certain portions of climbing. In addition, he initially lowers his basal rates by 25 percent, but if the activity is prolonged, he lowers them by 50 percent total, along with bolusing 50 percent less for meals and giving rapid-acting insulin slowly over a few hours (with an extended bolus on a pump) instead of all at once.

Tania Knappich of Brampton, Ontario, finds that she has to disconnect her pump while rock climbing and have a snack. She has frequent lows if she doesn't do both.

For Jimmy Dodson of North Carolina, ice climbing requires him to cut his basal rates to 30 percent of normal, and many days when he's climbing, he can eat up to 30 grams of carbohydrate per hour without taking any bolus insulin. The cold experienced when doing the activity increases his body's use of blood glucose to try to stay warm.

While walking the approach to where he'll be ice climbing, Edwin Sherstone of Southport in the United Kingdom has to increase his carbohydrate intake by 30 to 50 grams and reduce his fast-acting insulin by 1 to 2 units. During the actual climbing portion, he doesn't need to supplement at all.

SAILING

Sailing is mainly an anaerobic activity, requiring short, powerful movements like pulling a rope to adjust a sail. Little movement occurs between pulls except to maintain your balance while standing on the deck. The intensity of your activities may also vary with the size of the boat, the number of crew members, and the strength of the wind. Strong winds may not affect larger boats, which usually carry more crew members and thus require less work of each person. Particularly in smaller boats, strong winds will require more effort and more directional changes to control your course. For most recreational sailing, you will usually need no changes in your insulin or food intake. But for intensive sailing involving more physical labor, you may need to reduce your insulin doses by 10 to 25 percent and take in 10 to 15 grams of carbohydrate per hour.

Athlete Examples

Most sailing requires few regimen changes, but it depends on the level of competition and the duration of the activity.

Diet Changes Alone

For sailboat races lasting all day and sometimes overnight, Greg Cutter of Virginia checks his blood sugars frequently and errs on the high side (greater than 150 mg/dl, or 8.3 mmol/L) because getting low during this activity can be dangerous.

SCUBA DIVING

Scuba (self-contained underwater breathing apparatus) diving is a low-intensity aerobic activity that involves slow kicking and some arm movement. The main concern, as far as your diabetes goes, is the high environmental pressure experienced underwater. This pressure can increase your absorption of insulin and may cause an underwater hypoglycemic reaction, which can go unrecognized or be difficult to treat. Historically, insulin users have not been allowed to obtain National Association of Underwater Instructors (NAUI) certification to allow them to scuba dive legally, although you usually can be certified through the Professional Association of Diving Instructors, or PADI, which has allowed many diabetic athletes to dive safely.

Guidelines for safe diving focus primarily on your blood glucose levels. If you use insulin, you should determine whether your predive blood glucose levels are stable, rising, or falling by testing 60 minutes, 30 minutes, and immediately beforehand. Aim for them to be slightly higher than normal, such as 150 to 180 mg/dl (8.3 to 10 mmol/L) and stable. If they're lower but rising, don't dive until they reach at least 145 mg/dl (8.1 mmol/L). Under no circumstances should you start your dive if they're dropping. Consume carbohydrate until your blood sugars are stable or rising and carry some with you in a waterproof container (e.g., gels or cake frosting) to eat when you surface, if you need to. Injecting lower doses of insulin before dives can also lower your risk of underwater lows.

To dive safely, you should also be able to recognize and treat your own lows, have no advanced diabetic complications (especially active proliferative retinopathy, because increases in your intraocular pressures may cause hemorrhaging), and dive with a buddy educated in your diabetes care. If you develop hypoglycemia while underwater, signal your buddy with an "L" sign using your thumb and forefinger, and attempt to surface. A dive depth limit of 90 feet (27.4 meters) is recommended to help you avoid becoming confused between symptoms of nitrogen narcosis and low blood sugars and to avoid ever needing decompression therapy. Keep in mind that colder water will increase your metabolic rate while diving, even if you wear a wetsuit, and may require you to make greater changes in insulin or carbohydrate intake before diving than you would in warmer water. See table 12.7 for further instructions on scuba diving.

Table 12.7   Scuba Diving

Insulin: insulin pump	Insulin: basal-bolus regimen	Diet: insulin pump	Diet: basal-bolus regimen
• Remove your insulin pump during dives and give a bolus when reconnecting if you have had it off for longer than an hour. • Take little or no rapid-acting insulin before diving to reduce your risk of developing lows while underwater.	• If you take morning basal insulin doses, reduce them by up to 50% before diving. Correct any hyperglycemia later with doses of rapid-acting insulin as needed. • Minimize your use of rapid-acting insulin before diving because it can be absorbed more quickly underwater, possibly causing hypoglycemia.	• Consume enough carbohydrate (at least 15 grams) to ensure that your blood sugars are stable or rising before you dive.	• Consume 15–30 grams of extra carbohydrate before starting your dive to prevent drops underwater, depending on how much you reduced your insulin doses (bolus and basal).

Athlete Examples

The following examples show that most people try to reduce their insulin level and raise their blood sugars during a dive by taking less insulin and eating more beforehand.

Diet Changes Alone

For scuba diving, Arizona resident Jared Sibbitt runs his blood sugars slightly higher than normal to avoid any chance of becoming hypoglycemic underwater. He tests frequently before diving to get an idea of his blood sugars trends, and he eats additional snacks if he needs to.

Before Renée McNulty of Japan started using a pump, when she scuba dived she had to start with her blood sugars near 300 mg/dl (16.7 mmol/L) to end up near 100 (5.6) when she surfaced.

Combined Regimen Changes

For Jim Moore of Flagler Beach, Florida, starting out a dive with a blood sugar at or above 160 mg/dl (8.9 mmol/L) is optimal. He disconnects from his pump when diving and breathes Nitrox (instead of compressed air) because it causes less fatigue and allows shorter surface intervals. His open-water certification is through PADI, and his Nitrox one is through SSI (Scuba Schools International); both required his endocrinologist to sign off on them, which his doctor was willing to do as long as dives don't require decompression, which they don't because he follows the dive tables and dives no deeper than his PADI certification allows (90 feet, or 27.4 meters).

To scuba dive safely, Greg Cutter of Virginia checks his blood sugars before diving and eats enough snacks to raise his sugars to over 150 mg/dl (8.3 mmol/L) to avoid dangerous lows while underwater. Before diving, he takes a 50 percent reduced dose of Humalog for breakfast because he prefers to err on the high side than to be too low during submersion.

SKATEBOARDING

This activity is mainly anaerobic, involving short bursts of intense activity such as jumping, and more prolonged and aerobic use of postural muscles to maintain balance. Usually, you will need minimal changes in your insulin or carbohydrate intake for recreational skateboarding (depending on how long you skate), but if you use it as a form of transportation, the activity is more aerobic in nature and may require greater adjustments to compensate. You may need a 10 to 20 percent reduction in your insulin doses before the activity, combined with extra carbohydrate (0 to 15 grams per hour).

Athlete Examples

The following example shows that skateboarding after a meal can cause lows, especially if you don't adjust to compensate.

Diet Changes Alone

For New Jersey resident Michael Luzzi, skateboarding usually makes his blood sugars go low. Because he usually skateboards after breakfast when his insulin levels are high, he can do this activity for only 45 minutes or so without becoming symptomatic. If it's hot, he has to check more frequently because he may not notice his lows as easily.

SKYDIVING AND PARASAILING

These activities mainly involve the muscular contractions required to hold on to your parachute lines or parasail, which have little or no effect on your blood sugars. But these activities may cause an increase in your anxiety level and a release of adrenaline, which can raise your blood sugar levels. Skydivers in particular should monitor their blood sugars before and after diving. If your blood sugars increase, you may need some insulin to lower them. Neither decreases in insulin beforehand nor carbohydrate intake during these activities is usually necessary. The only exception is if you have to carry your parasail or parachute a long distance after landing, in which case you may need to eat some extra carbohydrate to compensate for that aerobic activity.

SNORKELING

Snorkeling is a low-intensity aerobic exercise. This activity is slower and less intense than regular swimming because you don't use your upper body as much to snorkel, but kicking with swim fins is a harder workout for your legs. The intensity of snorkeling can vary somewhat with your kicking speed and whether you spend time floating or doing minimal kicking. Because of its low intensity, you will need few, if any, regimen changes to maintain your blood sugars. The most important variable is how long you snorkel. For short durations you may not need to make any changes, but if you snorkel for an hour or longer you may have to increase your carbohydrate intake and decrease your insulin somewhat. Also, if you're kicking hard for a long time, expect a drop in blood sugars and make adjustments to prevent lows. See table 12.8 for further instructions on snorkeling.

Table 12.8   Snorkeling

Insulin: insulin pump	Insulin: basal-bolus regimen	Diet: insulin pump	Diet: basal-bolus regimen
• If your insulin pump is not waterproof, remove it while snorkeling and take a small bolus when reconnecting after an hour or more. • If your pump is on, reduce your basal rates by 0–50% during the activity, depending on how hard and long you're kicking in the water. • Reduce your boluses by 0–20% for short-duration snorkeling and by 10–30% for longer activity, particularly if your pump will be on.	• Reduce your insulin doses by 0–20% before short-duration snorkeling and by up to 30–40% for prolonged activity. • You probably don't need to change your basal insulin doses before doing this activity.	• Increase your carbohydrate intake by 0–10 grams per hour during short-duration activity and by 10–20 grams per hour for prolonged snorkeling.	• Consume 0–30 grams of carbohydrate per hour depending on how long and hard you snorkel and how much you reduced your preactivity insulin doses.

SNOWMOBILING

Snowmobiling is primarily an anaerobic activity that involves holding on while you're riding, but it also involves more aerobic use of your postural muscles. Therefore, how hard you're working and how long you snowmobile will affect your blood sugar responses, especially if the activity becomes more aerobic as its duration increases. You may need to eat more carbohydrate and possibly reduce insulin doses for this activity when it lasts for longer than an hour. Your responses may also be affected by how cold it is. Generally, colder temperatures and lower windchill will increase your body's glucose use and require greater regimen changes.

Athlete Examples

For snowmobiling, making special preparations may be as important for maintaining diabetes control as making changes in diet and insulin.

Combined Regimen Changes

Utah resident Sean Busby tries to be well prepared when going snowmobiling in the backcountry. He takes extra precautions, such as bringing extra insulin, food, and water with him, and he checks his blood sugars frequently to see how the elements (along with the exercise) are affecting him. Bringing extra batteries for his insulin pump is also important because he has found that cold weather drains them more quickly.

SNOWSHOEING

Snowshoeing is usually slower than regular walking, but it can be more intense because of the resistance of pulling your snowshoe up and out of the snow with each step, especially in powdery snow conditions. The terrain covered is similar to what you might encounter when hiking, backpacking, or cross-country skiing. How much you alter your insulin or carbohydrate intake will depend on the duration of the activity and other environmental factors. High altitude and low temperatures can affect your blood sugars.

Athlete Examples

For most people engaging in moderate snowshoeing, a combination of diet and insulin changes appears to work best to maintain blood sugars.

Diet Changes Alone

For snowshoeing, Deb Martin of Michigan finds that she needs to eat at least 30 grams of carbohydrate during the first 60 to 90 minutes of the activity. In addition, she eats an additional 15 grams per hour after that to keep her blood sugars stable.

A type 2 diabetic exerciser who uses no medications for control, Debra Simons from Georgia tests her blood sugars more often when she goes on winter snowshoe vacations. If she experiences a low related to this activity, she treats it with regular soda.

Combined Regimen Changes

Alisa Krakel of Conifer, Colorado, goes on long snowshoeing outings during which she tries to eat some additional carbohydrate every hour. She also reduces her basal rate on her pump to 30 to 40 percent of normal because this activity is strenuous and prolonged.

Although Bob Paxson of California generally doesn't make adjustments in his basal rate for snowshoeing, he eats more carbohydrate during the activity. He lowers his basal somewhat when he's experiencing a low blood sugar that won't go away, even with food and glucose, which usually happens during extremely cold weather.

For backcountry ski touring, which combines elements of snowshoeing with skiing and snowboarding, Sean Busby of Utah is extremely strict with his diabetes management because he travels to remote areas. He usually lets his sugars run a little higher (up to, but not over, 200 mg/dl, or 11.1 mmol/L) because climbing and hiking in the cold with snowshoes on lowers them quickly.

SURFING AND BOOGIEBOARDING

Surfing and boogieboarding both require you to use your postural muscles, an activity that is more aerobic in nature, to maintain your balance while riding a wave. A more anaerobic component arises when you paddle hard with your arms to get out to the waves or quickly recruit additional muscles to help you adjust to changes in the waves while surfing. The duration of a ride can be rather short, making these activities more intermittent than continuous. You may need to make regimen changes depending on how long you're active, as well how large and how rough the waves are. Riding on or paddling against stronger waves for a longer period will use more of your blood sugar than riding or paddling in calmer conditions. See table 12.9 for further instructions on surfing and boogieboarding.

Athlete Examples

These examples show that you can manage these activities with any type of regimen change (diet, insulin, or both).

Insulin Changes Alone

While surfing, Jamie Flanagan of Oregon takes his pump off. He generally checks his blood sugars every 20 to 30 minutes during the activity.

For surfing every week or two, Benny Privratsky of Carlsbad, California, takes his pump off during the activity, which he finds easier to do than using the waterproof case for the pump. He adjusts by checking his blood sugars before disconnecting. If he starts with his blood sugars at a good level, he can usually surf or body surf for 30 to 40 minutes without many changes in his readings. He always takes some snacks with him to the beach, just in case.

Table 12.9 Surfing and Boogieboarding

Insulin: insulin pump	Insulin: basal-bolus regimen	Diet: insulin pump	Diet: basal-bolus regimen
• Remove your pump during these activities or reduce your basal rate by 25–50%. Take a bolus when reconnecting to your pump if you are disconnected for an hour or more. • For surfing or boogieboarding after a meal, reduce your boluses by 20–50% depending on how long you plan to be active.	• Reduce your rapid-acting insulin by 20–50%, depending on how big the waves are and how long you plan to surf or boogieboard.	• Consume an extra 0–20 grams of carbohydrate per hour, depending on your insulin reductions and wave conditions.	• Consume 10–30 grams of carbohydrate per hour for surfing or boogieboarding when ocean conditions are rough, depending on your insulin levels.

Diet Changes Alone

For California resident Alexis Pollak, surfing requires her to monitor her blood sugars more closely because she is less aware of lows while she is in the water. She generally likes to start with a higher glucose level (around 200 mg/dl, or 11.1 mmol/L), because the water and waves make lows more dangerous. To raise her blood sugars beforehand, she usually eats some glucose tablets and keeps Gu on hand to treat low blood sugars.

Combined Regimen Changes

A professional surfer, Hawaii resident Scott Dunton takes his pump off before he goes surfing, and he tries to have his blood sugars at 140 mg/dl (7.8 mmol/L) or higher. His sugars are usually relatively stable during this activity, although how long he surfs varies depending on what the waves are like. He doesn't adjust his basal rates before or after this activity. When he first started surfing, his blood sugars dropped a lot during the activity, and he used to keep his pockets full of candy bars to eat when they dropped during the first 15 minutes of surfing. His body has adjusted to doing up to 3 hours of surfing at a time, and his blood sugars seldom drop anymore.

Darcy Hughes of Geelong, Victoria (Australia), finds that he has to snack during surfing to keep his blood sugars elevated. Before he surfs, he generally eats a normal breakfast without lowering his NovoLog injection. Just before he hits the water, he snacks on about 50 grams of carbohydrate in the form of sultanas, bananas, or other natural sugars. When he eats additional snacks during prolonged surfing, he doesn't take any NovoRapid to cover them. He uses Lantus for basal insulin coverage, but he doesn't adjust his doses at all for surfing.

WATERSKIING

Waterskiing mainly involves prolonged muscular contractions while you hold onto the rope and stabilize your body on the skis, but it includes a more intense component when you push with your legs to get up on your skis or when you have to deal with crossing a wave. Unless you ski for an extended period, you will usually need only minimal changes to regulate your blood sugars because of the brief, intense nature of this activity. If you take insulin, you may want to reduce your premeal insulin dose by 0 to 20 percent, in which case you may not need extra carbohydrate. If you are a pump user, you may choose to remove your pump during this activity and take a bolus when you reconnect if it has been off for an hour or more.

Athlete Examples

Regimen changes for water skiing vary depending on how long you ski and how accustomed to the activity you are.

Combined Regimen Changes

For water skiing for 45 to 60 minutes or longer, AnneLisa Butcher from California usually lowers her basal rate by 35 percent. If her blood sugars are in a normal range when she starts this activity, she eats a snack, but not if they're higher.

WHITEWATER SPORTS (CANOEING, KAYAKING, AND RAFTING)

Whitewater water sports usually have both aerobic and anaerobic aspects to them and may be quite prolonged. For low-level paddling (i.e., going downstream without much effort), you will need to make only minimal changes in your diabetes regimen. For longer or more intense paddling, however, you may need more carbohydrate or lower insulin levels to prevent hypoglycemia, even if a greater release of adrenaline in the short run keeps your sugars higher during the activity. For multiday trips, you may need to reduce basal insulin doses by 10 to 25 percent, especially afterward because more glycogen depletion will occur in your upper-body muscles from engaging in repeated days of this glycogen-depleting activity.

Athlete Examples

These examples show that required changes depend on the intensity and duration of your whitewater paddling activity.

Combined Regimen Changes

For whitewater paddling in cold water, Jennifer Roche of Melbourne, Australia, has to make adjustments to prevent lows. Usually, she eats jellybeans throughout the day when she's doing this activity. She needs fewer of them during the trickier parts of the paddling, however, probably because of greater release of adrenaline then.

Oregon resident Jamie Flanagan cuts his basal rate by about 20 percent when whitewater kayaking. He finds that his blood sugars don't drop as rapidly as they do during more aerobic sports. He likes his sugars to be around 180 mg/dl (10 mmol/L) when kayaking because going low during this activity would be life threatening and he has few opportunities to get out of his kayak and dry off his hands to test his sugars. In addition, he supplements with snacks throughout this activity to prevent lows.

For Alisa Krakel of Colorado, whitewater rafting trips lasting several days can be challenging to her blood glucose control. The heat, constant exercise, and adrenaline highs all affect her responses in varying ways. To compensate, she usually has to adjust both her insulin and her food intake.

Lisa Seaman of Colorado finds that the stress of doing whitewater kayaking causes enough adrenaline release for her blood sugars to rise during the activity. To compensate, she either increases her basal rate or keeps it the same, whereas she would normally lower it during other physical activities.

WINDSURFING

This activity usually involves prolonged muscular work to hold onto the sail and stand upright on the board without losing your balance. Windsurfing is similar to isometric resistance training, which uses static (fixed-length) muscle contractions. You mainly use anaerobic energy sources, with some fat and carbohydrate for the sustained contractions of postural and upper-body muscles. The intensity of this activity will depend on wind conditions and your skill level, while the adjustments that you need to make will be the result of how long you do the activity and how hard you're working. Stronger wind will increase the intensity of your workout and the amount of blood glucose and muscle glycogen that you use. You may need adjustments in your insulin and your carbohydrate intake under these more challenging conditions if you windsurf for more than 30 minutes at a time. Lighter winds or shorter bouts of windsurfing will reduce your blood glucose use and require minimal changes to prevent lows.

YARD WORK AND GARDENING

The effect of these activities on your blood sugars can vary. In general, working outdoors in your yard requires you to use postural muscles to maintain your balance (an aerobic activity) and other muscles to perform repetitive motions, such as raking, mowing with a push mower, weeding, and watering. If you're just weeding or watering, your blood sugars will probably remain stable, but doing harder work can have a greater glycemic effect. When you perform more forceful activities like carrying or chopping wood, shoveling snow, digging a hole, hoeing, or mowing high grass, your blood sugars are likely to decrease if you do any of these for long, and you'll likely have to take in some carbohydrate or lower your insulin levels to compensate. See table 12.10 for further instructions on yard work and gardening.

Table 12.10 Yard Work and Gardening

Insulin: insulin pump	Insulin: basal-bolus regimen	Diet: insulin pump	Diet: basal-bolus regimen
• Reduce your basal rates by 0–50%, depending on how long you'll be working and how hard the activity is (e.g., less for weeding, more for strenuous yard work). • Lower your preactivity meal boluses by 0–25%.	• For light gardening, reduce your preactivity insulin doses by 0–20%, but for strenuous activity, cut back by 10–30%.	• Increase your carbohydrate intake by 0–25 grams per hour, depending on how hard you're working.	• Consume 5–30 grams of carbohydrate per hour when doing strenuous yard work or gardening.

Athlete Examples

The following examples show that yard work and gardening can be compensated for in various ways, depending on how long and how hard you work.

Insulin Changes Alone

When doing yard work for a couple of hours straight or shoveling out horse paddocks, Lorri Sargent from New Hampshire suspends her pump because these intense activities would otherwise cause her blood sugars to decrease.

Diet Changes Alone

For doing lawn care (e.g., using a weed eater), snow blowing, or shoveling snow, Eagle Bend, Minnesota, resident Gary Taylor simply eats some extra carbohydrate before and during these activities because he doesn't do any of them regularly.

Type 2 diabetic exerciser Donna L. Johnson of Knoxville, Tennessee, finds that she usually underestimates the exercise intensity of gardening and landscaping work. She often has to stop midway through her planned activity to treat low blood sugars. For other activities like running and swimming, she actually lowers the dose of Starlix that she takes before breakfast and dinner.

D. Hollander of Westchester, New York, finds that doing any outdoor work like chopping wood, planting, or doing physical labor around his property drops his blood sugars quickly. To prevent lows, he "tops the tank" by drinking orange juice or milk to start with blood sugars in the range of 175 to 200 mg/dl (9.7 to 11.1 mmol/L) because he anticipates a decrease of 50 to 100 (2.8 to 5.6) in the first 30 minutes of working out. He prefers to eat only when he's hungry, so he reduces his basal rate or disconnects from his pump if his blood sugars start to decrease too much.

Combined Regimen Changes

Florian Menninger Jr. of Northborough, Massachusetts, finds that doing yard work, gardening, mowing, pruning, and more requires him to decrease his basal rates and eat more carbohydrate to compensate. He eats a good breakfast before most of these activities and tries to start with his blood sugars between 150 and 200 mg/dl (8.3 to 11.1 mmol/L). Eating half an english muffin with peanut butter helps prevent lows, and he controls highs with basal rate adjustments.

For shoveling gravel, dirt, and mulch or doing other intense yard work, Sheri Ochs of Virginia decreases her preactivity Humalog injection by 20 percent. She additionally eats 15 to 20 grams of extra carbohydrate per hour after the first hour and monitors her blood sugars more closely the rest of the day after doing these activities for two to three hours continuously.

From this chapter and the second half of this book, you can see that diabetes does not keep people from participating in every conceivable sport and recreational physical activity! In this second edition, you even learned what to do if you take up dog mushing. So go ahead—learn how to water ski, climb a mountain, ski the Alps, do an adventure race, or just try something new to test the limits of your physical ability. The important point is to stay physically active despite having diabetes. Your mind and body will thank you.

Athlete Profile

Name: Bruce Linton

Hometown: Kasilof, Alaska, USA

Diabetes history: Type 1 diabetes diagnosed in 1993 (at age 30)

Sport or activity: Dog mushing, triathlons, running

Greatest athletic achievement: Completing the Iditarod dog sled race for the first time in 2007 in 15 days, 23 hours, 38 minutes, and 30 seconds and then finishing more than 4 days faster on my second try in 2008. I have also finished 14 marathons and 3 full Ironman triathlons with diabetes. I even qualified for the Boston Marathon, which I have completed three times. Both the Iditarod and triathlons are extremely challenging, but for different reasons.

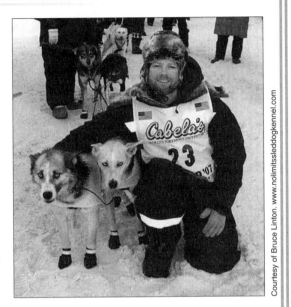

Courtesy of Bruce Linton. www.nolimitssleddogkennel.com

Current insulin and medication regimen: Insulin pump

Training tips: You don't want to be worried about your blood sugar going low during a race, so figure out beforehand how much insulin you need to cut out to keep it stable. It is incredible that your body doesn't need much insulin and becomes sensitive to it when you are exercising all day long!

Typical daily and weekly training and diabetes regimen: The Iditarod race is a 1,150-mile (1,850-kilometer) dog sled race across Alaska from Anchorage to Nome that occurs day and night and has taken mushers from less than 9 days to more than 32 days to complete. I basically just adjust my insulin intake based on the run and rest schedule of my dogs. When I am out there on the sled, I take less insulin because I am exercising (and I eat unrestricted amounts of carbohydrate without bolusing), and I also lower it for an all-night run (to avoid going low in the middle of the night while running the sled).

After completing a few marathons, I have found that for this event it is best for me not to take any insulin until the race is over. Most marathons are run in the morning, so I will not take any insulin beforehand, and after 26 miles (42 kilometers), my blood sugars are usually pretty good even though I have not taken any insulin and have ingested a lot of carbohydrate along the way. I learned this the hard way during my first Ironman triathlon when I took about half of the insulin that I normally take. That time, I had too much insulin on board when I got about 15 miles (24 kilometers) into the run, after already completing the 2-mile (3.2-kilometer) swim and 112-mile (180-kilometer) cycling portions, and I could not get my blood sugar up no matter how much carbohydrate I ingested. The next two Ironmans I did were the only 2 full days in my life in the last 14 years with diabetes that I did not take any insulin, and I completed them with blood sugars of 135 and 140.

Sample training day: I use a basal of 1.1 units of Humalog per hour and then bolus with a ratio of 1 unit of insulin for every 10 grams of carbohydrate. In an endurance event or training, I reduce my bolus intake when ingesting food to compensate for the exercising that I am doing. I also reduce my basal dose as well if the endurance event occurs over a long period (like the Iditarod or Ironmans).

Other hobbies and interests: Running and taking care of my dogs now takes up almost all my time! I like to go fishing here on the Kenai Peninsula in Alaska.

Good diabetes and exercise story: As I mentioned, 15 miles (24 kilometers) into my 26.2-mile (42-kilometer) run in my first Ironman triathlon, my blood sugar was below 70. My body was so tired that after every aid station, I would test my blood sugar and ingest more food and liquid. For a long while, no matter how much I ate, my blood sugar would not rise. Finally, after gorging myself with more than 200 grams of carbohydrate, I was able to get my blood sugar to rise a little bit. It was scary that I was not responding to my food intake. When I finished that race, I was probably the only person in the field to have gained weight after exercising for 13 hours! I learned that day that you really have to lower your insulin a lot when your event extends over a long time.

Diabetes and Athletic Organizations

American College of Sports Medicine (ACSM)

Street address: 401 W. Michigan Street, Indianapolis, IN 46202-3233

Mailing address: P.O. Box 1440, Indianapolis, IN 46206-1440

Phone: 317-637-9200

Fax: 317-634-7817

Web site: www.acsm.org

American Diabetes Association (ADA)

Address: 1660 Duke Street, Alexandria, VA 22314

Phone: 800-DIABETES (800-342-2383)

Fax: 703-549-1715

E-mail: AskADA@diabetes.org

Web site: www.diabetes.org

Children With Diabetes, Inc.

Address: 5689 Chancery Place, Hamilton, OH 45011

Web site: www.childrenwithdiabetes.com

Diabetes Education & Camping Association (DECA)

Address: P.O. Box 385, Huntsville, AL 35804

Phone: 902-479-0857

Fax: 902-431-0680

E-mail: labramson@eastlink.ca

Web site: www.diabetescamps.org

Diabetes Exercise and Sports Association (DESA)

Address: 10216 Taylorsville Road, Suite 900, Louisville, KY 40299

Phone: 502-261-8346

Fax: 615-673-2077

E-mail: desa@diabetes-exercise.org

Web site: www.diabetes-exercise.org

Diabetes Sports & Wellness Foundation (DSWF)

Address: 7241 North Avenue, Middleton, WI 53562

E-mail: jay@dswf.org

Web site: www.dswf.org

Diabetes Training Camp

Web site: www.diabetestrainingcamp.com

Dr. Sheri Colberg (author of *Diabetic Athlete's Handbook*)

E-mail: sheri@shericolberg.com

Web site: www.shericolberg.com

Fit4D (Personalized Diabetes Coaching)

Phone: 866-411-0254

Web site: www.fit4d.com

HypoActive (Australia)

E-mail: Monique@hypoactive.org

Web site: www.hypoactive.org

Insulin Dependence

E-mail: peter@insulindependence.org

Web site: www.insulindependence.org

Insulin Factor

E-mail: info@insulinfactor.com

Web site: www.insulinfactor.com

Integrated Diabetes Services

333 E. Lancaster Avenue, Suite 204, Wynnewood, PA 19096

Phone: 877-SELF-MGT (877-735-3648) or 610-642-6055

Fax: 610-642-8046

E-mail: gary@integrateddiabetes.com

Web site: www.integrateddiabetes.com

Juvenile Diabetes Research Foundation International (JDRF)

Address: 120 Wall Street, New York, NY 10005-4001

Phone: 800-533-CURE (2873)

Fax: 212-785-9595

E-mail: info@jdrf.org

Web site: www.jdrf.org

Lifelong Exercise Institute (LEI)

E-mail: info@lifelongexercise.com

Web site: www.lifelongexercise.com

Mountains for Active Diabetics (United Kingdom)

E-mail: webmaster@friendsinhighplaces.org

Web site: www.diabetic.friendsinhighplaces.org

B

Diabetes, Sport, and Nutrition Web Sites

acefitness.org

This site is the official Web site of the American Council on Exercise, a nonprofit organization targeting personal fitness trainers that offers fitness facts applicable to all active people.

ars.usda.gov/ba/bhnrc/ndl

This site provides access to USDA's food nutrient data laboratory, where you can access data about the nutritional content of any food or drink.

calorieking.com

This site, partnered with the Joslin Diabetes Center, allows you to download a food search toolbar that can even work from your mobile phone; it also contains recipes and articles of interest.

childrenwithdiabetes.com

Ever expanding, the Children With Diabetes organization offers a variety of conferences and events aimed at parents and type 1 diabetic youth, as well as lots of other information.

diabetes-exercise.org

The Diabetes Exercise and Sports Association (DESA), the premier organization for diabetic exercisers, posts newsletters, upcoming conferences, and other information on its site.

diabetesincontrol.com

This site reviews all the latest diabetes, fitness, and nutrition news on a weekly basis and posts articles about these research findings; you can search for archived articles by topic as well.

diabetestrainingcamp.com

Founded in 2006 by Dr. Matt Corcoran, Diabetes Training Camp offers a variety of sports training camps around the United States for adults with diabetes.

dLife.com

Started to enhance diabetes education on a wider scale with a TV show and Web site, dLife—For Your Diabetes Life—offers educational information, expert columns, and recipes on its site.

dswf.org

The Diabetes Sports and Wellness Foundation features diabetic athletes on its site. The organization also offers certain diabetes camps (e.g., snowboarding), which are listed on the site.

fit4d.com

A recent addition to the diabetes world, this site provides personalized fitness and nutritional coaching to people with diabetes, whether their goals are weight loss or serious exercise training.

gssiweb.com

This site is the official Web site of the Gatorade Sports Science Institute, which is proactive in its research in sports supplements and training-related issues.

hypoactive.org

Based in Australia, HypoActive promotes an active lifestyle for people with type 1 diabetes. The site includes profiles of inspirational athletes, links to exercise research, and more.

insulindependence.org

This nonprofit organization promotes adventure travel and expeditions for active people with diabetes, along with diabetic team participation in endurance-based events such as the Ironman Wisconsin in 2008.

insulinfactor.com

This group encourages people to join an athletic team of people with diabetes who compete in an array of athletic events like triathlons, marathons, century rides, and more.

lifelongexercise.com

The goal of the Lifelong Exercise Institute (LEI), of which Dr. Sheri Colberg is the executive director, is to be the premier resource for educational materials and take-charge, action plans with the potential for lifelong adherence that combat the health effects of diabetes, prediabetes, obesity, and unhealthy lifestyles.

diabetic.friendsinhighplaces.org

This site is for MAD—Mountains for Active Diabetics—a United Kingdom–based group of diabetic mountaineers who help other people with diabetes enjoy active, outdoor challenges.

nat.uiuc.edu/mainnat.html

This site contains the Nutrition Analysis Tools and System (NATS) 2.0, a free, online tool for dietary analysis of what you consume (including many brand name and fast-food items).

olympic-usa.org

This site, the official Web site of the United States Olympic team, contains updated information about all Olympic sports and athletes.

shericolberg.com

On Dr. Sheri Colberg's Web site, you can find articles about exercise, diabetes, fitness and more, along with links to her exercise blog, information about her books, and contact information.

sportsci.org

This site contains *SportScience*, a peer-reviewed site for sport research with up-to-date information and links to related topics.

tcoyd.org

The Taking Control of Your Diabetes organization offers informational conferences around the United States, as well as newsletters, a TV program, books, and additional educational materials.

thedietchannel.com

This site provides many links to articles on weight loss, sports nutrition, diet analysis tools, ideal body weight, body fat and exercise calorie calculators, and healthy living.

Suggested Reading

Becker, Gretchen. *The First Year—Type 2 Diabetes: An Essential Guide for the Newly Diagnosed* (2nd edition). New York: Marlowe & Company, 2006.

Brand-Miller, Jennie, et al. *The New Glucose Revolution* (3rd edition). New York: Marlowe & Company, 2007.

Colberg, Sheri. *Diabetes-Free Kids: A Take-Charge Plan for Preventing and Treating Type 2 Diabetes in Children.* New York: Avery, 2005.

Colberg, Sheri, and Steven V. Edelman. *50 Secrets of the Longest Living People with Diabetes.* New York: Marlowe & Company, 2007.

Colberg, Sheri. *The 7 Step Diabetes Fitness Plan.* New York: Marlowe & Company, 2006.

Edelman, Steven V. *Taking Control of Your Diabetes* (3rd edition). Caddo, OK: Professional Communications, Inc., 2007.

Hayes, Charlotte. *The "I Hate to Exercise" Book for People With Diabetes* (2nd edition). Alexandria, VA: American Diabetes Association, 2006.

Ivy, John, and Robert Portman. *Nutrient Timing: The Future of Sports Nutrition.* Laguna Beach, CA: Basic Health Publications, 2004.

Morley, John E., and Sheri R. Colberg. *The Science of Staying Young.* New York: McGraw-Hill, 2007.

Nathan, David, and Linda Delahanty. *Beating Diabetes (A Harvard Medical School Book).* New York: McGraw-Hill, 2005.

Peters, Anne. *Conquering Diabetes: A Cutting-Edge, Comprehensive Program for Prevention and Treatment.* New York: Hudson Street Press, 2005.

Porter, Kay. *The Mental Athlete: Inner Training for Peak Performance in All Sports.* Champaign, IL: Human Kinetics, 2003.

Price, Joan. *The Anytime, Anywhere Exercise Book.* Avon, MA: Adams Media Corporation, 2003.

Ruderman, Neil, ed. *Handbook of Exercise in Diabetes.* Alexandria, VA: American Diabetes Association, 2002.

Scheiner, Gary. *Think Like a Pancreas: A Practical Guide to Managing Diabetes With Insulin.* New York: Marlowe & Company, 2004.

Scheiner, Gary. *The Ultimate Guide to Accurate Carb Counting: Featuring the Tools and Techniques Used by the Experts.* New York: Marlowe & Company, 2007.

Walsh, John, and Ruth Roberts. *Pumping Insulin: Everything You Need for Success on a Smart Insulin Pump.* San Diego, CA: Torrey Pines Press, 2006.

Selected Bibliography

Chapter 1

American College of Sports Medicine. 2006. *ACSM's Guidelines for Exercise Testing and Prescription*, 7th ed. Baltimore, MD: Lippincott, Williams & Wilkins.

Fuchsjager-Mayrl, G., J. Pleiner, G.F. Wiesinger, A.E. Sieder, M. Quittan, M.J. Nuhr, C. Francesconi, H.P. Seit, M. Francesconi, L. Schmetterer, and M. Woltz. 2002. Exercise training improves vascular endothelial function in patients with type 1 diabetes. *Diabetes Care* 25:1795-1801.

Haskell, W.L., I.-M. Lee, R.R. Pate, K.E. Powell, S.N. Blair, B.A. Franklin, C.A. Macera, G.W. Heath, P.D. Thompson, and A. Bauman. 2007. Physical activity and public health: Updated recommendation for adults from the American College of Sports Medicine and the American Heart Association. *Medicine and Science in Sports and Exercise* 39:1423-1434.

Kubukeli, Z.N., T.D. Noakes, and S.C. Dennis. 2002. Training techniques to improve endurance exercise performances. *Sports Medicine* 32:489-509.

Johnson, S.T., L.J. McCargar, G.J. Bell, C. Tudor-Locke, V.J. Harber, and R.C. Bell. 2006. Walking faster: Distilling a complex prescription for type 2 diabetes management through pedometry. *Diabetes Care* 29(7):1654-1655.

Nelson, M.E., W.J. Rejeski, S.N. Blair, P.W. Duncan, J.O. Judge, A.C. King, C.A. Macera, and C. Castanedasceppa. 2007. Physical activity and public health in older adults: Recommendation from the American College of Sports Medicine and the American Heart Association. *Medicine and Science in Sports and Exercise* 39:1435-1445.

Penedo, F.J., and J.R. Dahn. 2005. Exercise and well-being: A review of mental and physical health benefits associated with physical activity. *Current Opinions in Psychiatry* 18:189-193.

Winett, R.A., J.R. Wojcik, L.D. Fox, W.G. Herbert, J.S. Blevins, and R.N. Carpinelli. 2003. Effects of low volume resistance and cardiovascular training on strength and aerobic capacity in unfit men and women: A demonstration of a threshold model. *Journal of Behavioral Medicine* 26:183-95.

Chapter 2

Bak, J., U. Jacobsen, F. Jorgensen, and O. Pedersen. 1989. Insulin receptor function and glycogen synthase activity in skeletal muscle biopsies from patients with insulin-dependent diabetes mellitus: Effects of physical training. *Journal of Clinical Endocrinology and Metabolism* 69:158-164.

Bergman, B.C., G.E. Butterfield, E.E. Wolfel, G.D. Lopaschuk, G.A. Casazza, M.A. Horning, and G.A. Brooks. 1999. Muscle net glucose uptake and glucose kinetics after endurance training in men. *American Journal of Physiology* 277:E81-92.

Borghouts, L., and H. Keizer. 2000. Exercise and insulin sensitivity: A review. *International Journal of Sports Medicine* 21:1-12.

Bruce, C., and J. Hawley. 2004. Improvements in insulin resistance with aerobic exercise training: A lipocentric approach. *Medicine and Science in Sports and Exercise*, 36:1196-1201.

Bussau, V.A., L.D. Ferreira, T.W. Jones, and P.A. Fournier. 2006. The 10-s maximal sprint: A novel approach to counter an exercise-mediated fall in glycemia in individuals with type 1 diabetes. *Diabetes Care* 29:601-606.

Bussau, V.A., L.D. Ferreira, T.W. Jones, and P.A. Fournier. 2007. A 10-s sprint performed prior to moderate-intensity exercise prevents early postexercise fall in glycaemia in individuals with type 1 diabetes. *Diabetologia* 50:1815-1818.

Colberg, S.R., J.M. Hagberg, S.D. McCole, J.M. Zmuda, P.D. Thompson, and D.E. Kelley. 1996. Utilization of glycogen but not plasma glucose is reduced in individuals with NIDDM during mild-intensity exercise. *Journal of Applied Physiology* 81:2027-2033.

Coyle, E., A. Coggan, M. Hemmert, and J. Ivy. 1986. Muscle glycogen utilization during prolonged strenuous exercise when fed carbohydrates. *Journal of Applied Physiology* 61:165-172.

Briscoe, V.J., D.B. Tate, and S.N. Davis. 2007. Type 1 diabetes: Exercise and hypoglycemia. *Applied Physiology, Nutrition, and Metabolism* 32:576-582.

De Feo, P., C. Di Loreto, A. Ranchelli, C. Fatone, G. Gambelunghe, P. Lucidi, and F. Santeusanio. 2006. Exercise and diabetes. *Acta Biomedica* 77:14-17.

Galassetti, P., D. Tate, R.A. Neill, S. Morrey, D.H. Wasserman, and S.N. Davis. 2003. Effect of antecedent hypoglycemia on counterregulatory responses to subsequent euglycemic exercise in type 1 diabetes. *Diabetes* 52:1761-1769.

Galassetti, P., D. Tate, R.A. Neill, S. Morrey, D.H. Wasserman, and S.N. Davis. 2004. Effect of sex on counterregulatory responses to exercise after antecedent hypoglycemia in type 1 diabetes. *American Journal of Physiology* 287:E16-E24.

Galassetti, P., D. Tate, R.A. Neill, A. Richardson, S.Y. Leu, and S.N. Davis. 2006. Effect of differing antecedent hypoglycemia on counterregulatory responses to exercise in type 1 diabetes. *American Journal of Physiology* 290:E1109-E1117.

Guelfi, K.J., T.W. Jones, and P.A. Fournier. 2005. The decline in blood glucose levels is less with intermittent high-intensity compared with moderate exercise in individuals with type 1 diabetes. *Diabetes Care* 28:1289-1294.

Guelfi, K.J., T.W. Jones, and P.A. Fournier. 2005. Intermittent high-intensity exercise does not increase the risk of early postexercise hypoglycemia in individuals with type 1 diabetes. *Diabetes Care* 28:416-418.

Guelfi, K.J., N. Ratnam, G.A. Smythe, T.W. Jones, and P.A. Fournier. 2007. Effect of intermittent high-intensity compared with continuous moderate exercise on glucose production and utilization in individuals with type 1 diabetes. *American Journal of Physiology* 292:E865-E8670.

Hernandez, J.M., T. Moccia, J.D. Fluckey, J.S. Ulbrecht, and P.A. Farrell. 2000. Fluid snacks to help persons with type 1 diabetes avoid late onset postexercise hypoglycemia. *Medicine and Science in Sports and Exercise* 32:904-910.

Hirsch, I.B., J.C. Marker, J. Smith, R. Spina, C.A. Parvin, J.O. Holloszy, and P.E. Cryer. 1991. Insulin and glucagon in the prevention of hypoglycemia during exercise in humans. *American Journal of Physiology* 260:E695-E704.

Houmard, J.A., C.J. Tanner, C.A. Slentz, B.D. Duscha, J.S. McCartney, and W.E. Kraus. 2004. Effect of the volume and intensity of exercise training on insulin sensitivity. *Journal of Applied Physiology* 96:101-106.

Kjaer, M., C. Hollenbeck, B. Frey-Hewitt, H. Galbo, W. Haskell, and G. Reaven. 1990. Glucoregulation and hormonal responses to maximal exercise in non-insulin-dependent diabetes. *Journal of Applied Physiology* 68:2067-2074.

Koivisto, V.A., T. Sane, F. Fyhrquist, and R. Pelkonen. 1992. Fuel and fluid homeostasis during long-term exercise in healthy subjects and type I diabetic patients. *Diabetes Care* 15:1736-1741.

Kreisman, S.H., J.B. Halter, M. Vranic, and E.B. Marliss. 2003. Combined infusion of epinephrine and norepinephrine during moderate exercise reproduces the glucoregulatory response of intense exercise. *Diabetes* 52:1347-1354.

Lisle, D.K., and T.H. Trojian. 2006. Managing the athlete with type 1 diabetes. *Current Sports Medicine Reports* 5:93-98.

McMahon, S.K., L.D. Ferreira, N. Ratnam, R.J. Davey, L.M. Youngs, E.A. Davis, P.A. Fournier, and T.W. Jones. 2007. Glucose requirements to maintain euglycemia after moderate-intensity afternoon exercise in adolescents with type 1 diabetes are increased in a biphasic manner. *Journal of Clinical Endocrinology and Metabolism* 92:963-968.

Mitchell, T.H., G. Abraham, A. Schiffrin, L.A. Leiter, and E.B. Marliss. 1988. Hyperglycemia after intense exercise in IDDM subjects during continuous subcutaneous insulin infusion. *Diabetes Care* 11:311-317.

Poirier, P., S. Mawhinney, L. Grondin, A. Tremblay, T. Broderick, J. Cleroux, C. Catellier, G. Tancrede, and A. Nadeau. 2001. Prior meal enhances the plasma glucose lowering effect of exercise in type 2 diabetes. *Medicine and Science in Sports and Exercise* 33:1259-1264.

Price, T.B., D.L. Rothman, R. Taylor, M.J. Avison, G.I. Shulman, and R.G. Shulman. 1994. Human muscle glycogen resynthesis after exercise: Insulin-dependent and -independent phases. *Journal of Applied Physiology* 76:104-111.

Raguso, C.A., A.R. Coggan, A. Gastaldelli, L.S. Sidossis, E.J. Bastyr 3rd, and R.R. Wolfe. 1995. Lipid and carbohydrate metabolism in IDDM during moderate and intense exercise. *Diabetes* 44:1066-1074.

Richter, E., L. Turcotte, P. Hespel, and B. Kiens. 1992. Metabolic responses to exercise: Effects of endurance training and implications for diabetes. *Diabetes Care* 15:1767-1776.

Sandoval, D.A., D.L. Guy, M.A. Richardson, A.C. Ertl, and S.N. Davis. 2004. Effects of low and moderate antecedent exercise on counterregulatory responses to subsequent hypoglycemia in type 1 diabetes. *Diabetes* 53:1798-1806.

Sandoval, D.A., D.L. Guy, M.A. Richardson, A.C. Ertl, and S.N. Davis. 2006. Acute, same-day effects of antecedent exercise on counterregulatory responses to subsequent hypoglycemia in type 1 diabetes mellitus. *American Journal of Physiology* 290:E1331-E1338.

Sigal, R.J., C. Purdon, S.J. Fisher, J.B. Halter, M. Vranic, and E.B. Marliss. 1994. Hyperinsulinemia prevents prolonged hyperglycemia after intense exercise in insulin-dependent diabetic subjects. *Journal of Clinical Endocrinology and Metabolism* 79:1049-1057.

Trout, K.K., M.R. Rickels, M.H. Schutta, M. Petrova, E.W. Freeman, N.C. Tkacs, and K.L. Teff. 2007. Menstrual cycle effects on insulin sensitivity in women with type 1 diabetes: A pilot study. *Diabetes Technology and Therapeutics* 9:176-182.

Tuominen, J., P. Ebeling, H. Vuorinen-Markkola, and V. Koivisto. 1997. Postmarathon paradox in IDDM: Unchanged insulin sensitivity in spite of glycogen depletion. *Diabetic Medicine* 14:301-308.

Zander, E., W. Bruns, P. Wulfert, W. Besch, D. Lubs, R. Chlup, and B. Schulz. 1983. Muscular exercise in type 1-diabetics: I. Different metabolic reactions during heavy muscular work is dependent on actual insulin availability. *Experimental and Clinical Endocrinology* 82:78-90.

Zander, E., B. Schulz, R. Chlup, P. Woltansky, and D. Lubs. 1985. Muscular exercise in type 1-diabetics: II. Hormonal and metabolic responses to moderate exercise. *Experimental and Clinical Endocrinology* 85:95-104.

Chapter 3

Aas, A.M., I. Bergstad, P.M. Thorsby, O. Johannesen, M. Solberg, and K.I. Birkeland. 2005. An intensified lifestyle intervention programme may be superior to insulin treatment in poorly controlled Type 2 diabetic patients on oral hypoglycaemic agents: Results of a feasibility study. *Diabetic Medicine* 22:316-322.

Admon, G., Y. Weinstein, B. Falk, N. Weintrob, H. Benzaquen, R. Ofan, G. Fayman, L. Zigel, N. Constantini, and M. Phillip. 2005. Exercise with and without an insulin pump among children and adolescents with type 1 diabetes mellitus. *Pediatrics* 116:e348-e355.

Ashwell, S.G., J. Gebbie, and P.D. Home. 2006. Optimal timing of injection of once-daily insulin glargine in people with type 1 diabetes using insulin lispro at meal-times. *Diabetic Medicine* 23:46–52.

Bischof, M.G., E. Bernroider, C. Ludwig, S. Kurzemann, K. Kletter, W. Waldhäusl, and M. Roden. 2001. Effect of near physiologic insulin therapy on hypoglycemia counterregulation in type-1 diabetes. *Hormone Research* 56:151–158.

Bond, A. 2006. Exenatide (Byetta) as a novel treatment option for type 2 diabetes mellitus. *Proceedings* (Baylor University Medical Center) 19:281–284.

Chokkalingam, K., K. Tsintzas, L. Norton, K. Jewell, I.A. Macdonald, and P.I. Mansell. 2007. Exercise under hyperinsulinaemic conditions increases whole-body glucose disposal without affecting muscle glycogen utilisation in type 1 diabetes. *Diabetologia* 50:414–421.

Cryer, P.E. 2006. Hypoglycemia in diabetes: Pathophysiological mechanisms and diurnal variation. *Progress in Brain Research* 153:361–365.

DeVries, J.H., I.M. Wentholt, N. Masurel, I. Mantel, A. Poscia, A. Maran, and R.J. Heine. 2004. Nocturnal hypoglycaemia in type 1 diabetes: Consequences and assessment. *Diabetes/ Metabolism Research and Reviews* 20:S43–S46.

Everett, J. 2004. The role of insulin pumps in the management of diabetes. *Nursing Times* 100:48–49.

Feinglos, M., and M. Bethel. 1999. Oral agent therapy in the treatment of type 2 diabetes. *Diabetes Care* 22:C61–C64.

Gomis, R., and E. Esmatjes. 2004. Asymptomatic hypoglycaemia: Identification and impact. *Diabetes/Metabolism Research and Reviews* 20:S47–S49.

Green, B.D., P.R. Flatt, and C.J. Bailey. 2006. Dipeptidyl peptidase IV (DPP IV) inhibitors: A newly emerging drug class for the treatment of type 2 diabetes. *Diabetes & Vascular Disease Research* 3:159–165.

Henderson J.N., K.V. Allen, I.J. Deary, and B.M. Frier. 2003. Hypoglycaemia in insulin-treated type 2 diabetes: Frequency, symptoms and impaired awareness. *Diabetic Medicine* 20:1016–1021.

Herman, W.H., L.L. Ilag, S.L. Johnson, C.L. Martin, J. Sinding, A. Al Harthi, C.D. Plunkett, F.B. LaPorte, R. Burke, M.B. Brown, J.B. Halter, and P. Raskin. 2005. A clinical trial of continuous subcutaneous insulin infusion versus multiple daily injections in older adults with type 2 diabetes. *Diabetes Care* 28:1568–1573.

Hirsch, I.B. 2005. Intensifying insulin therapy in patients with type 2 diabetes mellitus. *American Journal of Medicine* 118:21S–26S.

Joy, S.V., P.T. Rodgers, and A.C. Scates. 2005. Incretin mimetics as emerging treatment for type 2 diabetes. *Annals of Pharmacotherapy* 39:110–118.

Linkeschova, R., M. Raoul, U. Bott, M. Berger, and M. Spraul. 2002. Less severe hypoglycaemia, better metabolic control, and improved quality of life in type 1 diabetes mellitus with continuous subcutaneous insulin infusion (CSII) therapy; an observational study of 100 consecutive patients followed for a mean of 2 years. *Diabetic Medicine* 19:746–751.

Moon, R.J., L.A. Bascombe, and R.I. Holt. 2007. The addition of metformin in type 1 diabetes improves insulin sensitivity, diabetic control, body composition and patient well-being. *Diabetes Obesity and Metabolism* 9:143–145.

Peter, R., S.D. Luzio, G. Dunseath, A. Miles, B. Hare, K. Backs, V. Pauvaday, and D.R. Owens. 2005. Effects of exercise on the absorption of insulin glargine in patients with type 1 diabetes. *Diabetes Care* 28:560–565.

Peterson, G.E. 2006. Intermediate and long-acting insulins: A review of NPH insulin, insulin glargine and insulin detemir. *Current Medical Research and Opinion* 22:2613–2619.

Ratner, R.E., I.B. Hirsch, J.L. Neifing, S.K. Garg, T.E. Mecca, and C.A. Wilson. 2000. Less hypoglycemia with insulin Glargine in intensive insulin therapy for type 1 diabetes. *Diabetes Care* 23:639–643.

Rave, K., S. Bott, L. Heinemann, S. Sha, R.H. Becker, S.A. Willavize, and T. Heise. 2005. Time-action profile of inhaled insulin in comparison with subcutaneously injected insulin lispro and regular human insulin. *Diabetes Care* 28:1077–1082.

Ruegemer, J.J., R.W. Squires, H.M. March, M.W. Haymond, P.E. Cryer, R.A. Rizza, and J.M. Miles. 1990. Differences between prebreakfast and late afternoon glycemic responses to exercise in IDDM patients. *Diabetes Care* 13:104–110.

Sandoval, D.A., D.L. Guy, M.A. Richardson, A.C. Ertl, and S.N. Davis. 2006. Acute, same-day effects of antecedent exercise on counterregulatory responses to subsequent hypoglycemia in type 1 diabetes mellitus. *American Journal of Physiology* 290:E1331–E1338.

Sonnenberg, G., F. Kemmer, and M. Berger. 1990. Exercise in type 1 (insulin-dependent) diabetic patients treated with continuous subcutaneous insulin infusion: Prevention of exercise induce hypoglycemia. *Diabetologia* 33:696–703.

Yamakita, T., T. Ishii, K. Yamagami, T. Yamamoto, M. Miyamoto, M. Hosoi, K. Yoshioka, T. Sato, S. Onishi, S. Tanaka, and S. Fjuii. 2002. Glycemic response during exercise after administration of insulin lispro compared with that after administration of regular human insulin. *Diabetes Research and Clinical Practice* 57:17–22.

Chapter 4

Albarracin, C., B. Fuqua, J. Geohas, V. Juturu, M.R. Finch, and J.R. Komorowski. 2007. Combination of chromium and biotin improves coronary risk factors in hypercholesterolemic type 2 diabetes mellitus: A placebo-controlled, double-blind randomized clinical trial. *Journal of the Cardiometabolic Syndrome* 2:91–97.

Bahrke, M.S., and W.P. Morgan. 1994. Evaluation of the ergogenic properties of ginseng. *Sports Medicine* 18:229–248.

Bischof, M.G., E. Bernroider, M. Krssak, M. Krebs, H. Stingl, P. Nowotny, C. Yu, G.L. Shulman, W. Waldhausl, and M. Roden. 2002. Hepatic glycogen metabolism in type 1 diabetes after long-term near normoglycemia. *Diabetes* 51:49–54.

Brand-Miller, J., S. Hayne, P. Petocz, and S. Colagiuri. 2003. Low-glycemic index diets in the management of diabetes: A meta-analysis of randomized control trials. *Diabetes Care* 26:2261–2267.

Burani, J., and P.J. Longo. 2006. Low-glycemic index carbohydrates: An effective behavioral change for glycemic control and weight management in patients with type 1 and 2 diabetes. *Diabetes Educator* 32:78–88.

Bursell, S.-E., A.C. Clermont, L.P. Aiello, L.M. Aiello, D.K. Schlossman, E.P. Feener, L. Laffel, and G.L. King. 1999. High-dose vitamin E supplementation normalizes retinal blood flow and creatinine clearance in patients with type 1 diabetes. *Diabetes Care* 22:1245–1251.

Bussau, V.A., T.J. Fairchild, A. Rao, P. Steele, and P.A. Fournier. 2002. Carbohydrate loading in human muscle: An improved 1 day protocol. *European Journal of Applied Physiology* 87:290–295.

Cantorna, M.T., Y. Zhu, M. Froicu, and A. Wittke. 2004. Vitamin D status, 1,25-dihydroxyvitamin D3, and the immune system. *American Journal of Clinical Nutrition* 80:1717S–1720S.

Clapp, J.F., III, and B. Lopez. 2007. Low- versus high-glycemic index diets in women: Effects on caloric requirement, substrate utilization, and insulin sensitivity. *Metabolic Syndrome and Related Disorders* 5:231–242.

Clarkson, P.M. 1996. Nutrition for improved sports performance: Current issues on ergogenic aids. *Sports Medicine* 21:293–401.

Coyle, E.F. 1994. Fluid and carbohydrate replacement during exercise: How much and why? *Sports Science Exchange* 7(3):1–6.

Chiesa, G., M.A. Piscopo, A. Rigamonti, A. Azzinari, S. Bettini, R. Bonfanti, M. Viscardi, F. Meschi, and G. Chiumello. 2005. Insulin therapy and carbohydrate counting. *Acta Biomedica* 76:44-48.

Desbrow, B., and M. Leveritt. 2007. Well-trained endurance athletes' knowledge, insight, and experience of caffeine use. *International Journal of Sports Nutrition and Exercise Metabolism* 17:328-339.

Faure, P., P.Y.. Benhamou, A. Perard, S. Halimi, and A.M. Roussel. 1995. Lipid peroxidation in insulin-dependent diabetic patients with early retina degenerative lesions: Effects of an oral zinc supplementation. *European Journal of Clinical Nutrition* 49:282-288.

Faure, P., A. Roussel, C. Coudray, M.J. Richard, S. Halimi, and A. Favier. 1992. Zinc and insulin sensitivity. *Biological Trace Element Research* 32:305-310.

Foster, T.S. 2007. Efficacy and safety of alpha-lipoic acid supplementation in the treatment of symptomatic diabetic neuropathy. *Diabetes Educator* 33:111-117.

Foster-Powell, K., S. Holt, and J. Brand-Miller. 2002. International table of glycemic index and glycemic load values: 2002. *American Journal of Clinical Nutrition* 76:5-56.

Francescato, M.P., M. Geat, S. Fusi, G. Stupar, C. Noacco, and L. Cattin. 2004. Carbohydrate requirement and insulin concentration during moderate exercise in type 1 diabetic patients. *Metabolism* 53:1126-1130.

Gillespie, S.J., K.D. Kulkarni, and A.E. Daly. 1998. Using carbohydrate counting in diabetes clinical practice. *Journal of the American Dietetics Association* 98:897-905.

Kanter, M.M. 1994. Free radicals, exercise, and antioxidant supplementation. *International Journal of Sport Nutrition* 4:205-220.

Lane, J.D., M.N. Feinglos, and R.S. Surwit. 2008. Caffeine increases ambulatory glucose and postprandial responses in coffee drinkers with type 2 diabetes. *Diabetes Care* 31:221-222.

Larsson, S.C., and A. Wolk. 2007. Magnesium intake and risk of type 2 diabetes: A meta-analysis. *Journal of Internal Medicine* 262:208-214.

Lefavi, R.G., R.A. Anderson, R.E. Keith, G.D. Wilson, J.L. McMillan, and M.H. Stone. 1992. Efficacy of chromium supplementation in athletes: Emphasis on anabolism. *International Journal of Sport Nutrition* 2:111-112.

Legwold, G. 1994. Hydration breakthrough! A sponge called glycerol boosts endurance by super-loading your body with water. *Bicycling* 35:72-74.

Maughan, R.J. 1995. Creatine supplementation and exercise performance. *International Journal of Sport Nutrition* 5:94-101.

Mehdi, M.Z., S.K. Pandey, J.F. Theberge, and A.K. Srivastava. 2006. Insulin signal mimicry as a mechanism for the insulin-like effects of vanadium. *Cell Biochemistry and Biophysics* 44:73-81.

McKewen, M.W., N.J. Rehrer, C. Cox, and J. Mann. 1999. Glycaemic control, muscle glycogen and exercise performance in IDDM athletes on diets of varying carbohydrate content. *International Journal of Sports Medicine* 20:349-353.

Nielsen, F.H., and H.C. Lukaski. 2006. Update on the relationship between magnesium and exercise. *Magnesium Research* 19:180-189.

Norris, J.M., X. Yin, M.M. Lamb, K. Barriga, J. Seifert, M. Hoffman, H.D. Orton, A.E. Barón, M. Clare-Salzler, H.P. Chase, N.J. Szabo, H. Erlich, G.S. Eisenbarth, and M. Rewers. 2007. Omega-3 polyunsaturated fatty acid intake and islet autoimmunity in children at increased risk for type 1 diabetes. *Journal of the American Medical Association* 298:1420-1428.

Perrone, C., O. Laitano, and F. Meyer. 2005. Effect of carbohydrate ingestion on the glycemic response of type 1 diabetic adolescents during exercise. *Diabetes Care* 28:2537-2538.

Pittas, A.G., J. Lau, F.B. Hu, and B. Dawson-Hughes. 2007. The role of vitamin D and calcium in type 2 diabetes. A systematic review and meta-analysis. *Journal of Clinical Endocrinology and Metabolism* 92:2017-2029.

Rosenfalck, A.M., T. Almdal, L. Viggers, S. Madsbad, and J. Hilsted. 2006. A low-fat diet improves peripheral insulin sensitivity in patients with Type 1 diabetes. *Diabetic Medicine* 23:384–392.

Rosenthal, M.J., D. Smith, L. Yaguez, V. Giampietro, D. Kerr, E. Bullmore, M. Brammer, S.C. Williams, and S.A. Amiel. 2007. Caffeine restores regional brain activation in acute hypoglycaemia in healthy volunteers. *Diabetic Medicine* 24:720–727.

Thornalley, P.J., R. Babaei-Jadidi, H. Al Ali, N. Rabbani, A. Antonysunil, J. Larkin, A. Ahmed, G. Rayman, and C.W. Bodmer. 2007. High prevalence of low plasma thiamine concentration in diabetes linked to a marker of vascular disease. *Diabetologia* 50:2164–2170.

Vuksan, V., J.L. Sievenpiper, V.Y. Koo, T. Francis, U. Beljan-Zdravkovic, Z. Xu, and E. Vidgen. 2000. American ginseng (Panax quinquefolius L.) reduces postprandial glycemia in nondiabetic subjects and subjects with type 2 diabetes mellitus. *Archives of Internal Medicine* 160:1009–1013.

Williams, M.H. 1998. *The Erogenics Edge: Pushing the Limits of Sports Performance*. Champaign, IL: Human Kinetics.

Wolever, T.M., S. Hamad, J.L. Chiasson, et al. 1999. Day-to-day consistency in amount and source of carbohydrate associated with improved blood glucose control in type 1 diabetes. *Journal of the American College of Nutrition* 18:242–247.

Zunino, S.J., D.H. Storms, and C.B. Stephensen. 2007. Diets rich in polyphenols and vitamin A inhibit the development of type I autoimmune diabetes in nonobese diabetic mice. *Journal of Nutrition* 137:1216–1221.

Chapter 5

American Diabetes Association. 2000. Diabetes mellitus and exercise. *Diabetes Care* 23:S50–S54.

Colberg, S.R. 2000. Use of clinical practice recommendation for exercise by individuals with type 1 diabetes. *Diabetes Educator* 26:122–126.

Davidson, J. 2005. Strategies for improving glycemic control: Effective use of glucose monitoring. *American Journal of Medicine* 118:27S–32S.

Dela, F., M.E. von Linstow, K.J. Mikines, and H. Galbo. 2004. Physical training may enhance beta-cell function in type 2 diabetes. *American Journal of Physiology* 287:E1024–E1031.

Garg, S., and L. Jovanovic. 2006. Relationship of fasting and hourly blood glucose levels to HbA1c values: Safety, accuracy, and improvements in glucose profiles obtained using a 7-day continuous glucose sensor. *Diabetes Care* 29:2644–2649.

Houmard, J.A., N.J. Bruno, R.K. Bruner, M.R. McCammon, and R.G. Israel. 1993. Effects of exercise training on the chemical composition of plasma LDL. *Atherosclerosis and Thrombosis* 14:325–330.

Ivy, J.L., S.L. Katz, C.L. Cutler, W.M. Sherman, and E.F. Coyle. 1988. Muscle glycogen synthesis after exercise: Effect of time of carbohydrate ingestion. *Journal of Applied Physiology* 64:1480–1485.

MacDonald, M.J. 1987. Postexercise late-onset hypoglycemia in insulin-dependent diabetic patients. *Diabetes Care* 10:584–588.

McCall, A.L., D.J. Cox, J. Crean, M. Gloster, and B.P. Kovatchev. 2006. A novel analytical method for assessing glucose variability: Using CGMS in type 1 diabetes mellitus. *Diabetes Technology and Therapeutics* 8:644–653.

Roberts, L., T.W. Jones, and P.A. Fournier. 2002. Exercise training and glycemic control in adolescents with poorly controlled type 1 diabetes mellitus. *Journal of Pediatric Endocrinology and Metabolism* 15:621–627.

Zinman, B., N. Ruderman, B.N. Campaigne, J.T. Devlin, and S.H. Schneider. 2003. American Diabetes Association. Physical activity/exercise and diabetes mellitus. *Diabetes Care* 26:S73-S77.

Chapter 6

Allami, N., Y. Paulignan, A. Brovelli, and D. Boussaoud. 2008. Visuo-motor learning with combination of different rates of motor imagery and physical practice. *Experimental Brain Research* 184:105–113.

Hardy, J., C.R. Hall, and L. Hardy. 2005. Quantifying athlete self-talk. *Journal of Sports Science* 23:905–917.

Marsh, H.W., J.P. Chanal, and P.G. Sarrazin. 2006. Self-belief does make a difference: A reciprocal effects model of the causal ordering of physical self-concept and gymnastics performance. *Journal of Sports Science* 24:101–111.

Newmark, T.S., and D.F. Bogacki. 2005. The use of relaxation, hypnosis, and imagery in sport psychiatry. *Clinical Sports Medicine* 24:973–977.

Oishi, K., and T. Maeshima. 2004. Autonomic nervous system activities during motor imagery in elite athletes. *Journal of Clinical Neurophysiology* 21:170–179.

Papaioannou, A., E. Bebetsos, Y. Theodorakis, T. Christodoulidis, and O. Kouli. 2006. Causal relationships of sport and exercise involvement with goal orientations, perceived competence and intrinsic motivation in physical education: A longitudinal study. *Journal of Sports Science* 24:367–382.

Wang, J., D. Marchant, T. Morris, and P. Gibbs. 2004. Self-consciousness and trait anxiety as predictors of choking in sport. *Journal of Science and Medicine in Sport* 7:174–185.

Chapter 7

Arroll, B., and F. Goodyear-Smith. 2005. Corticosteroid injections for painful shoulder: A meta-analysis. *British Journal of General Practice* 55:224–228.

Balci, N., M.K. Balci, and S. Tüzüner. 1999. Shoulder adhesive capsulitis and shoulder range of motion in type II diabetes mellitus: Association with diabetic complications. *Journal of Diabetes and Its Complications* 13:135–140.

Cosca, D.D., and F. Navazio. 2007. Common problems in endurance athletes. *American Family Physician* 76:237–244.

Cymet, T.C., and V. Sinkov. 2006. Does long-distance running cause osteoarthritis? *Journal of the American Osteopathic Association* 106:342–345.

Fredericson, M., and A.K. Misra. 2007. Epidemiology and aetiology of marathon running injuries. *Sports Medicine* 37:437–439.

Ilahi, O.A., and H.W. Kohl, 3rd. 1998. Lower extremity morphology and alignment and risk of overuse injury. *Clinical Journal of Sport Medicine* 8:38–42.

Janghorbani, M., D. Feskanich, W.C. Willett, and F. Hu. 2006. Prospective study of diabetes and risk of hip fracture: The Nurses' Health Study. *Diabetes Care* 29:1573–1578.

Kimmerle, R., and E. Chantelau. 2007. Weight-bearing intensity produces charcot deformity in injured neuropathic feet in diabetes. *Experimental and Clinical Endocrinology and Diabetes* 115:360–364.

Mota, M., C. Panuş, E. Mota, V. Sfredel, A. Patraşcu, L. Vanghelie, and E. Toma. 2000-2001. Hand abnormalities of the patients with diabetes mellitus. *Romanian Journal of Internal Medicine* 38–39:89–95.

Vignon, E., J.P. Valat, M. Rossignol, B. Avouac, S. Rozenberg, P. Thoumie, J. Avouac, M. Nordin, and P. Hilliquin. 2006. Osteoarthritis of the knee and hip and activity: A systematic international review and synthesis (OASIS). *Joint Bone Spine* 73:442–455.

Wilder, R.P., and S. Sethi. 2004. Overuse injuries: Tendinopathies, stress fractures, compartment syndrome, and shin splints. *Clinical Sports Medicine* 23:55–81.

Chapters 8–12

Brubaker, P.L. 2005. Adventure travel and type 1 diabetes: The complicating effects of high altitude. *Diabetes Care* 28:2563–2572.

Fink, K.S., D.B. Christensen, and A. Ellsworth. 2002. Effect of high altitude on blood glucose meter performance. *Diabetes Technology and Therapeutics* 4:627–635.

Grimm, J.J., J. Ybarra, C. Berné, S. Muchnick, and A. Golay. 2007. A new table for prevention of hypoglycaemia during physical activity in type 1 diabetic patients. *Diabetes and Metabolism* 30:465–470.

Guelfi, K.J., T.W. Jones, and P.A. Fournier. 2007. New insights into managing the risk of hypoglycaemia associated with intermittent high-intensity exercise in individuals with type 1 diabetes mellitus: Implications for existing guidelines. *Sports Medicine* 37:937–946.

Rachmiel, M., J. Buccino, and D. Daneman. 2007. Exercise and type 1 diabetes mellitus in youth; review and recommendations. *Pediatric Endocrinology Reviews* 5:656–665.

Riddell, M.C., and K.E. Iscoe. 2006. Physical activity, sport, and pediatric diabetes. *Pediatric Diabetes* 7:60–70.

Toni, S., M.R. Reali, F. Barni, L. Lenzi, and F. Festini. 2007. Managing insulin therapy during exercise in type 1 diabetes mellitus. *Acta Biomedica* 77:34–40.

Valerio, G., M.I. Spagnuolo, F. Lombardi, R. Spadaro, M. Siano, and A. Franzese. 2007. Physical activity and sports participation in children and adolescents with type 1 diabetes mellitus. *Nutrition, Metabolism, and Cardiovascular Diseases* 17:376–382.

Index

Note: An *f* or *t* following a page number refers to a figure or table, respectively.

A

Abbott Freestyle Navigator 85*t*
Abbott monitor 84
acarbose 51*t*
Accel Gel 63*t*
acetaminophen 108
Achilles tendinitis 108, 111*t*, 122-123
Active Diabetes 79
active people. *See* resources for active people
activity adjustments
    aerobic conditioning machines 133*t*
    aerobic fitness classes 137*t*
    American football 191*t*
    aquatic exercise 150*t*
    backpacking 239*t*
    basal-bolus regimens 131, 159, 189, 216
    baseball 218*t*
    basketball 192*t*
    bodybuilding 220*t*
    boogieboarding 254*t*
    canoeing 234*t*
    cross-country running 161*t*
    cross-country skiing 162*t*
    cycling 164*t*
    dance 139*t*
    downhill skiing 235*t*
    field events 222*t*
    field hockey 195*t*
    golf 197*t*
    gymnastics 198*t*
    hiking 239*t*
    ice climbing 247*t*
    ice hockey 201*t*
    ice skating 142*t*
    indoor racket sports 202*t*
    inline skating 142*t*
    insulin pump users 130, 159, 188-189, 215-216
    intensity, duration, and other effects 131, 160, 189, 217, 230
    kayaking 234*t*
    kickboxing 143*t*
    lacrosse 195*t*
    marathons 169*t*
    martial arts 145*t*
    mountain biking 234*t*
    noninsulin and oral medication users 131, 159, 189, 217
    outdoor recreational activities 229-230
    rock climbing 247*t*
    rowing 204*t*
    rugby 191*t*
    running 172*t*
    scuba diving 250*t*
    snorkeling 252
    snowboarding 235*t*
    soccer (non-American football) 206*t*
    softball 218*t*
    sprinting 224*t*
    surfing 254*t*
    swimming 176*t*
    tennis 208*t*
    triathlons 180*t*
    ultraendurance events and training 184*t*
    volleyball and beach volleyball 225*t*
    walking and race walking 147*t*
    water aerobics 150*t*
    weight and resistance circuit training 152*t*
    wrestling 212*t*
    yard work and gardening 257*t*
Actos 51*t*, 52
Actrapid 46
acute injury, identifying 107-108
Adams, Jake 211
adhesive capsulitis 110, 114, 116
adrenaline 22, 99. *See also* epinephrine
adult-onset type 1 diabetes 4-5
adventure racing 231-232
Advil 108
aerobic activities 7-8, 14-16
aerobic conditioning machines 132-136
aerobic fitness classes 136-138
aerobic system 26-27
age
    guidelines for adults over 65 7*t*
    and injury 125-126
    and physical activity 6
    precautions for older athletes 126
Agnoli, Cristian 170
Ahern, Murray 174
airsoft 232-233
Airst, Malcolm 134
alanine 66*t*
Aleve 108
Alexander, Jen 178
All-Sport 60, 63*t*
alpha-glucosidase inhibitors 51*t*, 52
alpha-lipoic acid 72
alpinism 245
altitude extremes 230, 238, 246
Amaryl 51*t*, 52, 53
American College of Sports Medicine 6, 7*t*, 13, 261
American Diabetes Association 81, 261
American football 190-191
American Heart Association, physical activity recommendations 6, 7*t*
amino acids 65, 66*t*
amino acid supplements 68-69, 68*t*
amlyn 51*t*, 53
anaerobic activities, choosing 7-8
Anderson, Katrina 147
Andrews, Shirley 148, 149
ankle injuries 121-123
anterior cruciate ligament 119
anti-inflammatory medications 108
antioxidants 67*t*, 70-72
Apidra 46
aquatic exercise 150-151

arginine 66*t*
arm injuries 114-116
arthritis 125
Asherman, Sandy 138
asparagine 66*t*
aspart 46. *See also* NovoLog; NovoRapid
aspartic acid 66*t*
aspirin 108
athlete examples
    adventure racing 231-232
    aerobic conditioning machines 133-136
    aerobic fitness classes 136-138
    airsoft 233
    American football 190-191
    aquatic exercise 150-151
    baseball 218-219
    basketball 192-193
    bodybuilding 220-221
    boogieboarding 254-255
    canoeing 233-234
    competitive cheerleading and drill team 193-194
    cross-country running 160-161
    cross-country skiing 162-163
    cycling 164-168
    dance 139-140
    dog mushing 235
    downhill skiing 236-237
    extreme trail running 231-232
    fencing 221
    field hockey 194-195
    frisbee (ultimate) 196
    gaming (fishing, hunting, and shooting) 237
    golf 197-198
    gymnastics 199
    hiking and backpacking 238-241
    horseback riding, competitive 200
    housework 141
    ice hockey 201
    ice skating 142
    indoor racket sports 202-203
    inline skating 142
    kayaking 233-234
    kickboxing 142-144
    lacrosse 194-195
    marathons 169-171
    martial arts 144-146
    motorcycle riding and racing (off road) 242
    mountain biking 242-245
    mountaineering 246-247
    paintball 233
    physical education classes 146-147
    power lifting and Olympic weightlifting 223
    rock climbing and ice climbing 247-248
    roller derby 203
    rowing 204-205
    rugby 190-191
    running 172-175
    sailing 249
    scuba diving 250-251
    skateboarding 251
    snowboarding 236-237
    snowmobiling 252-253
    snowshoeing 253
    soccer (non-American football) 205-207
    softball 218-219
    sprinting 223-224
    surfing 254-255
    swimming 176-179
    tennis 208-210
    track events (400 to 1,600 meters) 210-211
    triathlons 179, 181-182
    ultraendurance events and training 183-184
    volleyball and beach volleyball 225
    walking and race walking 148-149
    water aerobics 150-151
    water polo 211
    waterskiing 255
    weight and resistance circuit training 151-153
    whitewater sports (canoeing, kayaking, and rafting) 256
    wrestling 211-212
    yard work and gardening 257-258
    yoga and stretching 153-154
athlete profiles
    Bruce Linton 259-260
    Chris Dudley 56
    Chris Jarvis 18-20
    Doug Burns 226-227
    Jake Sheldon 213-214
    Missy Foy 185-186
    Monique Hanley 98-99
    Nikki Wallis 78-79
    Robert L. Stewart 92-93
    Scott Dunton 42-44
    Sean Busby 120-121
    Zippora Karz 154-155
athletes
    about 95
    being 95-96
    competitive with selves and others 96-97
athletic shoulder issues 115-116
ATP (adenosine triphosphate) 24
ATP-CP system 24-25
autonomic neuropathy 88, 90
Avandamet 52
Avandaryl 52, 53
Avandia 51*t*, 52, 53

B
backcountry ski touring 253
backpacking 237-241
Band, Spencer 197, 201
basal insulins 47-48
baseball 217-219
basketball 192-193
beach volleyball 224-225
bedtime snacks 65
Beecroft, Spike 97, 167
Bell, Andy 96-97, 146, 212
Bell, Richard 209
Berg, Kris 178
Berg, Kyle 177
beta-carotene 71
Bethavas, Flip 196
biguanides 51*t*, 52
biking 163-168. *See also* mountain biking
biotin 75
Blackwell, Michael 195, 201
Blade, Ernest 124
Blatstein, Marc 146
blood glucose
    about 3-4
    and exercise 21-22
    exercise response and circulating plasma insulin levels 30*f*
    monitoring 82*t*, 83, 84, 87
    testing at different times 38
    variables affecting responses to exercise 22*t*
blood glucose meters 83, 230
blood pressure 93-94
bodybuilding 219-221
boogieboarding 254-255
Boren, Casey 181
Bostelman, Shiela 141
Boston Marathon 259
bowling 138
boxing 138
brain, effect of low blood sugars 40

Briel, Matthew 174
Brosnan, Gayle 219
Broussard, Jennifer 177
Bublitz, Brent 174
Burhoop, Kimberly 174
Burnham, Roy 184
Burns, Doug 221, 226-227
bursitis 115-116
Bursnall, Doug 79, 241
Busby, Sean 120-121, 236, 237, 253
Bussett, Meredith 199
Butcher, AnneLisa 234, 255
Byetta 54-55, 88
Byetta LAR 51t

C
caffeine 67t, 68t, 75-76
calcitriol 72
calcium 73-74
canoeing 233-234. *See also* white-water sports (canoeing, kayaking, and rafting)
carbohydrate
   about 57-58
   before, during, and after exercise 59-60
   body's use during exercise 28-29
   carbohydrate loading 64
   and fat, fueling activity 26-27
   fluids 60-62, 63t
   general increases for endurance sports 29t
   glycemic effect of 58-59
   intake guidelines 83-84
   taking in during exercise 29
carbohydrate loading 68t
cardiovascular problems 91, 93
carpal tunnel syndrome 110, 111t, 114, 115
catchers 217
Celebrex 108
Cerami, Patti Murphy 143, 144
cheerleading 193-194
Children with Diabetes, Inc. 261
chloropropamide 52. *See also* Diabinese
cholesterol
   and exercise 5-6
   and fats 65
   and zinc 74
chondromalacia patella 111t, 118
Chris Dudley Foundation Basketball Camp for kids 56

chromium 67t, 75
Clare, Todd 124
Clif Bars 60, 62, 63t
Clif Shot Bloks Chews 63t
climbing
   high-altitude climbing 246
   ice climbing 246, 247-248
   indoor climbing 139
   rock climbing 246, 247-248
Colberg, Sheri vii, viii, 264
cold extremes 230, 246
cold therapy 109
competitive cheerleading 193-194
complications, exercising safely with 89-91, 93-94
Connard, Adrian 221
continuous blood glucose monitoring 83, 84, 85t
cool-down, importance of 14, 16, 112
CoQ_{10} 70, 71
Corcoran, Matthew 54
cortisol 22, 23t, 99
cortisone injections 109
Craycraft, David 246
creatine 68t, 76-77
creatine monohydrate 77
creatine phosphate 24-25, 76-77
cross country running 160-161
cross-country skiing 88f, 162-163
cross-trainers 132
cross-training 112-113
Cunningham, Catherine 137
Cunningham, Kathryn 181
Cutler, Jay 187
Cutter, Greg 176-177, 242, 250-251
cycling 163-168. *See also* mountain biking
cycling sprints 39
cysteine 66t
Cytomax 60, 63t
Czerwonka, Carrie 244

D
Dalton, Candace 168
dance 139-140
Daypro 108
Dean, Alan 181
deBrauwere, Robert 153
dehydration 69, 88-89
delayed-onset muscle soreness 124-125
Delisio, J.P. 206, 218
Demma, Linda 167, 245
denagliptin 51t

DeNunzio, Ron 134
Depomedrol 109
Desbois, Martin 153, 174, 234
detemir 47. *See also* Levemir
DexCom STS 85t
Dex4 Glucose gel 63t
Dex4 Glucose tablets 63t
Dex4 Liquid Blast 62
DiaBeta 51t, 52, 87
diabetes
   about 3-4
   blood sugar balancing act 21
   heart disease risk 16
   proneness to overuse injuries 15
   types of 4-5
   willpower to survive 96
Diabetes Education & Camping Association 261
Diabetes Exercise & Sports Association (DESA) ix, 14, 95, 261
Diabetes Sports and Wellness Foundation (DSWF) 33, 261
Diabetes Training Camp 54, 262
The Diabetic Athlete (Colberg) vii, ix
Diabetic Athlete's Handbook (Colberg) vii, viii
diabetic athlete's Ironman experience 102-104
diabetic ketoacidosis 21, 82, 87
Diabinese 51t, 52, 87
DiCesare, Lorrie 153
dietary practices 57-64
Dodson, Jimmy 243, 245, 246-247, 248
dog mushing 234-235
downhill skiing 235-237
drill team 193-194
Drysch, Maggie 200
Dudley, Chris 56, 187
Duncan, Bob 223
Dunn, Charlie 233
Dunton, Scott 42-44, 237, 255
duration, in exercise training program 12-13
Dzebo, Sreten 149

E
Eggleston, Janis 54-55, 166
Eicholz, Robert 149
Eisen, Nicolas 173
electrolytes, replacing 61
elliptical striders 132
Elwood, John 190, 193, 218

endorphins 100
endurance-power sports 187
endurance sports 157
energy systems, and ATP use 23-27
Engelbrecht, Christiane 149
environmental extremes 230-231
epinephrine 22, 23t
exenatide 51t, 54. *See also* Byetta
exercise
  benefits of 3
  blood sugar responses to 21-22
  body's use of carbohydrate during 28-29
  carbohydrate before, during, and after 58, 59-60
  on dialysis 91
  duration and contribution of three energy systems 27f
  effect on insulin action 33-34
  health benefits of 5-6
  hormonal responses to 22-23
  and hypoglycemia, effect on hormonal responses 34-35
  insulin absorption increased by 50
  insulin levels importance during 30
  learning glycemic response to 83
  metabolic control before 82-83
  one step at a time 96
  preventing hypoglycemia or hyperglycemia 38-40, 87-88
  prior exercise decreases hormonal responses to next low 35
  regulating insulin levels during 31-32
  removing potential barriers 105
  staying motivated for 104-105
  timing of exercise and insulin levels 31
  tips for avoiding injury 113t
  variables affecting blood glucose responses 22t
exercise guidelines
  blood glucose monitoring 82t, 83, 84, 87
  food intake 82t, 83-84

metabolic control before exercise 82-83
preexercise medical evaluation 86
for type 1 diabetes 81-84, 82t
for type 2 diabetes 85, 86-87
exercise-induced hypoglycemia, dealing with 36-37
exercise intensity
  about 8-9
  hard and easy days 11-12, 112
  and interval training 9
  monitoring 9-11
  precompetition tapers 12
exercise precautions
  about 87
  exercising safely with complications 89-91, 93-94
  preventing dehydration and overhydration 88-89
  preventing hypoglycemia or hyperglycemia with exercise 87-88
exercise stress test 86
exercise training program
  about 7
  duration 12-13
  exercise intensity 8-12
  frequency 13
  mode 7-8
  progression 13-14
extreme trail running 231-232
Exubera 46

F
fat, and carbohydrate, fueling energy 26-27, 64-65
fatigue, from depletion of glycogen stores 28
fat loading 65, 68t
fatty acids 64
Faust, Sarah 182
Fedor, Marty 134
feet injuries 121-123
Feifer, Richard 225
fencing 221
Ferguson, Charles, Sr. 166
Ferreira, Betty 41
field events 222
field hockey 194-195
Fiorucci, Joe 160, 195, 212
fishing. *See* gaming (fishing, hunting, and shooting)
Fit4D 86, 262
fitness activities
  about 129
  general adjustments by diet regimen 130-131

general recommendations 129-130
Flanagan, Jamie 232, 236, 241, 254, 256
flax seed 117
flexibility training, with resistance training 13
Fluen, Tommy 191
food intake 82t, 83-84
football. *See* American football; rugby; soccer (non-American football)
footwear, choosing proper 89-90, 113-114
Foy, Missy 183, 185-186
free radical formation, and antioxidant vitamins 71f
frequency, in exercise training program 13
frisbee (ultimate) 196
Frischmeyer, Linda 166-167, 240
Fritschi, Cynthia 41, 136
frozen shoulder 110, 114, 116, 117
fruit juices 61

G
Gallagher, Thomas 162, 165
Galvus 51t, 53
gaming (fishing, hunting, and shooting) 237
gardening 257-258
gastroparesis 90
Gatorade 60, 63t
Gehring, Jim 135
gels 60-62, 63t
gender, and hormonal responses 35
Gillespie, Carter 209, 233
ginseng 77
glargine 47. *See also* Lantus
Glass, Baylee 146-147, 193, 218
glimepiride 51t. *See also* Amaryl
glipizide 51t. *See also* Glucotrol
gliptins 51t
glitazones 51t, 52
glucagon 22, 23t
glucagon-like peptide-1 53
GlucoBurst gels 60, 63t
Glucophage 51t, 52
Glucophage XR 51t
glucose tablets 58-59
Glucotrol 51t, 52
Glucotrol XL 51t
Glucovance 53
Glufast 51t
glulisine 46
glutamic acid 66t
glutamine 66t

glyburide 51t, 52, 53. *See also*
 Glynase
glycemic index 58, 59
glycerol 67t, 69
glycine 66t
glycogen. *See* muscle glycogen
glycogenolysis 25
glycogen repletion 60, 87
glycolysis 25
Glynase 51t, 52
Glyset 51t, 52
Godfrey, Tim 231
Gohl, Tom 175
golf 196-198
Gomez, Patricia L. 150
Gordon, Monique 149
GPP-4 53
Green, Matt 236, 237
Greenback, Susan 149, 152, 203,
 208-209, 240
Grogger, Paul 149
growth hormone 22, 23t
Gu Energy gel 63t
guided imagery 101
gymnastics 198-199

H

Hall, Gary, Jr. 157
Hammer Gel 63t
Handy, Jay 33, 102-104, 182
Hanley, Monique 97, 98-99
Harlan, Lisa 220
Harper, Paula 14
Harter, Curtis 179
Hausmann, Herbert 79
Haverly, Julie 197
heart disease 91, 93
heart rate, target training range
 9-11
heart rate reserve 9-11
heat extremes 230, 238
heat therapy 109
Heverly, Julie 141
Heyer, Bobby 33
high-altitude climbing 246
hiking 237-241
Hilliard, Connie 209
histidine 66t
hitting the wall 28, 58
hockey. *See* field hockey; ice
 hockey
Hollander, D. 258
hormones
 blunted response of glucose-
 raising hormones 35
 and caffeine intake 76
 exercise and hypoglycemia
 34-35
 with glucose-raising effects
 during exercise 23t

and insulin levels 30
and mental stress 99
and training adaptations 32
Hornsby, Guy 151
horseback riding, competitive
 200
horseback riding, recreational
 241
housework 140-141
Hudson, Maggie 194, 199
Hughes, Darcy 167, 255
Humalog 46, 47, 50
humidity extremes 230, 238
Humulin 47
Humulin R 46
Hunter, Brandon 219, 237
hunting. *See* gaming (fishing,
 hunting, and shooting)
Hurley, Kameron 143
hydration
 and caffeine intake 76
 and glycerol 69
 tips for exercise 89t
 types of drinks and their
 effects 39-40, 60-62, 63t
hyperglycemia, preventing with
 exercise 87-88
hypertension 93-94
HypoActive 97, 99, 262
hypoglycemia
 about 3
 blood glucose and exercise
 21-22
 during exercise 31
 and exercise, effect on hormonal responses 34-35
 keys to prevention 38t
 as possible Symlin side effect
 53, 54
 preventing during and after
 exercise 38-40
 preventing postexercise, late-
 onset hypoglycemia 39
 preventing with exercise
 87-88
 prior hypoglycemia increases
 risk of recurrence during
 exercise 35
 recognizing symptoms 36-37
 testing for 37-40
 underwater hypoglycemic
 reaction 248
hypoglycemic unawareness 36,
 40

I

ibuprofen 108
ice climbing 246, 247-248
ice hockey 200-201
ice skating 141-142

ice therapy 109
Iditarod 234-235, 259
iliotibial band friction syndrome
 111t, 118
impingement syndrome
 115-116
incretins 51t
indoor climbing 139
indoor racket sports 202-203
inflammation 108-109, 110
infrapatellar tendinitis 108
inhaled insulin 46
injury
 to arms and shoulders
 114-116
 common overuse injuries
 110-112
 emotional recovery from
 105-106
 to feet and ankles 121-123
 identifying acute and overuse
 injuries 107-108
 to knees and shins 117-119
 and older athlete 125-126
 tips for avoiding 113t
injury risk 12, 15
injury treatment
 about 108
 cold therapies 109
 with heat 109
 reducing inflammation with
 meds 108-109
inline skating 141-142
insulin
 absorption increased by exercise 50
 action times 46t
 basal-bolus regimens 47-48
 basal insulins 47-48
 effect on spontaneity 45
 in extreme environments
 230
 general reductions for endurance sports 32t
 importance of levels during
 exercise 30
 intermediate-acting insulins
 47
 and pancreas 3-4
 rapid-acting insulins 46, 50
 regulating levels during exercise 31-32
 short-acting insulins 46
 timing of exercise and insulin
 levels 31
insulin action
 exercise effect on 33-34
 and menstrual cycles 41
 and oral contraceptives 41
insulin analogs 46

insulindependence.org 66, 262
insulin pumps 48-50, 49*t*
insulin release, downward during exercise 32-33
insulin resistance 5, 23
Integrated Diabetes Services 262
intensity. *See* exercise intensity
intermediate-acting insulins 47
International Diabetic Athletes Association ix
International Federation of Bodybuilders 220
interval training, and exercise intensity 9
iron 73
iron deficiency 73
Ironman experience, of diabetic athlete 102-104
Ironman triathlons 259, 260
ischemia 93
isoleucine 66*t*
ITBF. *See* iliotibial band friction syndrome

J
Januvia 51*t*, 53
Jarvis, Chris 18-20, 205
jet skiing 241
jogging 171-175
Johnson, Donna L. 178, 258
Johnson, Kathleen 138
Johnson, Katie 182, 196
Johnston, Marilyn 135
Jones, Carys 203
Jones, Spencer Lee 205
Juvenile Diabetes Research Foundation International 262

K
Kahn, Cynthia 175
Kaiserman, Kevin 44
Karz, Zippora 154-155
Kasza, Felix 224
kayaking 233-234. *See also* whitewater sports (canoeing, kayaking, and rafting)
Kenalog 109
ketones 82
Keysering, Chuck 134
kickboxing 142-144
kidney disease 91
kidneys, and creatine 77
King, Bill 53-54, 95, 169-170
King, Robert 165
Kingerey, Tom 170
Kinnunen, Vic 190
Kirkse, Sara 165
Knappich, Tania 225, 248

knee injuries 117-119
Knight, Keith 223
Konvisser, Marc 163
Korlewitz, Lynne 135-136
Kotsifakis, Juliana 199, 200
Krakel, Alisa 253, 256

L
lacrosse 194-195
lactic acid system 25-26
LADA (latent autoimmune diabetes of the adult) 4-5
Lanclos, Rachel 137
Land, Gayle 141
Lantus 47-48, 50
latent autoimmune diabetes of the adult 4-5
late-onset hypoglycemia 21
lateral collateral ligament 119
lateral epicondylitis 108, 114, 115
Latham, Kathryn 242
Lawrence, Chad 245
Leeuwenberg, Jay 187
LeMar, Keith 166
leucine 66*t*
Levemir 47, 48, 50
Lewis, Al 96
Liebowitz, Ed 153, 182
Lifelong Exercise Institute 262
ligament tears 118, 119
Limbourg, Andrea 239-240
Lindahl, Adelaide 137, 197, 240
Linton, Bruce 235, 259-260
lispro 46. *See also* Humalog
Little League elbow 108
liver, and blood glucose 4
LoCurcio, Joe 242-243
Loganbill, Kent 244
low-carbohydrate diet 60
Luzzi, Michael 207, 251
lysine 66*t*

M
MADiDEA event 124
magnesium 74
Mailing, Chris 165, 168
Majurin, Julie 177, 182, 225
Malone, Michael 167
marathons 168-171
martial arts 144-146
Martin, Deb 163, 253
Mathias, K. 135
Maxey, Randall 173
maximal oxygen consumption (VO₂max) 7-8
Mazer, Jeff 79, 236, 239
McCotter, Michelle 137
McCullen, Riley 191, 195

McFarland, Roy 193, 236
McGann, Michelle 187
McGill, Kelsey 194, 199
McKinnon, Scott 153, 175
McMahon, Mike 153, 237
McNulty, Renée 240, 244, 250
medial collateral ligament 119
medications
    keys to managing with physical activity 55
    new choices 53-55
    oral diabetic medications 51-53, 87-88
    reducing inflammation with 108-109
meditation 101
Medtronic MiniMed Guardian RT 85*t*
Medtronic MiniMed Paradigm Real-Time System 85*t*
Meltzer, Allan 135
Mendosa, David 240
meniscal tears 118, 119
Menninger, Florian, Jr. 258
menstrual cycles, and insulin action 41
mental rehearsal 101
mental stress
    effect on diabetes control and health 99-100
    endorphins lowered by 100
    relaxation techniques 100-101
    training mind and body 100
    yoga for peak performance 101
metatarsal fractures 110-111, 122
metformin 51*t*, 52, 53
methionine 66*t*
Meyers, Joyce 96, 150
Micronase 51*t*, 52, 87
miglitol 51*t*. *See also* Glyset
milk 59
Miller, Alan 165
mind, enhancing performance with 101
minerals
    about 73
    calcium 73-74
    chromium 75
    iron 73
    magnesium 74
    vanadium 75
    zinc 74
mineral supplements 70
Mitchell, Kirsteen 206, 207
mitiglinide 51*t*

mode, of exercise in training program 7-8
Moore, Jim 167, 250
Moore, John 183, 207
Morrison, Adam 187
Morrison, Lulu 137
motivation
    keys to building 106t
    staying motivated to exercise 104-105
    tips for daily physical activity 105t
motorcycle riding and racing (off road) 241-242
mountain biking 242-245
mountaineering 230, 245-247
Mountains for Active Diabetics 79, 124, 262
mountain sickness 246
Moyers, Anne 165
Mr. California title 227
Mr. Universe title 215, 221
Muirhead, Madison 206
multivitamins 70
Murphy, James 50
muscle cramps 123
muscle glycogen
    breakdown of 25-26
    as energy source 57-58
muscles, strengthening after injury 113
muscle soreness 123-125
muscle-strengthening activities 16-17
muscular damage, from long-distance events 34

N
Nairn, Jerry 170-171, 183
Naprosyn 108
naproxen 108
Narula, Svati 160-161, 210
nateglinide 51t
National Association of Underwater Instructors 249
National Outdoor Leadership School 240
Natural Mr. Universe Tall Class title 226, 227
Natural Mr. USA title 226, 227
Neal, Garrick 50, 240
Necoche, Sheryl 150
nephropathy 91
Nerothin, Peter 34, 165, 171, 173, 178
nerve compression syndromes 111-112
neuropathy-related joint disorders 111

nonsteroidal anti-inflammatory medications (NSAIDs) 108
norepinephrine 22, 23t
Novolin N 47
Novolin R 46
NovoLog 46
NovoRapid 46
NPH 47
Nuprin 108
nutritional supplements
    about 67-68
    amino acid supplements 68-69
    caffeine 75-76
    creatine 76-77
    ginseng 77
    glycerol 69
    minerals 73-75
    of potential benefit to diabetic athletes 67t
    of potential harm to diabetic athletes 68t
    vitamins 69-73

O
Ochs, Sheri 141, 149, 177, 178, 258
O'Hare, Lindsey 194
Okereke, Akachi 193
Okereke, Cheokie 193
Olson, Linda 166
Olympic weightlifting 222-223
Oppen, Alex 236, 242
oral contraceptives, and insulin action 41
organizations 261-262
orthostatic hypotension 86
Ortiz, Meryl 174
osteoarthritis 125
outdoor recreational activities 229
overhydration, preventing 88-89
overtraining syndrome, recognizing and treating 114
overuse injury
    identifying 107-108
    most common 110-112
    preventing 112-113
overworked pancreas 5

P
pain, never ignoring 107
paintball 232-233
pancreas 3-4, 5
Panofsky, David 79, 124, 166, 246, 248
parasailing 251
Parker, Emmy 148

patellofemoral syndrome 118. See also chondromalacia patella
Paxson, Bob 138, 153, 184, 253
pelican box 230
Pentescu, Christopher 197, 207
performance, enhancing with mind 101
peripheral neuropathy 89-90
phenylalanine 66t
Philbin, Rick 193
phosphagen system 24-25
physical activity
    daily motivation tips for 105t
    keys to managing medications 55
    as main cause of hypoglycemia 31-32
physical education classes 146-147
physical fitness, benefits of 5-6
physical stress, endorphins lowered by 100
physical training
    effect on fuel utilization 32-33
    effect on insulin action 34
Pintar, Thomas 181, 237
Pinto, Esther 135, 148
Pisano, Rose 197, 198
pitchers 217
plantar fasciitis 108, 111t, 122
Pollak, Alexis 144, 255
polyuria 88
posterior cruciate ligament 119
PowerAde 60, 63t
PowerBar gel 63t
PowerBars 60, 62, 63t
power lifting 222-223
power sports 215
pramlintide 51t, 53. See also Symlin
Prandin 51t
Precose 51t, 52
preexercise medical evaluation 86
pregnancy, diabetes, and activity 41-42
Privratsky, Benny 173, 254
Professional Association of Diving Instructors 249
progression, in exercise training program 13-14
proliferative retinopathy 90-91
proline 66t
protein, fueling activity 26-27, 65-67

protein supplements 68*t*
Protophane 47
Purcell, Nicole 134

Q
Quinn, Joel 207, 209, 219

R
Race Across America 95, 98, 243
race walking 147-149
rafting 256
range of motion, limitation of 116
rapid-acting insulins 46, 50, 82
rating of perceived exertion 11
Rayner, Elise 167-168, 244
Raynes, Nev 221
Reeser, Jedidiah 240
Reily, Doretta 224
Relafan 108
relaxation techniques 100-101
repaglinide 51*t*
resistance circuit training 151-153
resistance training
    with flexibility training 13
    getting the most out of 16-17
    in regular exercise routine 8
resources for active people
    Diabetes Exercise and Sports Association 14
    Diabetes Sports and Wellness Foundation 33
    Diabetes Training Camp 54
    Fit4D.com 86
    HypoActive 97
    insulindependence.org 66
    Mountains for Active Diabetics 124
Restis, Jude 241
retinopathy 90-91
Rice, Susan 134
RICE (rest, ice, compression, and elevation) 108
Riddell, Michael 203, 232
Roche, Jennifer 166, 256
rock climbing 246, 247-248
Rockenfield, Tyler 177, 190
roller derby 203
Rono, Elly 186
Rossini, Brenda 175
rotator cuff tendinitis 108, 111*t*, 114, 115-116
Rothweiler, Steffi 140, 210
Routh, Kateri 134
rowers 133
rowing 204-205
rugby 190-191

runner's knee 108, 118
running
    about 171-175
    cross-country running 160-161
    extreme trail running 231-232
    on loose sand 224
    sprinting 223-224
Ryan, Blair 160, 161, 181, 210

S
sailing 248-249
Sargent, Lorri 257
saturated fats 65
saxagliptin 51*t*
Scheiner, Gary 143, 193
Schrank, Robert 167
Schroeder, Chris 79
Schroeder, John 79
scuba diving 249-251
Scuba Schools International 250
Seabourne, Tom 55, 168
Seaman, Lisa 79, 163, 230, 247, 256
Seeley, Kim 220-221
selenium 71-72
self-confidence, keys to building 106*t*
self-esteem 97
serine 66*t*
Shaw, Susan 240
Shearer, Tom 144, 166
Sheldon, Jake 207, 213-214, 218
Shermer, Pat 240
Sherstone, Edwin 232, 248
shin injuries 117-119
shin splints 108, 111*t*, 119
Shisler, Debbie 219
shooting. *See* gaming (fishing, hunting, and shooting)
short-acting insulins 46
shoulder injuries 114-116
Shriver, Mark 134
Sibbitt, Jared 240, 247, 248, 250
Sidener, Scott 181
Siler, Stetson 173
Simes, Michael 161
Simmonds, Chris 218
Simmons, Kendall 187
Simons, Debra 149, 253
Sinclair, Jean 232
sitagliptin 51*t*. *See also* Januvia
skateboarding 251
skiing
    cross-country skiing 88*f*, 162-163
    downhill skiing 235-237

jet skiing 241
    waterskiing 255
ski machines 132-133
skydiving 251
Smith, B.A. 244
Smith, Sharon 149
snorkeling 251-252
snowboarding 235-237
snowmobiling 252-253
snowshoeing 253
soccer (non-American football) 205-207
socks, selecting 89
softball 217-219
Somma, Tom 140, 144
Soper, Sarah 140, 142, 196
Sormani, Mauro 79, 163, 248
Southern States Championships 227
spontaneity, insulin's effect on 45
sports bars 60-62, 63*t*
sports drinks 67*t*
Spracklen, Mike 18
sprinting 223-224
stair climbers 132
stair steppers 132
Stark, Karen 48, 174, 236
Starlix 51*t*
static stretching 15
stationary cycles 132
Steckel, Andrew 177, 207
Stevens, Samantha 205
Stewart, Robert L. 92-93
Stone, Claude 134
Strausbaugh, Troy 144, 146
stress. *See* mental stress; physical stress
stretching
    before and after exercise 15
    as relaxation technique 101
    slowing loss of flexibility 126
    and yoga 153-154
sulfonlyureas 51*t*, 52
sunlight, as vitamin D source 72
superoxide 70
surfing 42-44, 254-255
Swanson, Kaylee 177, 218
Sweeney, Joey 192
swimmer's shoulder 108
swimming 175-179
Switzer, Janet 152, 240
Symlin 51*t*, 53-54, 55

T
talk test 11

Tank, Karen 138
tapering 64
target heart rate training zones 10*t*
Taylor, Gary 258
Taylor, Justin 244
Teffeteller, Alan Kent 210
tendinitis 110, 114-115, 116
tennis 208-210
tennis elbow 108, 110, 111*t*, 114, 115
thiazolidenediones 51*t*, 52
Thomas, Hortense 208
Thompson, Peter 143
Thorn, Victoria 195
Thornton, Taylor 225
threonine 66*t*
Tinker, Abigail 203
track events (400 to 1,600 meters) 210-211
trans fatty acids 65
treadmills 132
trekking 246
triathlons 179-182
trigger fingers 111
Trigo, Matehus 146
Triller, Shannon 199
Tylenol 108
type 1 diabetes 4, 81-84
type 1.5 diabetes 4-5
type 2 diabetes 5, 85, 86-87
tyrosine 66*t*
TZDs. *See* thiazolidenediones

U
ultimate frisbee 196
ultraendurance events and training 183-184
Ultra Fuel 60, 63*t*
underwater hypoglycemic reaction 248

Unger, Judy 151
urea 69

V
valerian root 117
valine 66*t*
vanadium 67*t*, 75
Vandevelde, Jenny 193, 207, 225
Verity, Larry 135
Verplank, Scott 187
VIAject 46
vildagliptin 51*t*. *See also* Galvus
Vinall, Kerry 135
visualization techniques 101
vitamins
    about 69-70
    antioxidants 70-72
    mineral supplements 70
    multivitamins 70
    vitamin A 71
    vitamin B_1 72
    vitamin B_{12} 73
    vitamin C 70
    vitamin D 72
    vitamin E 70-71
volleyball 224-225
Vollin, Jeff 134
Voulon, Roberta 154, 173
Vranich, Nancy 233-234

W
walking 147-149
Wallis, Nikki 78-79, 124
Walton, David 171, 224
warm-up, importance of 14, 16, 112
water aerobics 150-151
water intoxication 61
water polo 211
waterskiing 255

web sites
    Active Diabetes 79
    diabetes, sport, and nutrition sites 263-264
    Diabetes Training Camp 54
    Fit4D 86
    HypoActive 97
    insulindependence.org 66
    Mountains for Active Diabetics 79, 124
Wehrly, Ethan 207
weightlifting 222-223
weight training 151-153, 219, 221
Weingard, David 154, 179, 182
whey protein 68
Whitcombe, Mark 149
White, Kerry 95-96, 163, 243
whitewater sports (canoeing, kayaking, and rafting) 256
Wiebold, Scott 170
Willard, Troy 243-244
windsurfing 256-257
Wiseman, Jillian 140
Witmer, Lynn 135
Witschen, Brian 201
women, special concerns for female athletes with diabetes 40-42
Worsley, Brian 152
wrestling 211-212
Wright, Delaine 117, 199, 200

Y
yard work 257-258
yoga 101, 153-154
Young, Jeanne 140

Z
Zender, Kate 219
zinc 67*t*, 74

About the Author

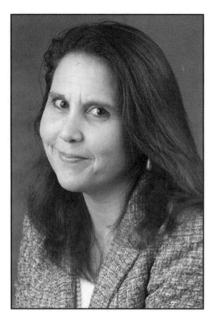

Sheri R. Colberg is an exercise physiologist and professor of exercise science at Old Dominion University in Norfolk, Virginia, and an adjunct professor of internal medicine at Eastern Virginia Medical School. She specializes in exercise and diabetes and conducts extensive research in these areas thanks to funding from the American Diabetes Association and other organizations.

Dr. Colberg has more than 40 years of practical experience as an athlete living with type 1 diabetes. She is the director of the Human Performance Laboratory at Old Dominion and is a fellow of the American College of Sports Medicine. She is also a professional member of the American Diabetes Association and serves on the board of directors for the Diabetes Exercise and Sports Association.

Dr. Colberg has written hundreds of articles on exercise and diabetes and is the author of six books: *Matt Hoover's Guide to Life, Love, and Losing Weight* (Skyhorse Publishing, 2008), *The Science of Staying Young* (McGraw-Hill, 2007), *50 Secrets of the Longest Living People with Diabetes* (Marlowe & Co., 2007), *The 7 Step Diabetes Fitness Plan* (Marlowe & Co., 2006), *Diabetes-Free Kids* (Avery, 2005), and *The Diabetic Athlete* (Human Kinetics, 2001). Her expertise on diabetes is also frequently shared in interviews and articles in popular magazines, including *Men's Health, Men's Fitness, Muscle & Fitness, Diabetes Health, Diabetes Forecast, Newsweek International,* and *USA Today.*

A resident of Virginia Beach, Virginia with her husband and three sons, she enjoys participating in myriad recreational sports and fitness activities, as well as exercising with and supporting the athletic endeavors of her growing boys.